AF386393

Current Topics in Pathology

Continuation of Ergebnisse der Pathologie

66

Editors

E. Grundmann W. H. Kirsten

Perinatal Pathology

Contributors

M. Bibbo, C. Bron, W.-W. Höpker, J. P. Kraehenbuhl
B. Ohlendorf, L. Olding, S. Panem, B. Sandstedt
H. Soma, B. Sordat

Editor

E. Grundmann

With 88 Figures

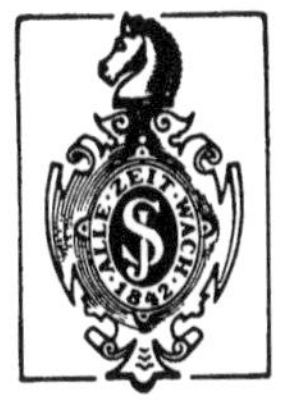

Springer-Verlag Berlin Heidelberg New York 1979

E. Grundmann, Professor Dr., Pathologisches Institut der Universität, Westring 17, D–4400 Münster/Westf., Germany

W.H. Kirsten, Professor Dr., Department of Pathology, The University of Chicago, 950 East 59th Street, Chicago, IL 60637, USA

ISBN-13: 978-3-642-67207-1   e-ISBN-13: 978-3-642-67205-7
DOI: 10.1007/978-3-642-67205-7

Library of Congress Cataloging in Publication Data. Main entry under title: Perinatal pathology. (Current topics in pathology; 66). Bibliography: p. Includes index. 1. Placenta–Diseases. 2. Maternal-fetal exchange. I. Bibbo, M. II. Grundmann, Ekkehard. III. Kirsten, Werner H. IV. Series: Current topics in pathology; v. 66. RB1.E6 vol. 66 [RG591] 616.07'08s [618.3] 79-450

2122/3130 – 543210

Contents

The Placenta and Low Birth Weight. With 26 Figures
B. Sandstedt 1

Placental Insufficiency. With 23 Figures
W.-W. Höpker, B. Ohlendorf 57

Interactions Between Maternal and Fetal/Neonatal Lymphocytes. With 1 Figure
L. Olding 83

Transfer of Humoral Secretory and Cellular Immunity from Mother to
Offspring. With 19 Figures
J.P. Kraehenbuhl, C. Bron, B. Sordat 105

Single Umbilical Artery with Congenital Malformations. With 4 Figures
H. Soma 159

C-Type Virus Expression in the Placenta. With 4 Figures
S. Panem 175

Transplacental Effects of Diethylstilbestrol. With 11 Figures
M. Bibbo 191

Subject Index 213

Indexed in ISR

List of Contributors

Bibbo, Prof. Dr. M.

Department of Obstetrics and Gynecology, The University of Chicago, 5841 Maryland Avenue, Chicago, Ill. 60637, USA

Bron, Prof. Dr. C.

Institut de biochimie, chemin des Boveresses, CH–1066 Epalinges

Höpker, Prof. Dr. W.-W.

Pathologisches Institut der Universität Münster, Westring 17, 4400 Münster, Fed. Rep. of Germany

Kraehenbuhl, Dr. J.P.

Institut de biochimie, chemin des Boveresses, CH–1066 Epalinges

Ohlendorf, Dr. Beate

Pathologisches Institut der Universität Münster, Westring 17, 4400 Münster, Fed. Rep. of Germany

Olding, Dr. L.

Department of Pathology, University of Göteborg, Sahlgrenska Sjukhuset, 41345 Göteborg, Sweden

Panem, Prof. Dr. S.

Department of Pathology, The University of Chicago, 950 East 59th Street, Chicago, Ill. 60637, USA

Sandstedt, Dr. B.

Patologavdelningen, Danderyds sjukhus, 18203 Danderyd, Sweden

Soma, Prof. H.

Department of Obstetrics and Gynecology, Tokyo Medical College Hospital, 1–7 Nishishinjuku 6, Sjinjuku, Tokyo 160, Japan

Sordat, Dr. B.

Institut de biochimie, chemin des Boveresses, CH–1066 Epalinges

The Placenta and Low Birth Weight

B. SANDSTEDT

I. Introduction 2
II. Factors Related to Low Birth Weight 3

   1. Maternal 3
   2. Placental 3
   3. Fetal 4
   4. Twinning 4
   5. Villitis 4

III. Material and Results 5
IV. Placental Outline and Gross Lesions in Low Birth Weight 7

   1. Configuration 8
   2. Placenta Extrachorialis 8
   3. Cord Insertion 9
   4. Infarction 9
   5. Subchorionic Thrombus 11
   6. Retroplacental Hematoma 11
   7. Chorangioma 12
   8. Single Umbilical Artery 12
   9. Unrelated Lesions 12

V. Placental Arterial Vasculature 13

   1. Definitions and Angiographic Method 13
   2. Arterial Vasculature in uncomplicated Term Pregnancy 14

      a) Allantochorial Vessels and Cotyledons 14
      b) Subcotyledons 17
      c) Intracotyledonary Arteries 17

   3. Arterial Vasculature of the Placenta in LBW 19

      a) Classification and Number of Cotyledons 19
      b) Subcotyledons and their Possible Relation to Maternal Arteries . . 26
      c) Abnormal Arterial Pattern — "Seaweed" Cotyledons 27

VI. Ultrastructure (SEM and TEM) of the Free Chorionic Villus 28

   1. Ultrastructure in Uncomplicated Pregnancies 28

      a) General Appearance 28
      b) Trophoblastic Layer 31
      c) Syncytial Microvilli 33
      d) Villous Core and Fetal Endothelium 38

   2. Ultrastructure in LBW 38

      a) General Appearance 40
      b) Trophoblastic Layer and Syncytial Microvilli 43

    c) Syncytium 44
    d) Placental "Glycocalyx" 46

VII. Conclusions 47
References 48

I. Introduction

In recent years the child with low birth weight (LBW) with or without signs of intrauterine malnutrition has attracted much attention. The condition has human as well as economic aspects since it scores high in perinatal deaths and brain damage (*Potter* and *Davies,* 1969; *Fitzhardinge* and *Steven,* 1972; *Bjerre* and *Östberg,* 1974). By gaining a better understanding of the extent to which placental changes could indicate the etiology of low birth weight, the pathologist can contribute to the prevention of this condition.

That the placenta, as a link between mother and child, can affect fetal development and postnatal adaption is certain. However, an infant with low birth weight and perhaps signs of fetal deprivation may be encountered without there being extensive lesions in the placental parenchyma. This often frustrates the pathologist, who inherits the task of looking for placental "insufficiency." He or she must realize that the condition is multifactorial and may be the result of premature delivery, multiple pregnancy, maternal disease and malnutrition and, less commonly, a primary disturbance in placental function. It is practical to think in terms of "fetal supply line" used by *Gruenwald* (1975a) which, schematically, can be divided into maternal, fetal, and placental aspects. These could act independently or together. All studies of the placenta must thus be related to clinical information from mother and child. The placental lesion might then fit as a piece of puzzle into the clinical picture and help explain and prevent future fetal distress and wastage.

All infants with low birth weight used to be called "premature". With the recognition of full-term infants having low birth weight and reflecting insufficient intrauterine growth, the terms "dysmaturity" (*Sjöstedt* et al., 1958), "pseudoprematurity" (*Söderling*, 1953), and "small for dates" (*Butler* and *Bonham*, 1958) have come into use. *Gruenwald* (1963) used the terms "chronic" and "subacute" fetal distress, which are not invariably present in these cases. More recently, it has become apparent that infants born prematurely by date can also be retarded in growth.

Before an accurate definition of terms can be achieved, there are two basic problems to be solved. The first is determination of the duration of gestation; the second has been the lack of knowledge about what is normal or pathologic growth in relation to length of gestation. Length of gestation can now be determined objectively by applying knowledge about the development of the fetal nervous system in conjunction with visible external signs of maturity (*Saint-Anne Dargassier*, 1962; *Koenigsberger*, 1966; *Usher* et al., 1966; *Harnack* and *v. Bernuth*, 1971). Efforts have been made to gain a better understanding of the problem of normal or abnormal intrauterine growth by the construction of statistical diagrams based on large populations and relating length and weight of infants to the length of gestation. The problems inherent in this have been reviewed by *Gruenwald* (1975b). The term low birth weight (LBW) in this review will be used for infants born with a birth weight of 2500 g or less. Furthermore, infants are designated as small (SGA) and appropriate (AGA) for gestational age with respect to borderlines set at the 10th and 90th percentiles of weight for the respective week of gestation. This SGA group can be divided clinically into two groups — "dysmature" (disproportionate-SGA) and "small for date" (SFD) (proportionate-SGA). See also discussion concerning this subject by *Rosso* and *Winick* (1974). This review is based on the author's experience with placentas from a clinical prospective study by *Enocksson* (1975) of infants with low birth weight. It will be restricted to the methods used and consider mainly shape and gross lesions of the placenta, angiography of the arterial vasculature, and ultrasturcture of the free chorionic villus.

II. Factors Related to Low Birth Weight

For the sake of completeness it is necessary to reconsider briefly some causes of low birth weight at different levels.

1. Maternal

These factors are mainly circulatory with impaired blood flow to the intervillous space and abnormalities in the mother such as anemia or nutritional deficiencies. It is difficult to ascertain whether genetic factors or immunologic interactions between mother and infant may cause reduced size, as some data from animal models (*Walton* and *Hammond,* 1938; *Billington,* 1964) and human pregnancies (*Ounsted* and *Ounsted,* 1968; *Warburton* and *Naylor,* 1971) indicate. *Barnes* (1963) showed that women with congenital or acquired heart disease tend to have small and even growth-retarded infants. It is known that uterine blood flow is reduced in pre-eclampsia and that this condition is associated with retarded fetal growth. Nonhypertensive mothers who have small, slowly filled uterine vessels in radioangiograms are also associated with fetal retardation (*Bieniarz* et al., 1966). Finally, low socioeconomic status, a badly defined term, includes several factors, each of which can influence intrauterine growth.

2. Placental

Primary placental causes leading to reduced fetal size seem to be unusual, especially because the functional capacity of the "placental membrane" in relation to the need of the fetus is not understood. Structural changes in the "membrane" must be judged carefully, because they are also influenced by maternal blood flow in the intervillous space. Infarcts, asynchronous maturation of chorionic villi, numerous syncytiocapillary membranes, and syncytial knots, fibrinoid changes, thick basement membrane etc., all should be related to impaired circulation of the intervillous space. Because the development and the function of the placenta are partly formed by fetal and local uterine factors, it is, from a functional point of view, reasonable to speak of the "utero-placental unit", which in a broad sense includes the two most important factors for fetal size, namely, the maternal blood supply and placental extension.

3. Fetal

These are arbitrary but may include chronic disease, e.g., infections or malformations having genetic or other causes. The fetus shows an inability to grow though adequately supplied.

There are two important conditions which intimately related to reduced fetal size that will not be considered extensively in the review, namely, multiple pregnancy and villitis.

4. Twinning

There is a well-documented tendency for twins to be smaller than singletons of the same gestational age in the last third of gestation (*Lubchenko* et al., 1963; *McKeown* and *Record*, 1953). The low incidence of gross lesions in the twin placentas of the author's study also points to the fact that multiple birth in itself constitutes a reduction in fetal growth rate. The finding that one twin was of normal size and the other underweight has also been noted by *Scott* and *Usher* (1966). The higher incidence of chorangiomas, single umbilical artera (SUA), and velamentous cord insertion in twinning is also well known. The placenta in itself is not a limiting factor, because it is proportionally larger in twins than in singletons. Unfortunately, there were few twins in the author's material. Otherwise, twin pregnancies provide a unique opportunity for making correlations between placental disease and fetal development. The subject has been considered in other publications (*Benirschke*, 1975; *Strong* and *Corney*, 1967).

5. Villitis

Altshuler and *Russel* (1975) recently provided an extensive and excellent review on this topic. It was their contention that villitis was of etiologic importance in the genesis of a significant percentage of SGA infants. In an earlier report, *Altshuler* et al. (1975) suggested an incidence of 25% in 63 placentas from infants small for gestational age. Similar figures were given by *Laga* et al. (1972) and *Dollman* (1973). In the material described below the incidence of focal and diffuse inflammation within villi was only 10%, which may find its explanation in differences in so-called socioeconomic factors of the populations studied.

III. Material and Results

From a clinically controlled consecutive series of 152 LBW infants (128 singletons and 24 twins) the placentas were studied to determine the possible role of grossly observable abnormalities in the pathogenesis of LBW syndromes. The clinical results and the clinical follow-ups are reported elsewhere (*Enocksson* et al., 1972; *Enocksson*, 1975). Special care was taken in evaluating duration of gestation and the degree of maturity of the infants. The mothers represented a fairly homogeneous population with a better-than-average socioeconomic status living in a limited area. More than 90% of the mothers attended prenatal units. The infants were divided into groups appropriate (AGA) and small for gestation age (SGA). The control series consisted of 200 placentas from "ideal" pregnancies and infants. The placentas were investigated fresh and after formalin fixation with standardized methods and definitions, principally according to the method described by *Benirschke* and *Driscoll* (1967). From some of the placentas, tissue pieces were taken for ultrastructural studies. Most of the placentas were also investigated by angiography (vide infra). In the present material, maternal factors, except toxemia, were not related to LBW or any placental lesion. A small number of mothers with LBW infants had had previous abortions and LBW infants with some association to placental configuration and cord abnormalities. The details are found elsewhere (*Sandstedt*, 1974).

The general results are found in Table 1. Placentas with none of the observed lesions are termed "normal." Apart from the gross lesions, the presence of villous inflammation and intervillous fibrin deposition (IVFD) with necrosis have been included

Table 1. Incidence (per cent) of placental lesions in 152 LBW infants and 200 normal term infants. "Normal" placentas without any of the listed lesions

	Singletons	Controls	Twins
"Normal" placentas	22	64	46
Abnormal configuration (including PE)	17	5.5	12.5
Acute/subactue infarct	34	3	8
Old infarct	13	9.5	21
Abnormal cord insertion	16.5	5	21
SUA	2	1	4
Chorangioma	1.5	0.5	8
RPH	15	0	0
IVT	18	20	4
Subchorial thrombus	5.5	0	0
Villitis	3	0	0
Mixed infarction	7	0.5	0

PE = Placenta extrachorialis; SUA = single umbilical artery; RPH = retroplacental hematoma; IVT = intervillous thrombus

Table 2. Distribution of abnormal placental configuration and extrachorial placentas in 128 LBW infants and 200 normal term AGA infants

	AGA		SFD		Dysmature	
	Preterm	Term	Preterm	Term	Preterm	Term
Normal	48	189	19	22	11	7
Abnormal configuration	2	3	1	2	0	0
Extrachorial	8	8	5	3	1	0
Total	58	200	25	27	12	7

Table 3. Cord insertion related to placental configuration and retroplacental hemorrhage

	Placental configuration			Retroplacental hematomas
	Ordinary	Bilobate, heart-shaped	PE	
Central	119	3	9	16
Marginal	9[a]	2	8[b]	1
Velamentous	4	1[c]	3	2

PE = placenta extrachorialis

[a] 2 twin placentas; [b] 2 twin placentas; [c] 1 twin placenta

Table 4. Distribution of placentas with acute and subactue infarction in 128 LBW infants and 200 controls (term AGA infants)

Placental volume (%)	AGA		SFD		Dysmature	
	Preterm	Term	Preterm	Term	Preterm	Term
0	41	194	12	20	7	6
1−5	7	6	8	5	2	1
6−15	7	0	3	1	2	0
16−100	2	0	2	1	1	0

when this was the only pathologic finding in the placenta. The distribution of placenta extrachorialis and other abnormal configurations are found in Table 2. Deviations in cord insertion in relation to the different groups of infants studied, placental configuration, and retroplacental hematomas are given in Table 3. There were 19 placentas in the LBW group with distinct retroplacental hematomas (RPH), three of which were associated with placenta praevia. In 15 placentas the hemorrhage was associated with acute or subacute infraction. The relation of placental infarction to separations was found to follow the size of the hemorrhage. The incidence and distribution of the different kinds of infarcts in the maturity groups are found in Tables 1, 4 and 5. No placenta contained more than five infarcts. The mean volume of the infarcts was low. When placentas with abnormal outline (PE included) and premature detachment are excluded, the difference in infarcted placental volume between the maturity groups was further diminished.

Table 5. Distribution of placentas with old infarction in 128 LBW infants and 200 controls (term AGA infants)

Placental volume (%)	AGA		SFD		Dysmature	
	Preterm	Term	Preterm	Term	Preterm	Term
0	52	181	19	24	9	6
1–5	5	19	6	2	2	1
6–15	0	0	0	1	1	0

IV. Placental Outline and Gross Lesions in Low Birth Weight

The gross lesions of the placenta are well recognized and have all been discussed in relation to "placental insufficiency;" however, there is no general agreement concerning the significance of each particular gross lesion. To overcome this, scoring systems have been developed (*Scott* and *Jordan*, 1972) which, with increasing experience, will probably be a good method for judging placental insufficiency. Since our knowledge of placental morphology and lesions is inadequate, it is still necessary to consider gross lesions for possible relationship with LBW. To apply sophisticated methods to study the placenta, it is necessary to know to what extent gross lesions are associated with LBW. Studies dealing with, e.g., electron microscopy, histochemistry, must hence also include a macro- and light-microscopic description of the placenta as well as a description of the area studied.

To judge placental functional capacity, *Gruenwald* (1963) used placental weight with the reservation that no better parameter existed. Most studies giving weight curves for the fetus and placenta have resulted in similar shapes of these curves but at different levels. This is mainly explained by the difference in the techniques used when weighin, as emphasized by *Garrow* and *Hawes* (1971). Placental mass may be reduced both in absolute terms and relative to the size of the fetus in cases of fetal growth retardation (*Younoszai* and *Haworth*, 1969).

A small reduction in placental weight has been found to be associated with a disproportionate reduction in birth weight (*Kloosterman* and *Huidekoper*, 1954). Alterations of the fetal–placental weight ratio have been said to be of no significance, but in dysmature infants, a ratio of less than 0.10 has been found (*Bazso*, 1966; *Little*,

1960b). Some controversy exists as to whether the gross examination revealing the different lesions should be done before or after fixation. Various methods have been suggested (*Bartholomew*, 1961; *Becker*, 1962; *Gruenwald*, 1964; *Benirschke* and *Driscoll*, 1967). It is important to realize that various results in different series might be due to the method used. Particularly, red infarcts and chorangiomas are difficult to see in fresh, unfixed placentas. The examiner must be consistent and record the method, including the method of weighing the placenta. Concerning size and dimensions, it can be noted that the cross-sectional area of the umbilical cord is related to fetal size and to certain complications of pregnancy (*Scott* and *Jordan*, 1972; *Coulter* and *Scott*, 1975). There is also some evidence that the size of the decidual surface is a good parameter of fetal size (*Younoszai* and *Haworth*, 1969; *Wulf* and *Becker*, 1975), though it is necessary to create rules on how to measure decidual surface in a malformed placenta.

1. Configuration

Abnormal placental configuration, what *Shanklin* (1970) calls "error in outline," is uncommon and, when it does occur, it is usually accompanied by normal fetal development. The most extreme variants, accessory lobes and membranous placentation, are so rare that they are irrelevant in the larger context of LBW. The more common bilobar variants, according to *Shanklin* (1970), are not a major cause of LBW. Among the 22 placentas with an accessory lobe described by him (1958), seven were associated with premature infants. In a similar series collected by *Torpin* and *Hart* (1941), the frequency of placentas with accessory lobes was the same (8%) at term as at premature birth. *Fujikura* et al. (1970) found a frequency of 4% but no association with birth weight or gestational age. In a study of SGA infants, *Dollman* (1973) found an incidence of 18% abnormal outline compared with 8% in the controls.

Taken as a whole, the studies cited do not closely relate abnormal configuration to LBW. In part, this is a question of definition, especially in the case of the slightest degree of bilobation, the heart or kidney-shaped placenta. In many instances, distinction from normal configuration is arbitrary.

2. Placenta Extrachorialis

There are wide differences in reported frequency of placenta extrachorialis (PE) (*Hobbs* and *Price*, 1940; *Pinkerton*, 1956; *Scott*, 1960; *Williams*, 1927; *Fox* and *Sen*, 1972; *Hunt*, 1953; *Morgan*, 1955). Some of these reflect different definitions — partial or total, circumvallate or circummarginate. PE has been associated with early abortion (*Hertig* and *Sheldon*, 1943; *Hunt*, 1953) and with hemorrhage during pregnancy (*Scott*, 1960). Some authors (*Fox* and *Sen*, 1972; *Benson* and *Fujikura*, 1969) have found a high frequency of premature labor and intrauterine growth retardation in association with placenta circumvallata, but they found the circummarginate placenta of no clinical importance. *Hunt* (1953) has seen a recurrence rate in subsequent pregnancies approaching 20% and, in some cases, repeated birth or premature infants. *Sexton* et al.

(1950) found PE to be overrepresented among prematurely separated placentas. A high frequency and great degree of circumvallation has been observed in a Guatemalan group of infants with low fetal and placental weight (*Laga* et al., 1972). Four examples of circumvallate placentation were recorded in a series of 63 SGA infants reported by *Altschuler* et al. (1975).

The significant difference in the author's material (Table 1) between the selected LBW children and the completely normal pregnancies is striking and indicates the importance of PE for LBW syndromes. On the other hand, *Scott* and *Jordan* (1972) did not find a significant association between PE or abnormal shape and "placental insufficiency" and malnutrition. In large series, such as those of *Scott* (1960) and of *Shanklin* and *Sotelo-Avila* (1966), the birth weight at term is the same for infants with PE as for their control infants. The confusing results must be due to the failure to distinguish between the circummarginate and circumvallate froms. PE (circumvallate) as a pathogenetic factor in fetal growth retardation and premature labor requires further study, especially as the pathogenesis of this condition is still unclear.

3. Cord Insertion

The frequency of marginal cord insertion in the author's study (Table 1) is not high in LBW in comparison with figures given by *Brody* et al. (1953), who observed 22 of 32 premature infants with marginal cord insertion.

Velamentous and marginal insertions of the cord have also been reported to associate with a tendency toward gestational prematurity by *Shanklin* (1958) and also a high frequency of fetal anomalies (*Krone* et al., 1965; *Monie*, 1965). On the other hand, no association between abnormal cord insertion and SGA infants was found by *Scott* and *Jordan* (1972). *Busch* (1972) observed battledore and velamentous insertion in 23% in a study of intrauterine growth-retarded infants. The association between velamentous insertion and twinning (*Benirschke*, 1965; *Benirschke* and *Driscoll*, 1967), abnormal placental shapes and an absent umbilical artery (*Benirschke* and *Brown*, 1955; *Little*, 1958) might in part add to a high frequency of LBW. The cited works and the present study indicate a strong association of abnormal cord insertion with the LBW syndrome and reflect a disturbed uteroplacental relation. The theories to explain the development of velamentous cord insertion have been discussed by *Grosser* (1927) and *Krone* (1961). The latter considered that these placentas are placed low in the uterus with a poorer uterovascular supply, which fits with the concept of "trophotropism," in which the author of this paper believes. This idea is supported by the finding that the site of membrane rupture is near the site of insertion in battledore and velamentous placentas (*Shanklin*, 1958).

4. Infarction

Placental infarction has long been discussed from the viewpoint of acute as well as chronic placental insufficiency. The incidence and volume of infarcts in the placenta reported by different authors show considerable variation and must be the result of

10

selection, different definitions, and examination techniques. The synonyms used by various authors can be summarized as follows:

Acute infarct: Corresponds to type E of *Bartholomew* (1961) and *Steigrad* (1952), to type II of *Zeek* and *Assali* (1952), to *Budlinger's* (1964) peracute and acute hemorrhagic infarct, and to types 2 and 3 of *Carter* et al. (1963).

Subacute infarct: Corresponds to type *C and D* of *Bartholomew*, to type II of *Zeek* and *Assali*, and to *Budlinger's* acute brown infarct.

Old infarct: Corresponds to types A and B of *Bartholomew*, to types IV and V of *Little* (1960a), to type 4 of *Zeek* and *Assali*, and to *Fox's* (1963) so-called genuine infarct (type 4).

Mixed infarct: Corresponds to *Shanklin's* (1970) mixed infarct and so-called diffuse fibrinosis. This lesion can be considered as extensive perivillous fibrin deposition (*Fox*, 1967), ischemic necrosis by fibrin deposition (*Wilkin*, 1965), and the static/villous lesion resulting from fibrin encasement (*Carter* et al., 1963).

Support for ischemia as a contributing cause of intrauterine growth retardation can be found in the occlusive and degenerative changes in uteroplacental vessels and the significantly increased rate of infarction in conjunction with maternal hypertension and toxemia (*Dixon* and *Robertson,* 1961; *Fox,* 1963; *Marrais,* 1962a, b; *Rumboltz* and *McGoodan*, 1953). The reserve capacity of the placenta, however, is apparently great since full-term AGA infants can have heavily infarcted placentas (*Shanklin,* 1970). *Beltran-Paz* and *Driscoll* (cited by *Benirschke* and *Driscoll,* 1967) found no clear evidence that infarction caused "dysmaturity" and *Shanklin* (1970) also considers infarction to be rarely implicated in low birth weight or premature deliveries.

The difficulty in this context is to ensure separation of toxemic and hypertensive mothers from normotensive mothers. Many toxemic mothers were included in the series of *Busch* (1972), *Dollman* (1973), *Wigglesworth* (1964), and *Reichwein* and *Vogel* (1972), in which extensive (more than 5% of placental volume) infarcts were associated with SGA infants. *Gruenwald* (1961) and *Clifford* (1954) selected only normotensive mothers and still found an association between SGA and placental infarcts.

In the present material, fresh infarcts were frequently found in conjunction with abruptio placentae and premature labor. The acute lesion was not related to growth retardation except in conjunction with hypertension and toxemia. There were few of the latter, however, in this material.

Experimental occlusion of the uteroplacental arteries does not result in demonstrable infarction before 23 h (*Wallenburg* et al., 1973), a possible explanation for negative findings in placentas with acute placental insufficiency.

Wigglesworth (1964) considers it unlikely that an occlusion of a single spiral vessel would be sufficient to cause placental infarction unless there is considerable reduction of blood flow through neighboring vessels. Thus, even a small area of infarction indicates a widespread reduction in retroplacental blood flow. In view of this consideration, the observed difference (Tables 4 and 5) in subacute and old infarction between the placentas from infants appropriate for gestational age and small for gestational age is more significant and points further to reduced uteroplacental circulation as the cause of the fetal complication.

Old and recent infarcts were more frequent in placentas of infants with LBW from a population with a low socioeconomic status (*Laga* et al., 1972), another complicating factor in comparing different series. With the definitions applied to the present series, there is evidence that the number, rather than the volume, of old infarcts is related to prematurity or intrauterine growth retardation. The small volume of placenta tissue involved in old infarcts can be explained by shrinking of infarcts and compensatory hyperplasia of surviving chorionic villi. In a few instances, SGA can be associated with widespread infarction of the diffuse fibrinous or mixed types (*Shanklin*, 1970; *Gruenwald*, 1963; *Reichwein* and *Vogel*, 1972).

5. Subchorionic Thrombus

This condition is here defined as an, at least 1 cm thick, layer of laminated thrombus extending over at least half the subchorial area. It seems that no thorough attempt has been made to investigate the nature of this lesion. In my opinion, the thrombus is probably not caused by slow maternal blood flow. The lesion is not common, but it has been found to be frequent in placentas from SGA infants by *Reichwein* and *Vogel* (1972).

6. Retroplacental Hematoma

When recording this lesion it is important to differentiate it from a simple, adherent postpartum clot. True hematoma, irrespective of age, cannot be removed by careful blotting, and it leaves a depression on the maternal surface. Retroplacental hematoma (RPH) with premature detachment is a well-known cause of prematurity with acute danger to the fetus. In *Hibbard* and *Jeffcoate*'s (1966) series, many infants weighed less than expected for their age, which was especially notable in the more premature babies. They also found a relatively large number of fetal malformations, a strong tendency for RPH to recur in subsequent pregnancies, and many perinatal deaths.

Sexton et al. (1950) noted an association not only with fresh but also with old infarction in premature separation. *Scott* and *Usher* (1966) found retroplacental hemorrhage associated with LBW. On the other hand, *Reichwein* and *Vogel* (1972) found that infants that were premature due to premature separation had normal weight. In their series of intrauterine growth-retarded infants, *Dollman* (1973) and *Busch* (1972) did not mention retroplacental hematomas as an etiologic factor. Finally, the fact that a circumvallate placenta may also initiate the premature separation has also been noted (*Sexton* et al., 1950; *Naftolin* et al., 1973). RPH emerges as one important and clearcut factor in LBW, including SGA, and indicates severely disturbed uteroplacental circulation.

12

7. Chorangioma

Chorangiomas are histologically similar to hemangiomas. They are vascular malformations rather than true neoplasms. They are said to be present in about 1% of placentas.
Chorangiomas, regardless of size, have on occasion been associated with low birth
weight (*Shanklin*, 1970). *Gruenwald* (1963) also related single or multiple chorangiomas to LBW or chronic fetal distress. In larger series, however, the frequency of chorangiomas was not greater for LBW infants than for control infants (*Froehlich* et al.,
1971; *Battaglia* and *Woolever*, 1968). In the material of *Froehlich* et al., more than
half the chorangiomas were less than 1 cm in diameter.

It has often been held that chorangiomas influence the fetus only if they displace
a major part of the placental substance (*De Costa* et al., 1956; *Marchetti*, 1939) and
that these tumors function as an arteriovenous shunt with an increased cardiac load on
the fetus. There seems to be little doubt that this lesion, particularly when multiple or
diffuse, is accompanied by a fairly high incidence of fetal hypoxia and low birth weight
(*Fox*, 1967).

8. Single Umbilical Artery

The frequency of single umbilical artery (SUA) is apparently higher in twins, and the
twin lacking one artery has been noted to be smaller (*Thomas*, 1959, 1961; *Froehlich*
and *Fujikura*, 1973). A veriety of associated malformations has been reported (*Bourne*
and *Benirschke*, 1960) with an overall frequency of 11% (*Wilson*, 1964). As *Faierman*
(1960), *Little* (1958), and *Benirschke* and *Brown* (1955) also have reported, a single
umbilical artery is likely to be accompanied by abnormalities of the placenta such as
velamentous insertion and circumvallate placentation. The higher incidence of infarction in placentas with a single artery reported by *Faierman* was also found in this series.
The peculiar vascularity (vide infra) seen in placentas with SUA and velamentous cord
insertion might be a common denominator. A causal relationship between SUA and
growth retardation was suggested by *Beyreiss* et al. (1968), and there is also experimental support for this (*Hobel* et al., 1970). In the absence of fetal malformation,
however, *Longo* (1972) did not find that lack of one umbilical artery affected fetal
growth.

9. Unrelated Lesions

Intervillous thrombosis is usually considered to result from rupture of fetal vessels.
There is no evidence in the present series or in others (*Shanklin*, 1970) that these
thrombi are associated with LBW. Small subchorionic thrombi, marginal lesions, calcif-
ications, and septal cysts likewise are not connected with LBW.

V. Placental Arterial Vasculature

The formation of the definite human placenta is tied in essence to the development of fetal arteries and the cotyledons. Inasmuch as the vascularity of the placenta is intimately related to its anatomy and function, it is not surprising that angiographic studies have classic traditions since the works of *Bumm* (1890, 1893). These were followed by the well-known publications of *Spanner* (1935) and *Stieve* (1941a) and later of *Wilkin* (1954) among others. Maternal placental circulation has been described by *Borell* et al. (1958, 1965). During the 1960s, in vivo angiography on subhuman primates was employed, sometimes simultaneously on fetal and maternal circulatory systems (*Ramsey* et al., 1967; *Freese*, 1966; *Freese* et al., 1966). The contrast media and techniques have differed and so have conclusions concerning the vascular pattern of the placenta. Some of the radiographic methods permit evaluation of flow dynamics (*Fernström*, 1955; *Dixon* et al., 1963), while quantitative and qualitative evaluation of the entire vascular patterns of the placenta require complementation of angiographic findings by light microscopy (*Krohn* et al., 1970).

1. Definition and Angiographic Method

Because of the various synonyms used in the literature it is necessary to define the terms that will be used subsequently.

Allantochorionic arteries are branches of the umbilical arteries running on the fetal side of the placenta between the amnion and chorion.

A dispersed pattern is formed by the allantochorionic arteries when each umbilical artery divides at once, dichotomously, with gradually diminishing caliber.

A magistral pattern is present when these arteries extend almost to the margin before their caliber diminishes, giving off small branches along their course.

A primary cotyledonary artery is a branch of an allantochorionic artery penetrating to the interior of the placenta. Synonyms: primary trunc (*Crawford*, 1962), truncus chorii (*Bøe*, 1953), subchorionic artery. The primary cotyledonary arteries divide into *secondary and tertiary branches* in different ways, and form a relatively uniform vascular structure, the fetal cotyledon, which is supposed to consists of subunits or subcotyledons (*Smart*, 1962); Synonym: lobules (*Gruenwald*, 1966).

The placental septa consists of more or less distinct grooves on the decidual surface and form wall-like projections from the basal plate toward the intervillous space (IVS) seen on the cut surface of the placenta.

Placental lobes are the projecting convex areas seen on the decidual surface of the placenta, which are separated by often indistinct grooves of variable depth.

The placentas were first washed with tepid physiologic saline through one umbilical artery and then injected with a 7.5% aqueous suspension of $BaSO_4$ at a continuous pressure of 100 mmHg for 1 h, while being kept in tepid physiologic saline. They were then submerged in 10% neutral formalin solution for at least two weeks. After fixation the whole placenta was X-rayed and sliced, and the slices were X-rayed (Figs. 1 and 2).

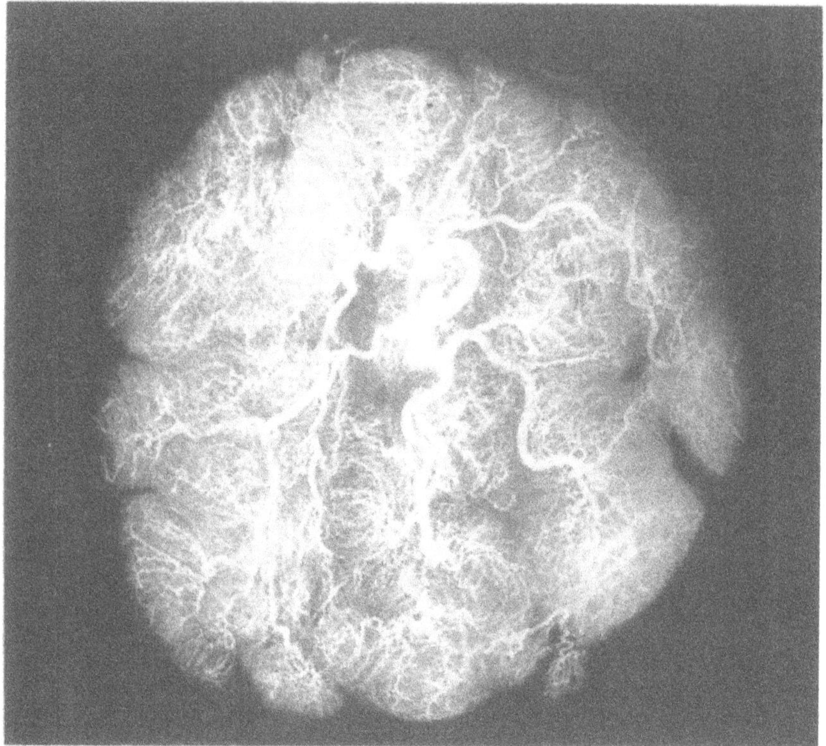

Fig. 1. Angiogram of a placenta predominantly of the disperse type

2. Arterial Vasculature in uncomplicated Term Pregnancy

The following description is based on angiography of the arterial vessels in placentas from normal, uneventful pregnancies that resulted in the birth of healthy infants.

a) Allantochorial Vessels and Cotyledons

In angiograms of the intact placenta, the *umbilical arteries* enter upon the fetal surface and divide both into the magistral and the disperse patterns, to use *Schordania*'s nomenclature. The former consists of a V and the latter of a stellate pattern. It is obvious that these represent two extremes, and there are mixed types.

The disperse placenta is the most common and is usually associated with a near-central cord insertion. The pure magistral placenta most often has a marginal or velamentous cord insertion. This finding is not new (*Bacsich* and *Smout,* 1938). The relationship between the pattern of these vessels and the type of division of the intraplacental vessels (vide infra) was also noted by *Crawford* (1962), who found by dissection that the magistral placenta contained larger and heavier cotyledons and that even the

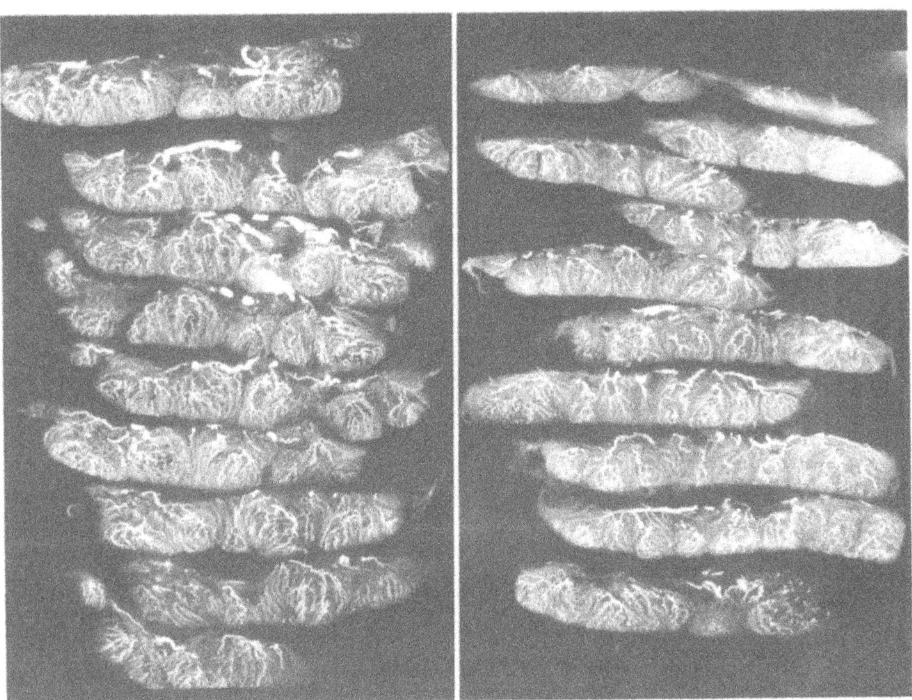

Fig. 2. Angiogram of the serially sliced placenta in Figure 1

villi seemed to be influenced. *Schordania* (1929) in fact, hypothesized that the magistral placenta should produce a better-developed fetus and that the vascular pattern was genetically determined by the vascular characteristics of the mother.

The allantochorionic arteries give off one primary cotyledonary artery to the central part of 10–30 spherical vascular units, which are seen in the angiogram and are called cotyledons by authors who have used angiographic techniques (barium sulfate, lipoid, pastoid, etc.) for the study of the fetal vasculature (*Romney* and *Reid*, 1951; *Lemtis*, 1955; *Panigel*, 1962). Most authors report similar results concerning size and number of cotyledons, irrespective of the method used. The high number of cotyledons reported by *Crawford* (1956a) and by *Gruenwald* (1966) can probably be explained by their defining subcotyledons as cotyledons.

The cotyledons are formed principally in two ways. The most common variety, often combined with dispersed vasculature, is the branching of the primary cotyledonary artery into 2–7 secondary arteries. These then divide into finer tertiary intracotyledonary branches that run toward the decidual plate and form a spherical vascular unit, the subcotyledon, with a diameter of 1–3 cm (Fig. 5). The subcotyledons in one cotyledon are centered around are larger subcotyledon or they have a circular arrangement. In the other variety, often present in the magistral placenta, the primary cotyledonary artery branches at once into arteries of the tertiary type and form a cotyledon without distinct subcotyledons (Fig. 5). The main pattern of the vascular units in the placenta with a primary cotyledonary artery, umbilical artery of tertiary order, which

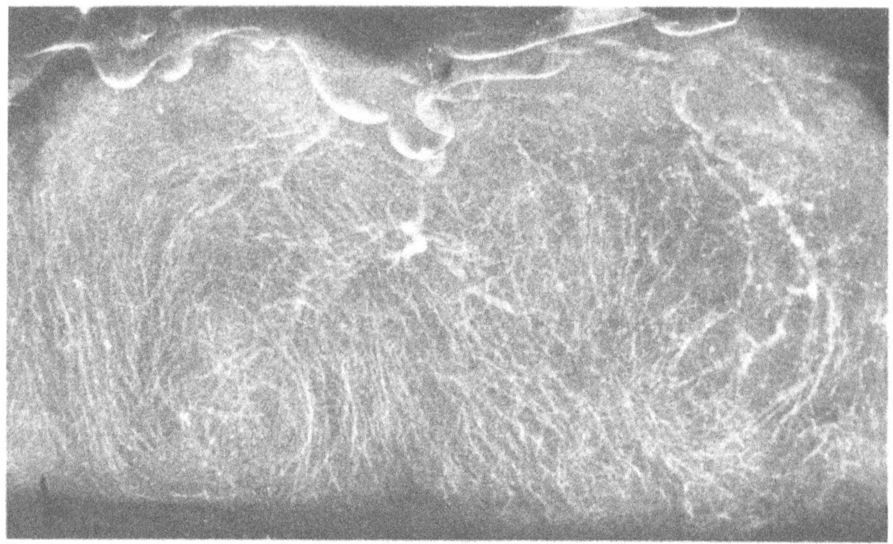

Fig. 3. Angiogram of a cotyledon, Type 1, with nonbranching slender arteries

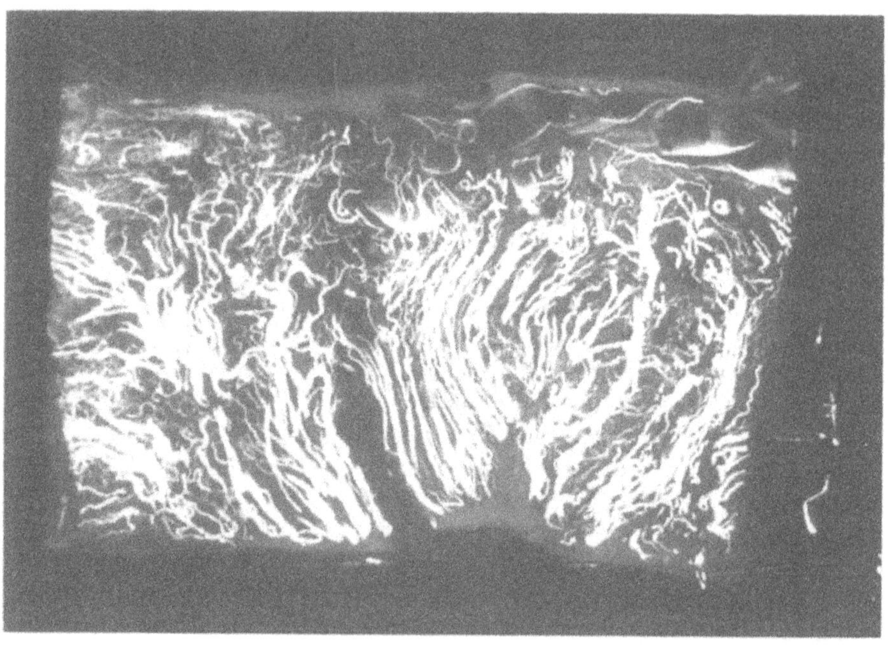

Fig. 4. Angiogram of a cotyledon, Type 2, partly inverted with coarse branching arteries

can divide into 2–5 subcotyledonary vessels forming round subcotyledons, is in line with findings of *Panigel* (1962), *Smart* (1962), *Wilkin* (1965), and *Strauss* (1964).

b) Subcotyledons

The existence of the subcotyledons has been stressed especially by authors using plastic casting of the fetal vasculature (*Panigel*, 1962; *Smart*, 1962). This method permits a better three-dimensional view. The subunits are more difficult to see in angiograms, also noted by *Lemtis* (1955), who used radiopaque oil suspension, though he considered that the cotyledons had several *Hauptbezirke.* The packing together of the subcotyledons makes them less evident even in the vertical angiogram because the arteries in the subcotyledons interdigitate in a more intimate fashion than the arteries of the cotyledons. However, the more friable villous tissue freely interdigitates. Thus, *Lemtis* (1955) found that ligation of one main artery did not lead to a well-delimitated contrast defect in his angiograms because of irregular interdigitation of chorionic villi from neighboring cotyledons.

Subcotyledons have been considered to be the true functional units of the placenta (*Smart*, 1962; *Freese*, 1966; *Boyd* and *Hamilton*, 1967) with a number and spacing corresponding to the maternal spiral arteries, as suggested by *Smart* (1962) and by *Marais* (1962a, b, c). *Wigglesworth* (1969) demonstrated that the site of the arterial opening is in the cavity of the fetal cotyledon. *Arts* (1961) did not find any definite position of the uteroplacental arteries relative to the cotyledons, but he denies the subdivision into subcotyledons and did not take them into account. Only occasionally is a duplicate arterial supply of marginal cotyledons found, which is not in line with the observation of *Romney* and *Reid* (1951) who maintained that the majority of peripheral cotyledons had a double arterial supply.

c) Intracotyledonary Arteries

Spiralization of chorionic and subchorionic arteries is often noted and has also been seen in cast preparations (*Romney* and *Reid*, 1951). According to *Reynolds* (1966), this is a manifestation of rapid growth under the trophic stimulus of steroid hormones. The intracotyledonary arteries are of different types but usually have a pattern that gives the cotyledon or subcotyledon a characteristic configuration (Fig. 5). They run toward the basal plate slightly bent in relation to the axis of the cotyledon. The arteries in the periphery of the cotyledon are narrow and have only a few branches that run in the same direction as the main artery. The central arteries have a larger diameter and a more irregular course. They give rise to several branches that leave at right or acute angles.

The arteries in the intermediate and peripheral parts of the cotyledon or subcotyledon reach the decidua as anchoring arteries and then take a horizontal course. They often run in or close to the septa (Fig. 5). In occasional cotyledons, the intracotyledonary arteries have a more horizontal course but the general pattern is the same as in a vertical angiogram. The horizontal cotyledons are often separated by very deep oblique fissures.

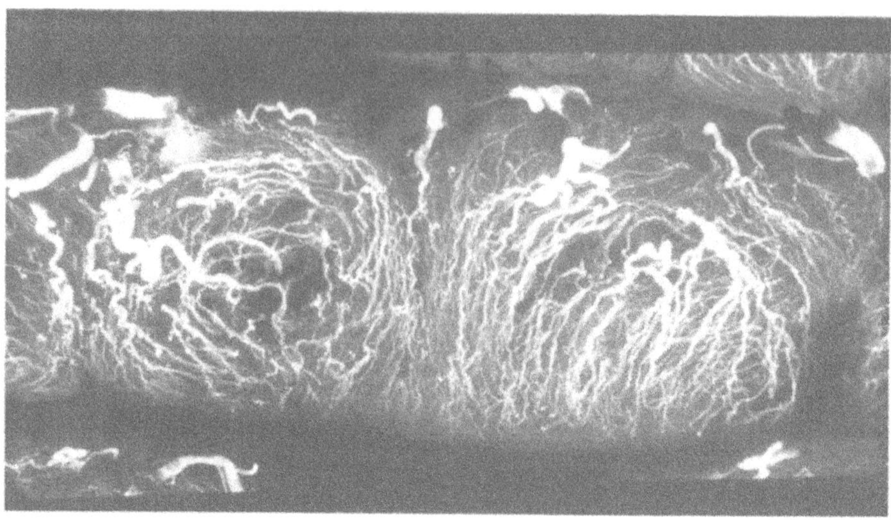

Fig. 5. Angiogram with Type 3 cotyledons. At *left* no clear subcotyledons, at *right* three subcotyledons

The different types of intracotyledonary arteries were described earlier by *Krohn* et al. (1970) and in part by *Romney* and *Reid* (1951). The branching of the arteries, predivision, and the reversed course have been described in detail by *Bøe* (1953) and by *Spanner* (1935). Whether the intracotyledonary arterial pattern is related to the dividing scheme of the allantochorionic arteries is not clear although this has been suggested by *Bacsich* and *Crawford* (1960). They also put forward the interesting question of whether a woman has the same particular vascular pattern in all her placentas.

In histologic sections from selected areas, the density of the villous tissue varies in both the single cotyledon and the subcotyledon, which was stressed by *Gruenwald* (1966). Within a circumferential area, the uniformly thin terminal villi are in close apposition and correspond to the cotyledons or subcotyledons seen macroscopically. Villous stems were found in this portion. The loose central area contains only few terminal thick and somewhat irregular villi. In the subchorionic area, the lobular arrangement is not seen. This part of the placenta contains many villous stems but only a few terminal villi, spread far apart. In the basal region, the lobular pattern is only partly evident. The central, loose areas are small or have disappeared. Terminal villi are large but not so abundant, and anchoring stems constitute the main bulk of tissue. The intercotyledonary zone is almost devoid of terminal villi, which are thin and far apart. In sections taken parallel to the placental surfaces, similar variations of villous structures are seen. This variability of the villous tissue and its relation to the arterial type is important to recognize, especially when taking only small pieces for microscopic studies.

3. Arterial Vasculature of the Placenta in LBW

The form and sturcture of the cotyledons, with their attachments to both the chorionic and basal plates, are conceivably controlled by genetic and local uterine factors. They may influence the development of the placenta and hence that of the fetus, and thus they may cause low birth weight. It is possible then that structural differences in fetal arteries as well as cotyledons exist in LBW infants. The qualitative and quantitative possibilities of the angiographic method employed have been utilized for the study of placentas of infants in the categories "appropriate" and "small" for gestational age.

a) Classification and Number of Cotyledons

The number of cotyledons and subcotyledons is found in Tables 6, 7 and 8. An attempt was also made to classify the cotyledons by their content of intracotyledonary arteries. Long and narrow arteries with few branches and running in the periphery of a cotyledon are called "A arteries." "B arteries" are coarser and more centrally placed in a cotyledon or subcotyledon and have numerous branches (Fig. 5). With these arterial types as the basis, cotyledons can be divided into four types:

1. A arteries only (Fig. 3)
2. B arteries only (Fig. 4)
3. Both A and B arteries. The A arteries always run along the periphery and B arteries in the central portion of a cotyledon (Fig. 5)
4. A composite type with both A and B arteries in an irregular pattern (Fig. 6)

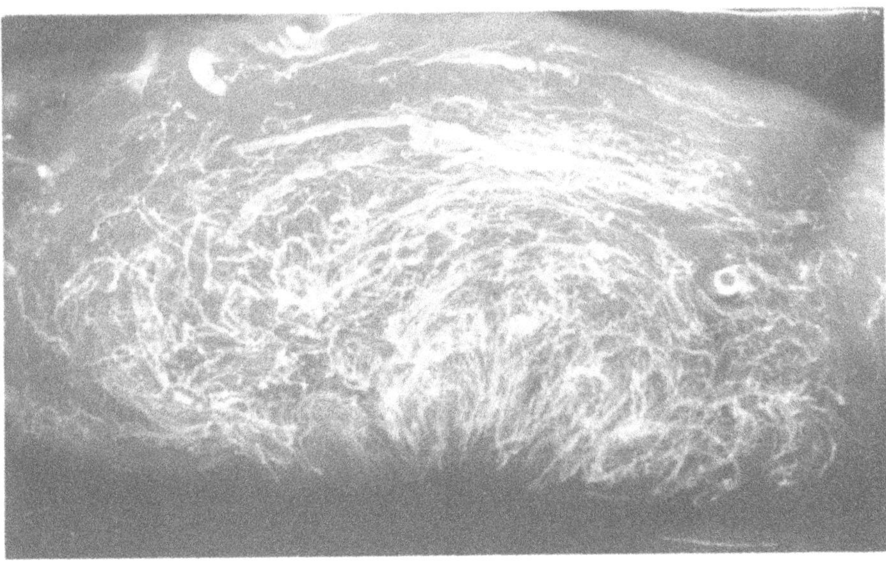

Fig. 6. Cotyledon of Type 4 with mixed arterial pattern

Table 6. Distribution of cotyledons with different arterial types and subcotyledons in 14 placentas from term pregnancies, appropriate for gestational age

Placenta No.	Arterial type				Not filled	Total	No. of sub-cotyledons	Decidual surface (cm^2)	Remarks
	1	2	3	4					
62	0	1	10	2	0	22	182	230	
64	0	1	14	3	0	18	176	215	
66	0	2	18	3	0	23	114	218	
70	0	1	15	0	0	16	134	203	Partial cir-cumvallate
69	0	0	17	0	0	17	142	230	
58	1	3	9	2	1	15	129	196	Marginal insertion
57	0	0	10	3	0	13	129	196	
51	0	1	8	3	0	12	98	163	Marginal insertion
48	0	2	23	4	0	29	187	196	
36	0	7	8	0	0	15	96	165	Heartshaped
20	0	1	18	4	0	23	138	175	
19	0	2	16	4	0	22	129	163	
18	0	2	15	1	0	19	96	172	Marginal insertion
13	0	2	9	1	0	12	111	152	Bilobate and extrachorial

The results of the classification of vessels and cotyledonic structures are given in Tables 6–8. The placentas are arranged according to gestational age, and the plain decidual surface (in cm^2) has been calculated. The source of errors and artifacts inherent in the methods and their possible effect on the classification of the arteries are discussed by *Krohn* et al. (1970) and *Sandstedt* (1974).

In some placentas there was a type of cotyledon that has to be described in detail since it does not fit into the definitions that were based on earlier results. This type is usually very large and the peripheral delimitation is diffuse. Distinct subcotyledons are

Table 7. Distribution of cotyledons with different arterial types and subcotyledons in 12 placentas from preterm infants, appropriate for gestational age

Placenta No.	Arterial type				Not filled	Total	No. of sub-cotyledons	Pregnancy (weeks)	Decidual surface (cm^2)	Remarks
	1	2	3	4						
684	1	2	6	1	1	11	43	28	134	Partial circumvallate
3115	7	2	13	4	0	26	62	32	164	Marginal insertion
2386	2	3	31	4	0	39	63	33	180	Accessory lobe
3051	2	1	17	2	0	22	62	33	148	
2920	3	1	12	1	2	19	98	35	149	Marginal insertion
2387	2	3	18	2	1	26	75	35	170	Twin
1163	0	1	11[a]	11	0	23	90	36	210	Marginal insertion
2206	0	0	12	2	1	15	106	36	170	
1248	1	0	7	5	0	13	56	36	175	
1329	0	3	12	2	0	17	80	36	155	
1843	3	1	14	0	0	18	71	36	175	
2041	1	0	7	2	0	10	(64)	37	173	Velamentous insertion, circumvallate

[a] Seaweed type

Table 8. Distribution of cotyledons with different arterial types and subcotyledons in 13 placentas from preterm and term infants, small for gestational age

Placenta No.	Arterial type				Not filled	Total	No. of sub-cotyledons	Pregnancy (weeks)	Decidual surface (cm^2)	Remarks
	1	2	3	4						
845	1[a]	7[a]	7[a]	0	0	15	45	32	144	One umbilical artery
2387	2	0	7	3	2	14	54	35	124	Twin
739	0	0	6[a]	0	0	6	23	36	113	Circumvallate
1074	2	1	14	0	0	17	55	36	144	Bilobate
2140	0	1	13	4	0	18	57	37	142	
738	0	4	12	1	0	17	62	37	146	
2139	1[a]	1[a]	3[a]	0	0	5	48	37	162	Circumvallate
2116	2	1	11	0	0	14	51	38	148	
2478	2	0	12	1	0	16	66	38	155	
1076	0	4[a]	3	1[a]	0	8	$-^b$	38	154	One umbilical artery, circum-vallate
3222	1	1	10	2	0	14	54	39	158	
4414	1	0	18	2	0	21	58	40	157	
2329	1	1	18	2	0	22	72	40	160	

[a] Seaweed cotyledons

[b] No distinct subcotyledons

difficult to see; the vessels are long and narrow and have a parallel, wavy arrangement running in different directions, often horizontal. The central part of the cotyledon can hardly be delimited. This cotyledon differs from the type 4 cotyledon by being larger and having longer vessels running in waves and bundles. The type 4 cotyledon is small and present in all placentas, usually at the periphery.

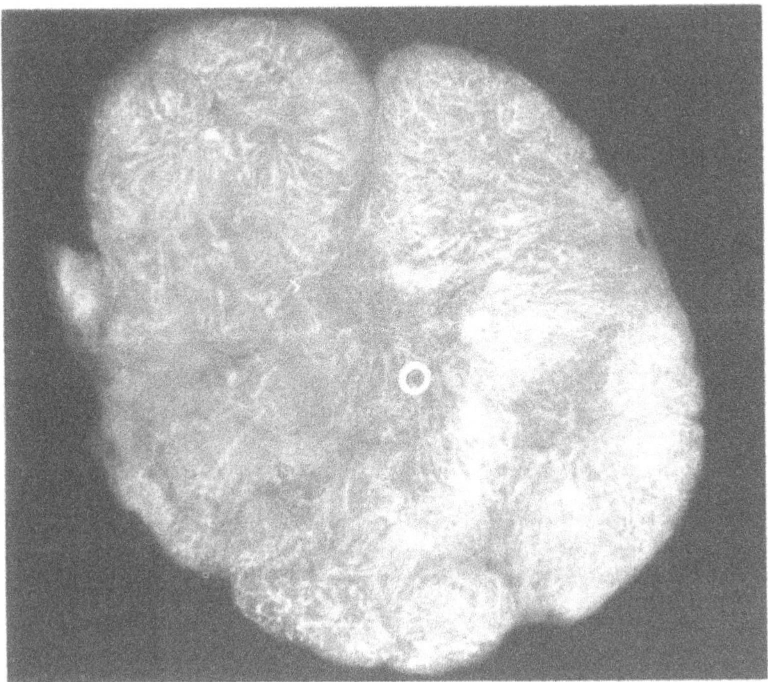

Fig. 7. Angiogram of a placenta with single umbilical artery and large cotyledons showing long vessels (seaweed) and no distinct subcotyledons

This larger, "seaweed" cotyledon predominated in one extrachorial placenta with a chorangioma, in two with a single umbilical artery each (Figs. 7 and 8) and in one "dumpy" placenta with extrachorial configuration (Fig. 9). In two placentas with marginal cord insertion there were a few cotyledons of this type also. It was also noted in placentas with marginal cord insertion or of "magistral" type that the intracotyledonary arteries often had a horizontal course and that the subcotyledons were ill-defined.

Since the material is limited and represents different gestational ages and categories of infants, and since there is a wide variation in the number of *cotyledons*, it is impossible to make a detailed statistical comparison between placentas from the different maturity groups. There was, however, a distinct tendency for the full-term AGA infants to have a more uniform number of cotyledons than the other groups. On the whole, the number of cotyledons agrees with that in other series (*Panigel*, 1962;

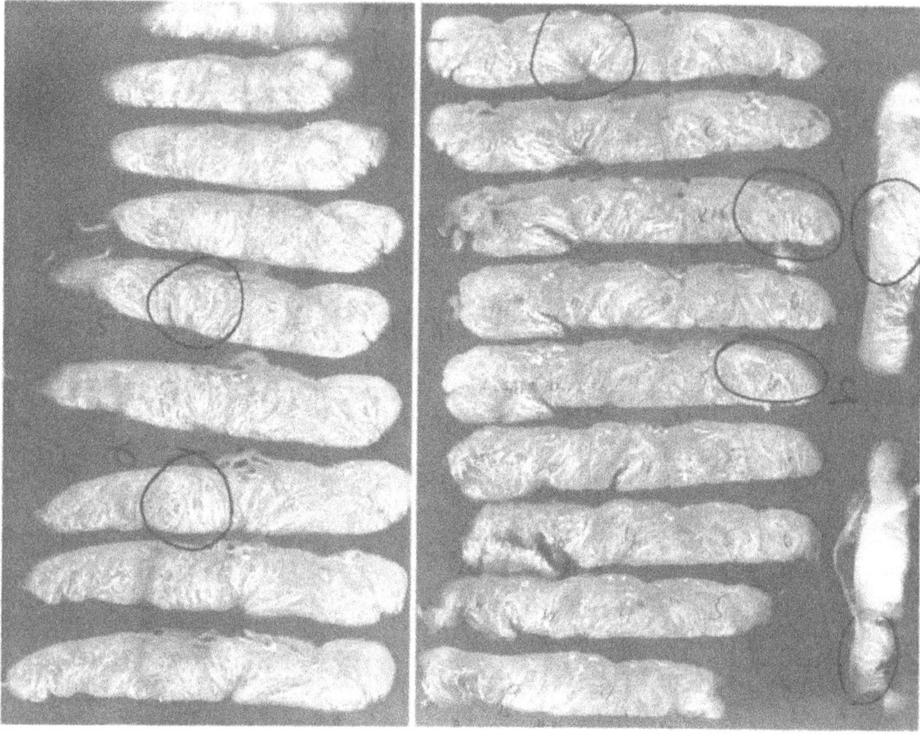

Fig. 8. Angiogram of the sliced placenta in Figure 7

Crawford, 1956a, 1962; *Krohn* et al., 1970). However, it should be remembered that the nomenclature applied to cotyledons is confusing.

Some points emerge from comparison of particular placentas with the profile of the whole or parts of the material. After exclusion of placentas with extremes in the number of cotyledons (one accessory lobe with many, and extrachorial with few), there is no clear difference in the number of cotyledons between preterm and term AGA infants. SGA infants, however, have somewhat fewer cotyledons. There was no increase in the number of cotyledons with increasing gestational age. As *Boyd* and *Hamilton* (1967) pointed out, the number of cotyledons is determined by the end of the first trimester. *Crawford* (1962) also considered the number of cotyledons to remain constant throughout pregnancy and observed that the dispersed or magistral arterial pattern is recognizable by the twelfth week of pregnancy.

The size and number of the cotyledons have been said to follow the pattern of the allantochorionic vessels as they divide, and also to influence the size of the infant. The cotyledons in the magistral placenta have been found to be larger and heavier (*Crawford*, 1962). In this context it is interesting to note that *Shanklin* (1970) mentions a condition with severe reduction in the number of vascular units, apparently cotyledons, in the absence of placenta extrachorialis, which he terms "insufficient vascular pattern."

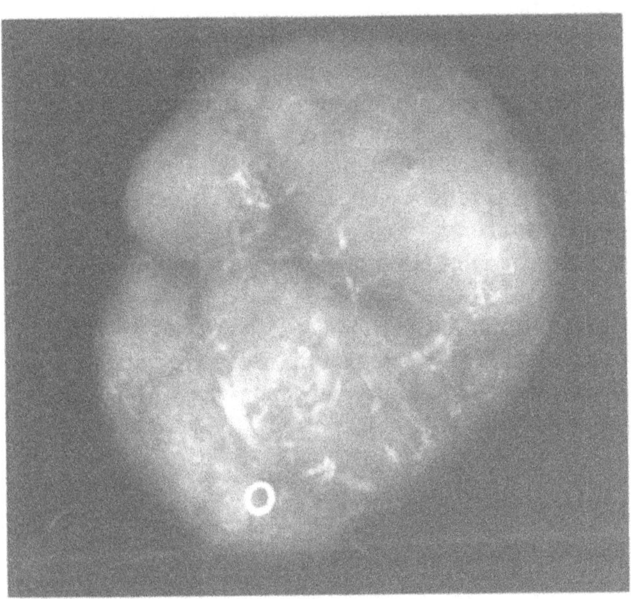

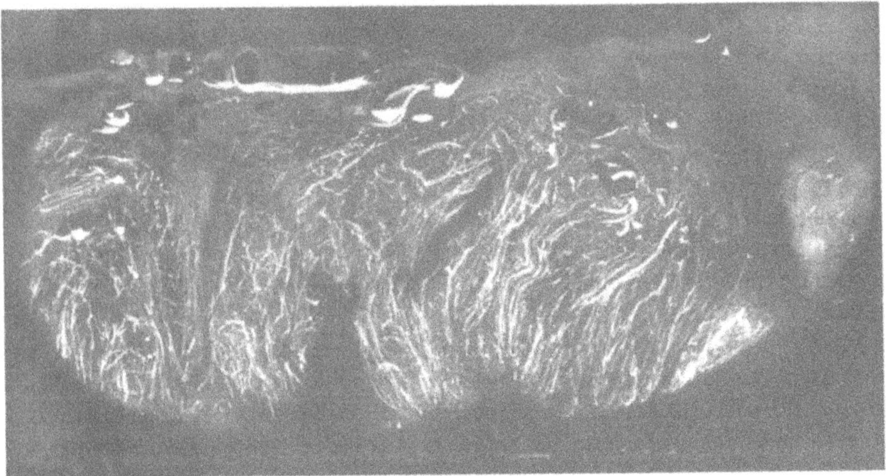

Fig. 9a and b. Angiogram (a) of extrachorial placenta (No. 739 in Table 8) with large cotyledons. Angiogram (b) of slice showing one large seaweed cotyledon and no distinct subcotyledons

Five of seven such cases were associated with appropriate birth weight at term. As was the case in the present series, *Shanklin* and *Sotelo-Avila* (1966) found the superficial branching of arteries in the chorion to be significantly less in PE than in normal placentas. PE with the fewest cotyledons were in the present SGA group, a possible indicator of an insufficient vascular pattern. Unfortunately, it was not always possible to relate the cotyledons in this material to magistral or disperse vessel pattern. The impression is that in many placentas, this pattern is mixed. In one battledore placenta with a typical magistral vessel pattern, there were few and consequently larger cotyledons as well as subcotyledons. Some placentas with marginal cord insertion, usually of magistral type, had few cotyledons.

Schordania's (1929) theory that the vascular pattern of the placenta is not a haphazard phenomenon but genetically determined by the vascular characteristics of the mother, finds additional support from *Bacsich* and *Crawford* (1960). They also believe that the vessel pattern of the chorionic plate influences the type of division of the free villi.

Since the number of cotyledons and the allantochorial vascular pattern are recognizable early in pregnancy, it seems logical to assume that the site of implantation and the endometrial arterioles influence their formation. Otherwise, the extreme number seen in PE or bilobate placentas would have to be determined by the genetics of the ovum.

b) Subcotyledons and Their Possible Relation to Maternal Arteries

Unlike the cotyledons, the small vascular units, i.e., the *subcotyledons*, increase in number during gestation until about the 36th week. They may follow the same growth pattern as the cell mass in the fetoplacental unit. If this is true, it could explain why subcotyledons are fewer and do not increase in number at the same rate in the SGA group. The placental cell mass is smaller in SGA infants and its growth parallels that of the fetus (*Winick*, 1967). An alternative explanation for the relative paucity of subcotyledons in the SGA group is that the subcotyledons are difficult to identify because of indistinct contours, but this seems less likely.

The number of subcotyledons has been assumed to be the same as that of the maternal spiral arteries (*Wilkin*, 1954; *Smart*, 1962). However, the number of spiral arterial openings into the intervillous space is unknown. Various figures have been given in the literature, i.e., 94 by *Spanner* (1935), 263 by *Franken* (1954), and 105 by *Marais* (1962d). The discrepancy in the figures given may be the result of the fact that one uterine artery can have several decidual openings through which blood spurts simultaneously. The subcotyledon could then correspond to a distal split-up branch and the cotyledon to the main artery. This suggestion fits with the 25 arteries emptying into the IVS found by *Borell* et al. (1965) in their radiographic study of uteroplacental circulation. *Wilkin* (1954) put forward the idea that there are about 100 arterial openings and that each of his "tambours" (subcotyledons) is centered over its own spiral arterial opening, a suggestion considered reasonable by *Boyd* and *Hamilton* (1967). In a serial section examination of an in situ placenta at term, *Brosens* and *Dixon* (1966) found one arterial opening per 2 cm² of basal plate. The occurrence of an increase in the number of spiral arterial openings during gestation into the IVS has been suggested (*Boyd* and *Hamilton*, 1967).

The general relation between the number of subcotyledons and the surface area of the basal plate in the placentas of the present series fits with the figures arrived at by *Wilkin* (1954) and by *Brosens* and *Dixon* (1966). The tendency for the AGA placentas to have a greater number of subcotyledons and a larger surface area than the SGA placentas could well imply a similar increase in nutritive maternal arteries since definitely discoid placentas grow mainly in diameter. The question of whether placentas from AGA infants with few subcotyledons have larger spiral arteries must be raised. The problem could perhaps be settled with in situ angiography of the uterus and placenta.

The significance of extrachorial implantation for the LBW syndrome has already been discussed. The few but large cotyledons in extrachorial placentas imply that mere largeness of cotyledons cannot be associated with better intrauterine fetal growth as suggested by *Crawford* (1965a, b) and *Schordania* (1929). The paucity of subcotyledons in extrachorial placentas is compatible with the primary cause of PE being faulty implantation, i.e., a local uterine factor. Because of its deeper but less extensive manner of growth, it is possible that PE makes contact with fewer spiral arteries. Supplied by fewer spiral arteries, PE may not be able to meet demans for increased blood flow, with LBW as a conceivable result. A similar explanation may hold for the placentas with abnormal cord insertion, single umbilical artery, and chorangioma, because an interrelationship seems to exist between these abnormalities (*Benirschke* and *Brown, Froehlich* et al., 1971; *Froehlich* and *Fujikura*, 1973).

c) Abnormal Arterial Pattern – Seaweed Cotyledons

Demonstration of the new intraplacentary seaweed vascular anomaly naturally suggests further exploration of the possibility that vascular anomalies involving the fetal-placental unit exist more commonly than is recognized at present. The association between SUA and cardiovascular and other anomalies in the fetus as described by *Froehlich* et al. (1971) is now accepted. SUA is also associated with velamentous insertion of the cord (*Le Marec* et al., 1972) and extrachorial placentas (*Benirschke* and *Brown*, 1955). In the present series, large placental cotyledons with the seaweed anomaly were, in turn, associated with SUA and velamentous insertion of the cord as well as with placenta extrachorialis. Through study of many more specimens of this type than included in the present consecutive series, it may be possible to establish additional links and ultimately understand their pathogenesis. The unusually large cotyledon with its horizontal vessels, the seaweed type, possibly represents a vascular malformation in some placentas from LBW infants. The most bizarre placenta in this respect also contained a small chorangioma. The tumor was poorly filled with contrast medium, possibly because of the viscosity of the medium. The abnormal vascular pattern was much more extensive than the tumor. Against this background of a generalized vascular abnormality, it would appear that the chorangioma itself is a vascular abnormality rather than a real tumor.

If the spiral arteries influence the size and type of cotyledon and subcotyledon, the seaweed type must be implanted in a uterus or a part of a uterus with abnormal arteries of some kind. To some extent the same can hold true for the placentas with marginal cord insertion and a horizontal vessel pattern. Alternatively, the primary reason for this kind of vascular anomaly must be sought in the fetoplacental unit.

VI. Ultrastructure (SEM and TEM) of the Free Chorionic Villus

The syncytial trophoblast, which constitutes a true syncytium, completely surrounds the villus as an uninterrupted layer, which is probably continuous from villus to villus. It is in contact with the maternal blood, and across it occurs the exchange of gases and other substances. Several hormones are synthesized in this layer. One morphologic expression for the activity of the syncytiotrophoblast is its "brush border" which, as observed by transmission electron microscopy (TEM), has a multitude of microvilli, first described by *Kastschenko* (1885).

However, thin sections for transmission studies do not generally reveal comprehensive information about the structure of biological surfaces. The scanning electron microscope (SEM) has overcome some of the limitations of the TEM and ligh microscope and is an excellent tool for the study of surface structure. Early attempts to examine the human placenta were made by *Herbst* et al. (1968). Recently, an atlas on SEM of the human reproductive system has appeared (*Ludwig* and *Metzger*, 1976). Apart from the more spectacular features in SEM, at the present stage of knowledge it is important to correlate the findings with conventional TEM. Problems concerning fixation, dehydration, drying, etc. are discussed elsewhere (*Echlin*, 1973; *Cohen*, 1974). The problem of charging in SEM is serious, with the coral-like chorionic tissue. It is necessary to investigate small pieces of tissue and coat the specimen several times with coal and gold. However, this might influence measurements because the metal coat can be very irregularly distributed on the surface. Some aspects concerning sampling of placental tissue merit attention. The placental parenchyma is not homogeneous. Moreover, it can contain lesions due to maternal disease, inflammation, etc., which probably will change the ultrastructure. Any study dealing with ultrastructure of the placenta must carefully take into account clinical factors, gross and light-microscopic changes as well as the cotyledonary structure.

1. Ultrastructure in Uncomplicated Pregnancies

This description will deal with the appearance of the free chorionic villus in SEM and some complementary findings in TEM. For a review of the ultrastructure, see e.g. *Wynn* (1972, 1975).

a) General Appearance

Preliminary inspection of the chorionic tissue by SEM reveals its coral-like structure. In the tissue from the *central part of the cotyledon* (Figs. 10 and 11) the following pattern was usually seen: From the coarser main stem villi the thinner terminal villi leave with a tapered base. Terminal villi have a fairly constant thickness with slight variation in their caliber. Short thumb-like daughter ends (growing ends) of different sizes branch out from the terminal villi. These growing ends, like their "mother" villi, have a bulb-like end. On the villous surface there are also slightly rounded or ridge-like elevations and somewhat higher spherical projections.

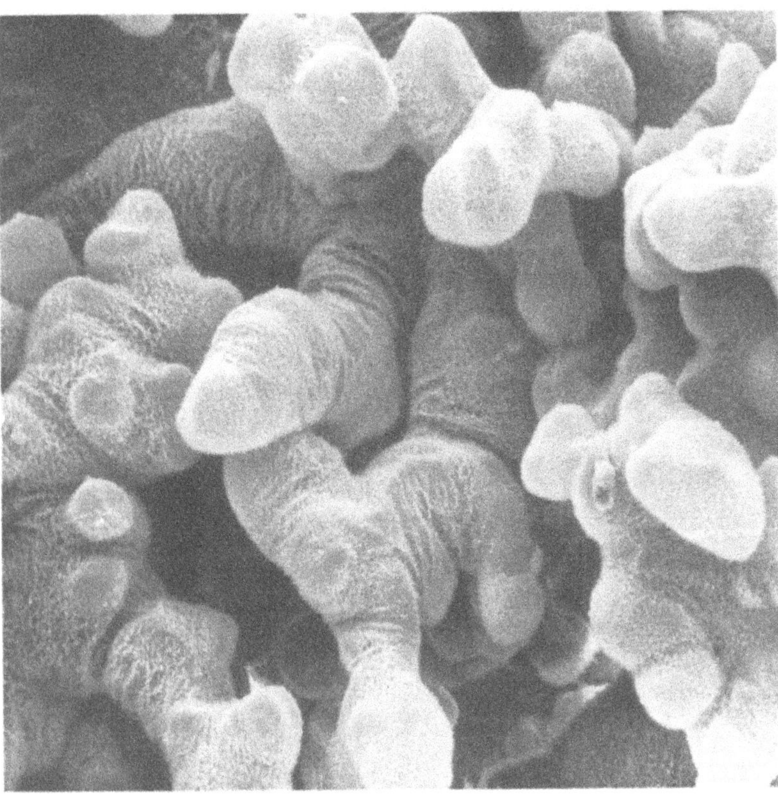

Fig. 10. Chorionic villi from central part of a cotyledon with coarse main villi, short distal villi, and buds. Note regular crests on syncytial surface carrying microvilli. SEM x 200

The chorionic tissue from the *dense part of the cotyledon* has more well-developed and longer terminal villi of equal thickness (Fig. 12). There are few short daughter ends. The general appearance is also more compact. The relative distance between terminal villi, which constitutes the intervillous space, is broadly comparable with that seen in ordinary sections and in the dissection microscope. Thus, the distance between the terminal villi is greater in the central area of the cotyledon. Terminal villi are in closest apposition at their origin from the main stem villi. Syncytial adhesions are sometimes evident between closely neighboring terminal villi (Fig. 13). The arrangement of the chorionic villi is not that of a lattice work.

Taking samples of fresh chorionic tissue for immersion fixation presumably results in the IVS not being properly visualized in all parts. *Ludwig* (1971), using perfusion fixation in his SEM studies, firmly states that the IVS constitutes a capillary space. However, in utero, the pressure of the maternal blood would change that. Furthermore, free villi are freely movable. Syncytial adhesions are quite evident but not so frequent as supposed by **Stieve** (1941a, b). Adhesions have been considered as a

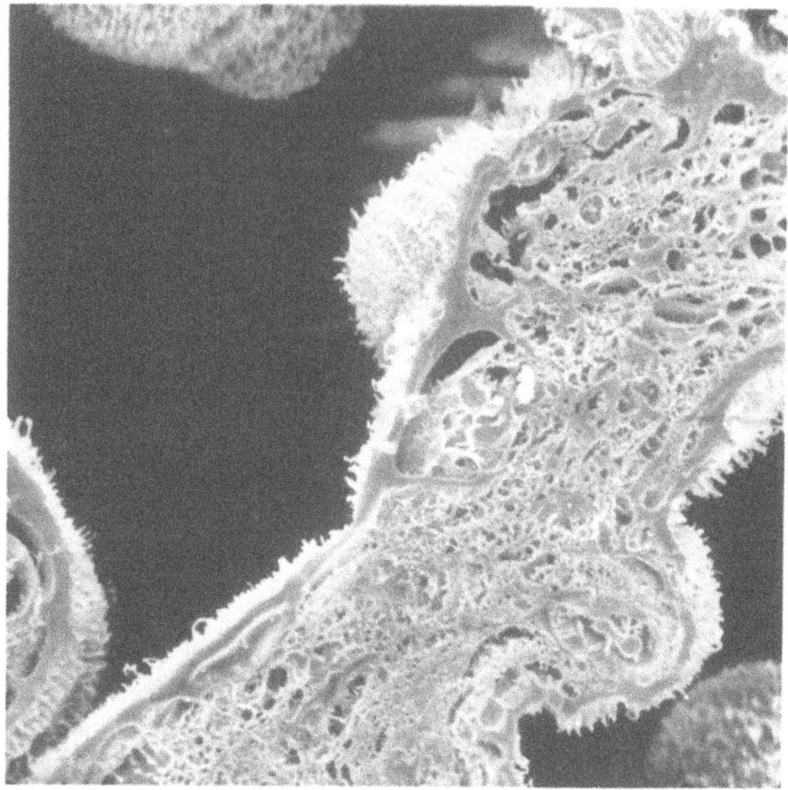

Fig. 11. Fracture through chorionic villus. In the stroma, fetal capillaries are visible. Note syncytial bud with fetal capillary. SEM x 250

momentary picture of an ameboid movement stopped by fixation. It has also been found that the cell membrane disappears in the border zone of the adhesions (*Geller*, 1962). A common cytoplasmatic zone is thus created that is still covered by microvilli (Fig. 14).

The different-sized, thumb-like branches of the terminal villi (see Fig. 10) correspond to *Crawford*'s (1956b) "growing ends" and *Boyd* and *Hamilton*'s (1967) "buds," which they considered responsible for the growth of the cotyledon. It is interesting to note that these are more frequent in the central area of the cotyledon, where immature chorionic villi have been described (*Gruenwald*, 1966; *Schuhmann* and *Wehler*, 1971). The appearance of these less-branched and somewhat coarser villi is compatible with the assumption that they are influenced by higher arterial pressure and faster blood flow. They have been considered as "young villi" responsible for regeneration of new villous tissue (*Schuhmann* and *Wehler*, 1971). The well-developed microvilli at the tips of the short "daughter" villi (Fig. 15) perhaps reflect a more active proliferation of this part. Studies with ^{3}H-thymidine uptake also indicate this (*Okudaira* et al., 1971). These tips or buds seem to play a role in the formation as well as in the elongation of

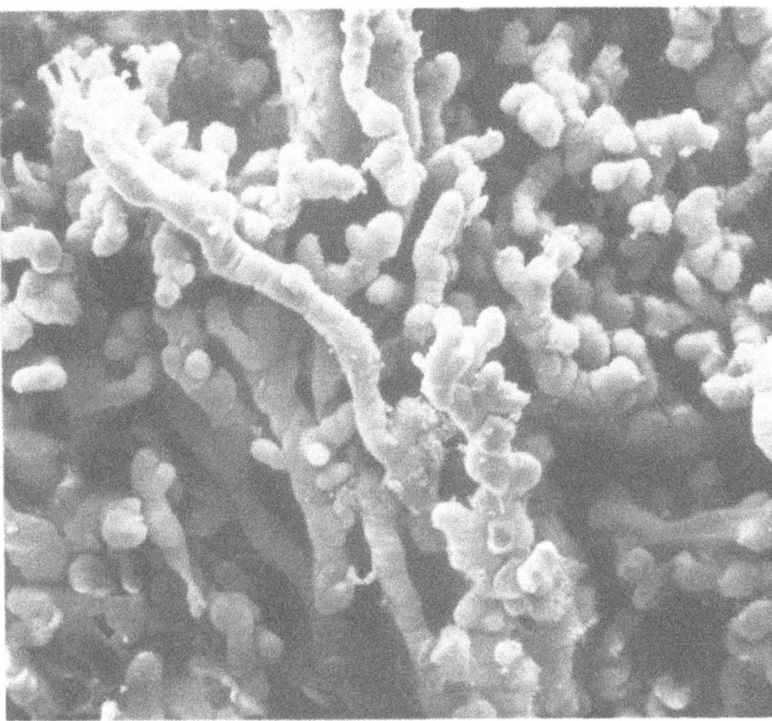

Fig. 12. Chorionic villi from the dense part of a cotyledon viewed from the intervillous space. Note freely branching villi. Term placenta from AGA infant. SEM immersion fixation, x 100

villi (*Boyd* and *Hamilton,* 1967). The presence of the growing ends does not necessarily indicate that the placenta still grows in the last weeks of pregnancy. *Winick* (1967) showed that there is no further increase in cell numbers after approximately the 36th week of gestation. The elongated slender types of growing ends, which are frequent in early pregnancy, are not present (*Ivemark* and *Sandstedt*, 1971; *Bergström*, 1971).

b) Trophoblastic Layer

Erythrocytes are occasionally present on the syncytial surface. They seem to adhere but are not enclosed in depressions or microvilli. Apart from cut and fractured lesions, the syncytial surface is intact. On the fractured surface, the trophoblast forms a homogeneous layer of varying thickness covering the villous core (see Figs. 11 and 16). It is not possible to see any basement membrane, which apparently is included in this layer. At low magnification, the syncytial surface has a finely granular appearance due to microvilli. These cover terminal as well as main stem villi. The surface frequently has rows of "tall" microvilli, giving it a wavy appearance (see Fig. 10). This is most

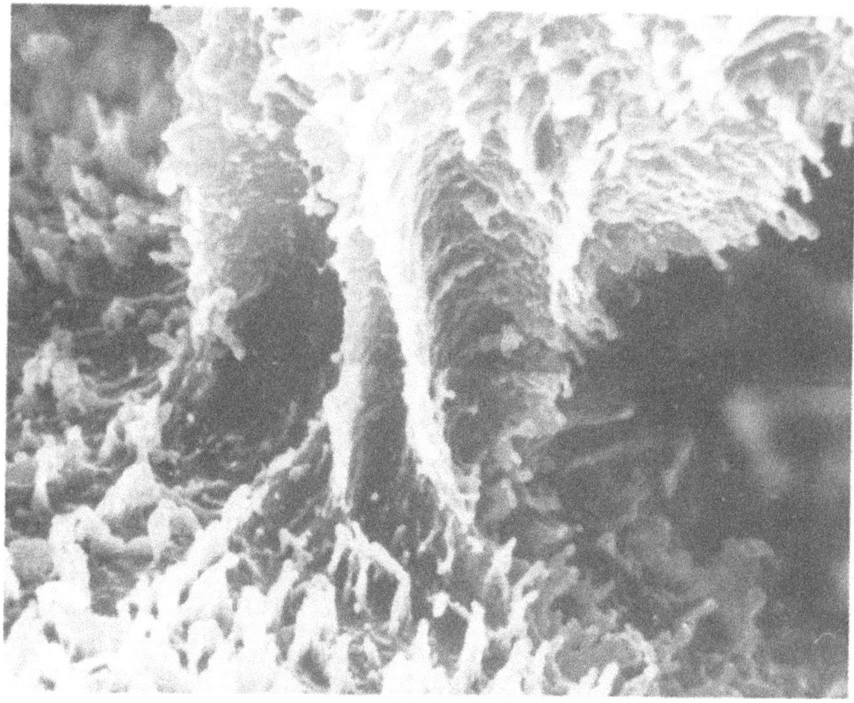

Fig. 13. Syncytial adhesion in SEM. Regular syncytial crests and mainly flat microvilli. x 9000

prominent on terminal villi close to the main stems. The waves or crests often have a parallel arrangement and are spaced with an almost periodic regularity. In other places, the crests cross or fuse to give a honey-comb appearance to the surface. In fractured specimens and in TEM pictures these waves correspond to syncytial projections carrying microvilli (Figs. 16 and 17). These syncytial crests, especially when periodic, have a fairly regular size and configuration. Their height is about 3 μ, the diameter 3–5 μ. Their length varies considerably because they often fuse. The shortest flat, leaf-like forms are approximately 2–3 μ long. When fused they may extend over half the circumference of the terminal villus. A similar, though not so pronounced waviness in the same phase can be traced on the trophoblastic underside. No definite differences in this respect could be seen between stem villi and terminal villi, or the different parts of the cotyledon.

The wave-like appearance of the syncytial surface, observed in TEM as well as in SEM, is certainly not an artifact. The periodic appearance of these was also noted by *Boyd* et al. (1968) in TEM. The reason for this "movement" is not clear. It could be due to a cytoplasmic movement spreading over the syncytial surface similar to the oscillating membrane seen in cultured cells studied in SEM. Another explanation could be that these ridges are formed mechanically and passively by the maternal

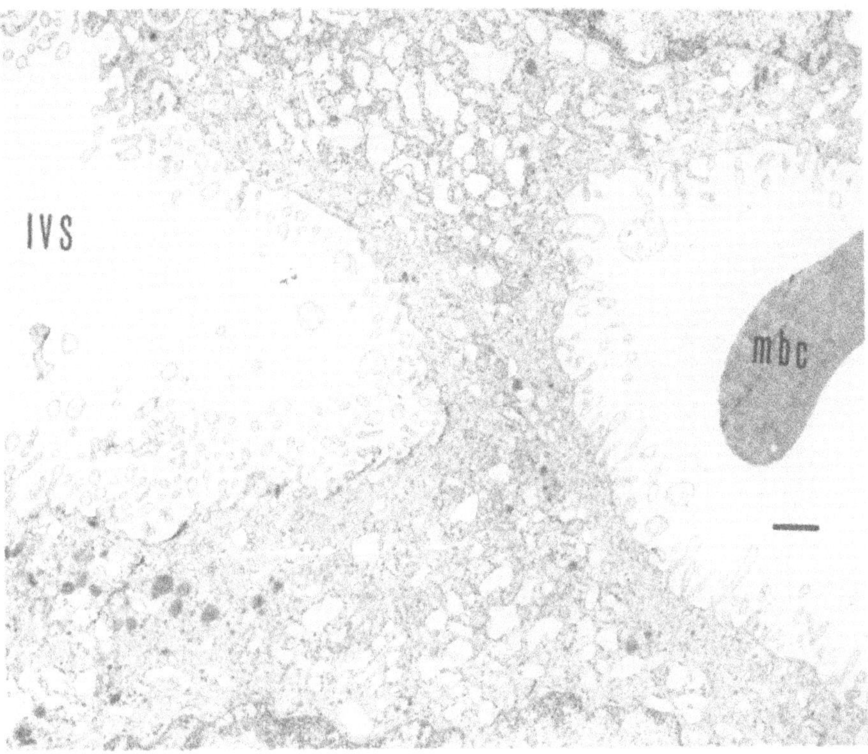

Fig. 14. Syncytial adhesion in TEM with a common cytoplasmatic zone and numerous dilated profiles. *MBC*, maternal red blood corpuscle in IVS. x 600

blood streaming over the surface. Where the depressions are uniform, they have measurements corresponding to the convexity of an erythrocyte.

c) Syncytial Microvilli

The configurations of the microvilli are most evident on fractured surfaces. Despite varying configuration and size, different main types can be distinguished, although transitional forms are seen. The various microvilli show a certain relationship to the syncytial ridges and to the interposed depressed areas. In the depressed or in the flat areas devoid of ridges, microvilli are fairly equal in hight but several types are represented. Most are cylindrical with tapered or bulbous ends. Others are conical and irregular with enlargements and constrictions. There are also flat, leaf-like forms with numerous small protrusions on the top. This form could as well be called a small syncytial projection. Ramifying microvilli are almost never seen in the depressions between ridges (Fig. 18). Small irregular areas free from microvilli are also present, measuring

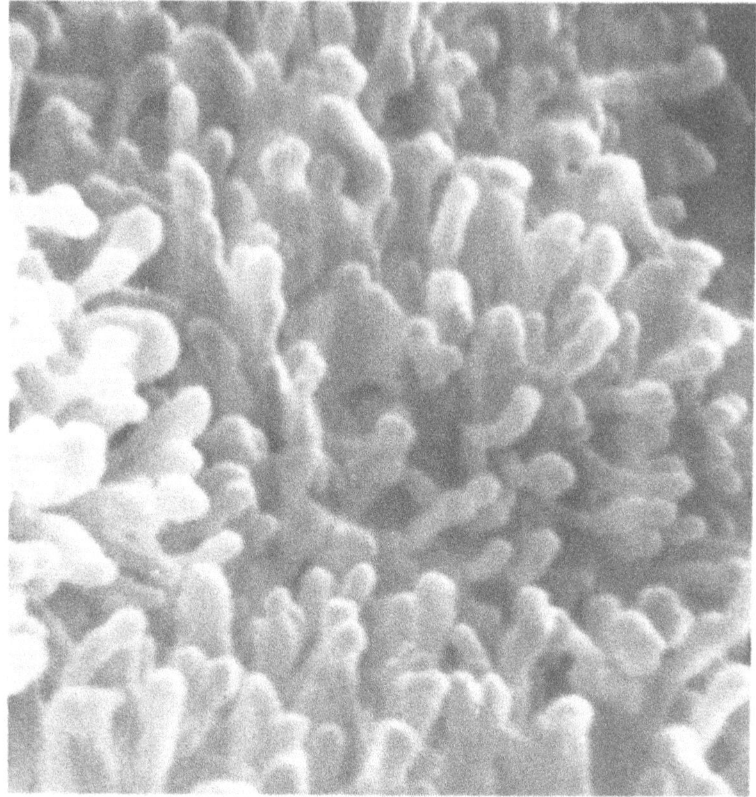

Fig. 15. Syncytial cylindrical microvilli on chorionic villus tip. SEM x 25,000

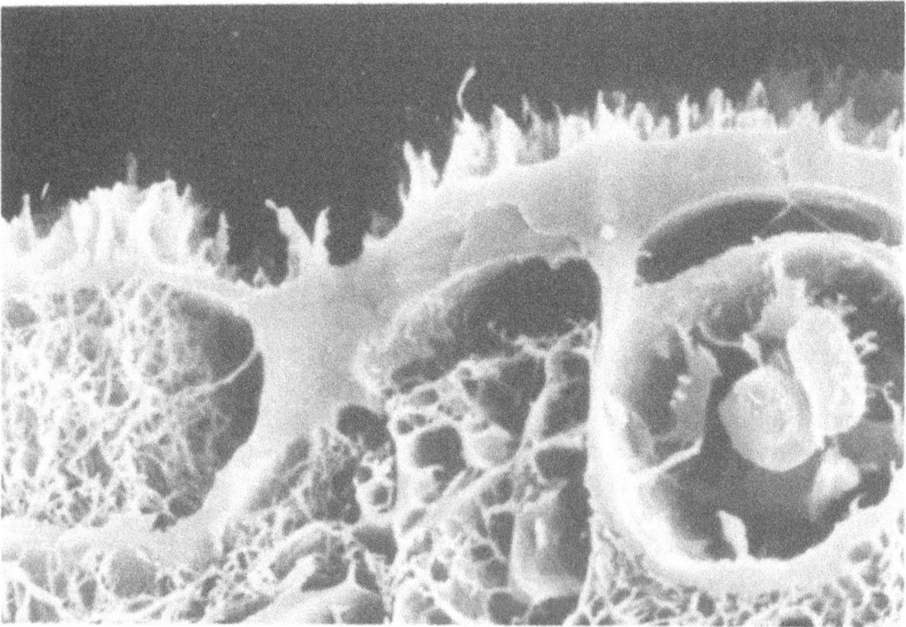

Fig. 16. (Legend see page 35)

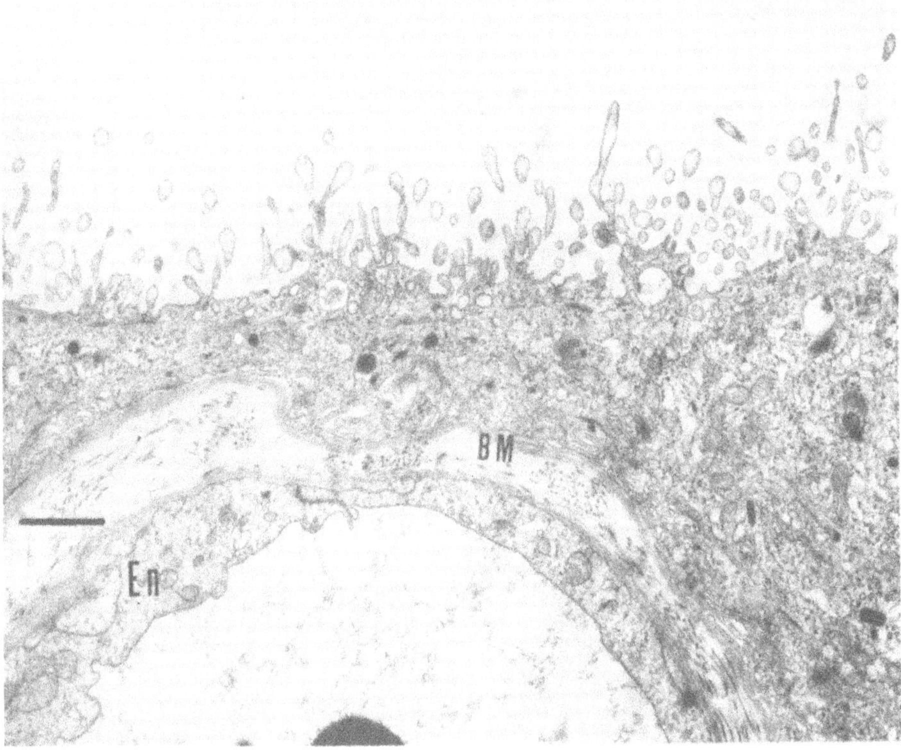

Fig. 17. Syncytium with microvilli and vesicles of varying sizes and densities. Basement membrane *(BM)*. Fetal capillary endothelium *(En)*. Cf. dilated extracellular space in Figure 16. TEM, x 10,000

at the most 3 μ. Along the crests, microvilli usually are cone-shaped with a broad base (1 μ) arising from the waves. Often, they have irregular enlargements and pseudopods. Large ramified, frond-like microvilli are often localized here. The height of the microvilli varied from 0.5 μ to almost 5 μ (frond-like) and the diameter from 0.2 μ to 0.4 μ.

In the flat, nonwavy areas, cylindrical microvilli dominate with sparse ramified forms (see Fig. 15). At the tips of the free chorionic villi, especially the short daughter ends, microvilli are always well developed, tall, cyclindrical, and closely packed. Viewed from the surface, the microvilli have a rounded configuration with slight variation of the diameter (0.4–0.5 μ). The branches of the frond-like microvilli are broader (5 μ), and, owing to their brightness, the neighboring branches seem to fuse. This, however, is a rare finding in the term placenta. The number of microvilli as calculated from SEM microphotographs varies from 10–12 x 10^6 per mm^2.

Fig. 16. Fracture through surface area of chorionic villus. Syncytial microvilli of various types and a subtrophoblastic dilated space. No internal structures seen in trophoblastic layer. Stroma and fetal capillary containing a fractured fetal red blood corpuscle. Note flat endothelial protrusions. Cf. Figure 17. SEM, x 400

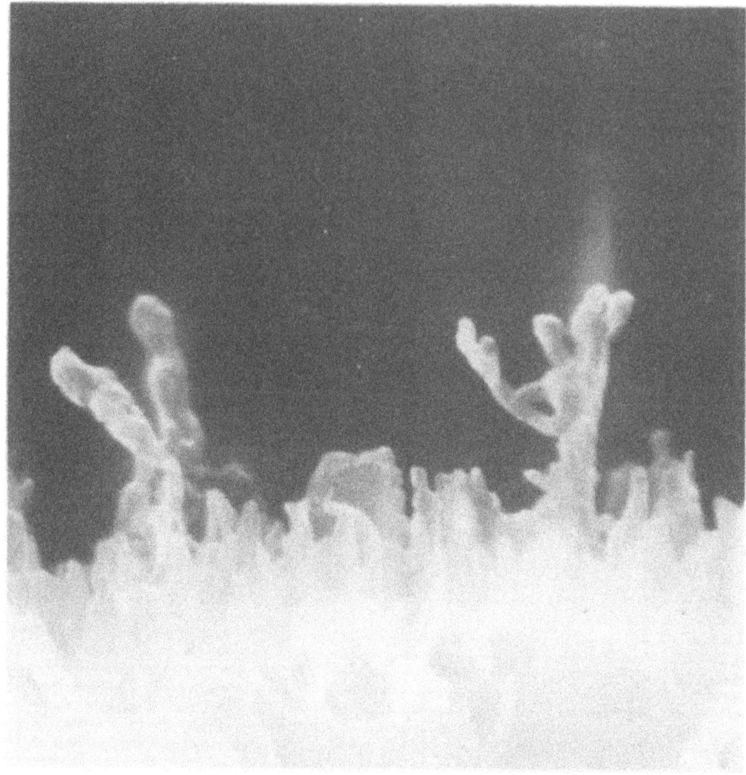

Fig. 18. Syncytial microvilli. Cylindrical, cone-shaped, flat, and frondlike forms. SEM, x 15,000

The SEM gives a clear view of the great variability and development of the microvilli in different regions of the syncytial surface. Just one view of a square centimeter area corresponds to thousands of ultrathin sections. The appearance of the syncytial surface gives the impression of constant changes in contour and is thus quite unlike other absorbing epithelial surfaces like those of the intestine and the kidney. This variablity might be associated with different local functions of the syncytium, as suggested by *Boyd* et al. (1968), who further postulated that maternal estrogens and progesterone were responsible for the presence and absence of the microvilli. The tall frond-like forms have been described in TEM and considered to be associated with secretion of gonadotropin (*Yoshida,* 1961).

The presence of the microvilli suggests considerable metabolic activity. Changes in their shape during pregnancy probably also indicate changes in absorption and excretion as an expression of altered placental metabolism. The number of microvilli found in this series as counted in several areas in SEM is similar to that found by *Geller* (1962) using horizontal surface sections studied in TEM. *Ikawa* (1959) found a similar number and also that the microvilli decrease in size and number, especially the frond-like forms, during the last trimester. This tallies well with the results of investigations of placentas from early pregnancies. The approximate size of microvilli found in TEM is similar to that given by different authors (*Ikawa,* 1959; *Widmaier,* 1969; *Herbst* et al., 1969; *Kaufmann* and *Stegner*, 1972). *Ikawa* (1959), and several other Japanese workers consider it possible to determine the age of the placenta by the changes in height and thickness of microvilli. The microvilli enormously increase the syncytial surface. The plain surface is usually calculated to be $11-13$ m^2 (*Aherne* and *Dunnill,* 1966). The size and number of microvilli encountered in the present study would increase this twentyfold.

The configuration of the microvilli in SEM corresponds to that in TEM. The difference in height and, above all, in the width between TEM and SEM is explained mainly by the preparative gold coat. The placental glycocalyx and the dissimilar processing techniques probably have a lesser influence in this respect.

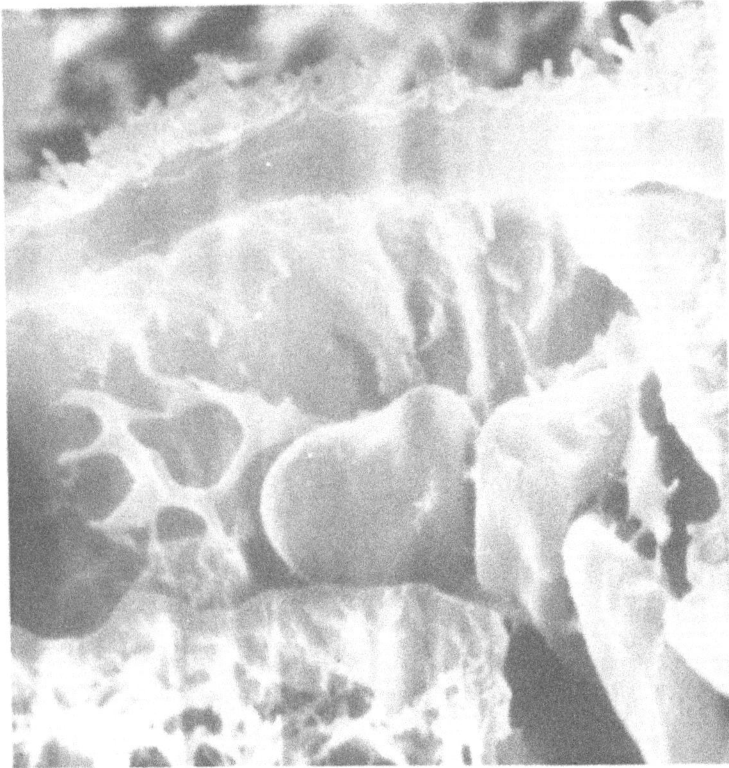

Fig. 19. Fracture through fetal capillary in chorionic villus. The thick homogeneous area covered by microvilli constitutes the "placental membrane." Inside fetal capillary are red blood corpuscles. The endothelium shows flat and microvilli-like protrusion. (Brighter and darker vertical lines are caused by charging effects). SEM, x 6000

38

d) Villous Core and Fetal Endothelium

The fractured tissue (see Figs. 11 and 16) demonstrates not only the surface layer but also the stromal part of the villus. The villous core is dominated by loose tissue interlaced by bars, probably corresponding to the collagen fibers. Individual cells are difficult to identify. Occasionally, nuclei are present but it is not possible to see whether these belong to fibroblasts, Hofbauer cells, or macrophages. The sinusoid fetal capillaries are prominent and are usually close to the trophoblastic basement membrane. The vessel caliber varies only slightly. The endothelial luminal surface has ridges and distinct microvilli-like protrusions of different sizes. These are not so prominent as the syncytial microvilli. There are no obvious differences in the number and size of the endothelial microvilli in capillaries close to or far from the syncytial surface (Figs. 19 and 20).

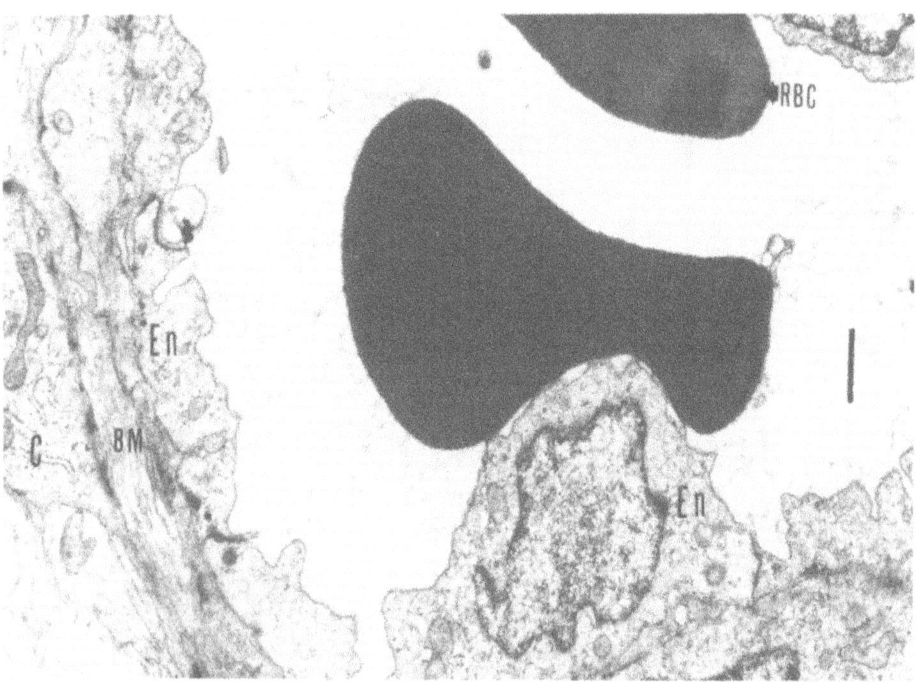

Fig. 20. Portion of fetal capillary wall. Thin basement membrane *(BM)*, cytotrophoblast *(C)*, endothelial cell *(RBC)*. Normal term placenta. AGA infant. Compare Figure 19. TEM x 12,000

2. Ultrastructure in LBW

Several descriptions are available of the ultrastructure of the placenta and particularly of the microvilli (*Boyd* et al., 1968; *Herbst* et al., 1969; *Kaufman* and *Stegner*, 1972).

Quantitative and qualitative differences have been noted at different stages of gestation (*Ikawa*, 1959). Only little attention has been paid to changes associated with intra-uterine growth retardation (*MacLennan* et al., 1972; *Lister*, 1968). Scanning electron microscopy makes it possible to study biological surfaces ultrastructurally over large areas. To utilize this tool effectively, however, scanning should be complemented by transmission electron microscopy. If morphologic changes in the placenta are associated with SGA infants, interest ought to be focused on peripheral villous structures, which constitute the bulk of the placenta. By using SEM with correlative TEM, sampling errors can be avoided to some extent.

The following description is based on the study of chorionic tissue from ten placentas. They were from SGA infants according to definitions given earlier. Four were term and two were preterm (28-30 weeks) deliveries. Placentas from four preterm AGA infants served as controls for the placentas from preterm infants. The placentas had normal configurations and did not contain any lesion occupying more than 5% of the placental parenchyma. The mothers were healthy and their pregnancies normal. No diabetes was known in the families. All mothers were taller than 155 cm.

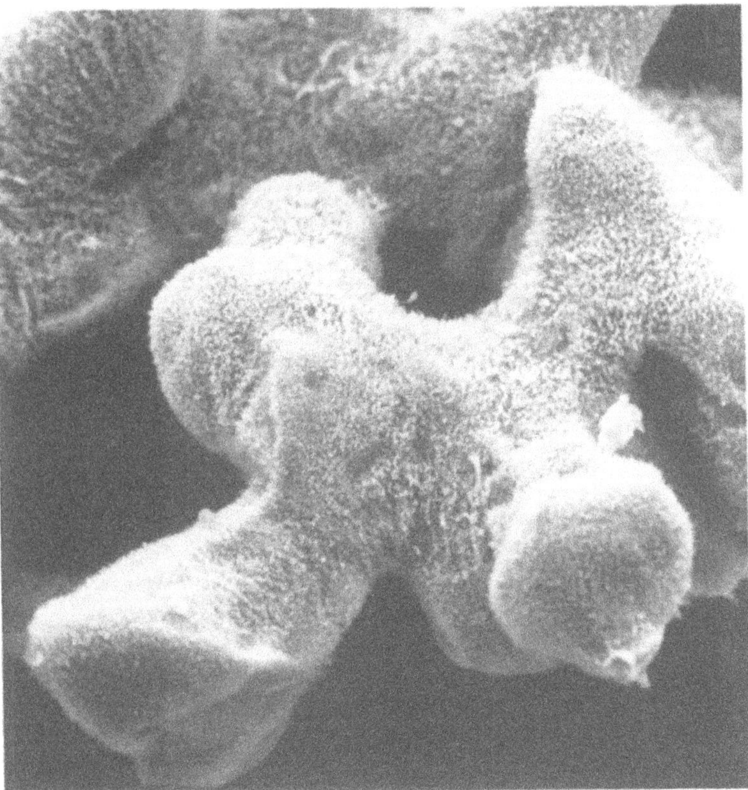

Fig. 21. Chorionic villi from central part of a cotyledon. Note luxurious microvilli and crests. Placenta from immature AGA infant. SEM, x 700

40

a) General Appearance in SEM

No clear differences could be recognized between the chorionic tissue from the *preterm placentas* from AGA and SGA infants. The chorionic tissue from the central part of the cotyledon had an irregular coral-like appearance (Figs. 21 and 23). The minor stem villi were coarse and rounded with somewhat varying calibers. The terminal chorionic villi branched off in an irregular way. The latter were mostly short and their caliber varied. One minor stem villus seldom gave rise to more than five branches (terminal villi). The average diameter of the minor stem villi and terminal villi of the different placentas ranged from 100 μ to 250 μ and from 40 μ to 60 μ respectively.

Chorionic tissue from the intermediate or dense part of the cotyledon has somewhat longer terminal villi, which had a more regular appearance and a more uniform caliber than terminal villi from the central part of the cotyledon (Fig. 22). Even from this area, few branches were almost always the rule. The general appearance of the chorionic villi in *term placentas* from the SGA infants was almost the same as that found in preterm placentas. The terminal villi were only somewhat longer than in the intermediate part of the cotyledon. However, in one placenta the terminal villi were

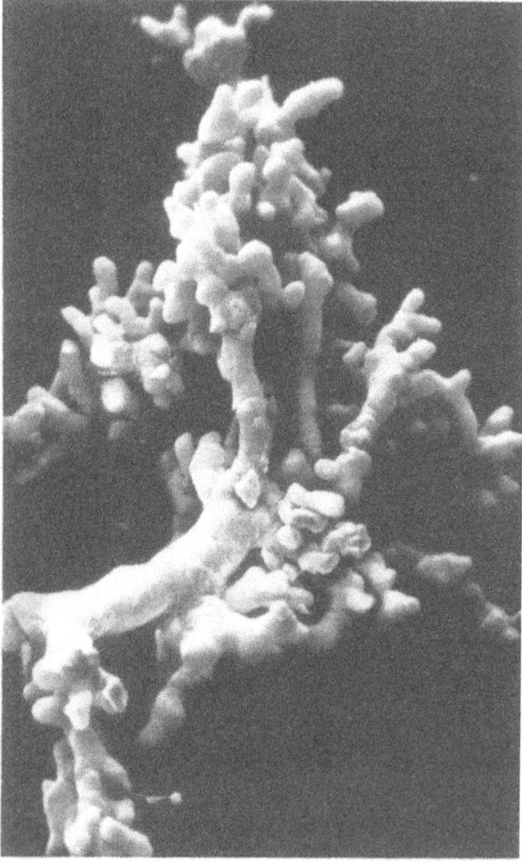

Fig. 22. Chorionic villi from dense part of a cotyledon with sparse branching. Placenta from immature AGA infant. SEM, x 140

long, more regular, and freely branching in tissue from the intermediate part of the cotyledon and, thus, similar to the finding in placentas from normal term infants. The calibers of stem and terminal villi were the same as found preterm. The intervillous space was somewhat wider, compared with that seen in normal term placentas. Syncytial adhesions were infrequent.

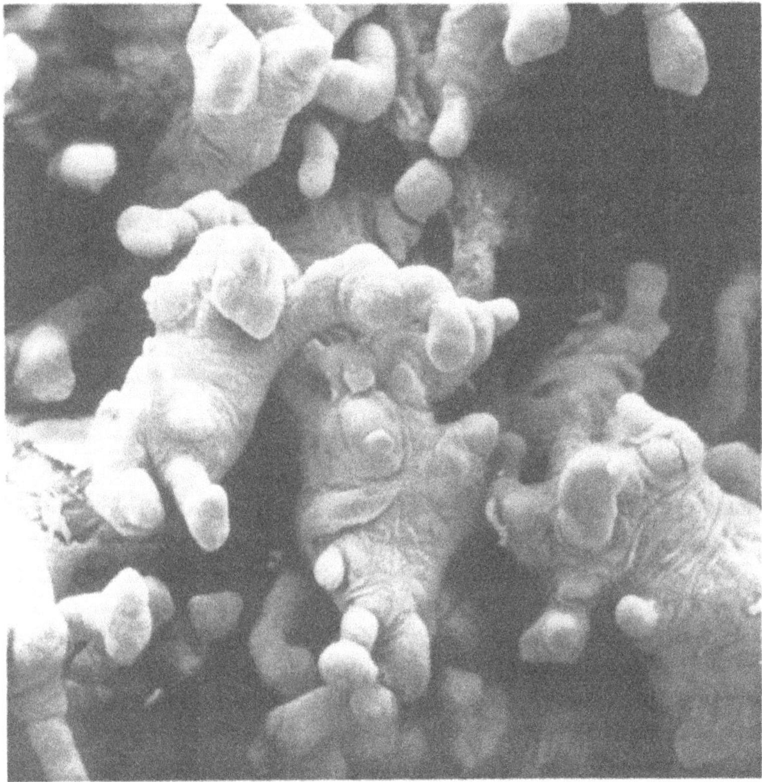

Fig. 23. Chorionic villi from central part of a cotyledon. Note short thumb-like distal villi and coarse stem villi. Placenta from a SGA infant 35 weeks of gestational age. SEM, x 150

Among alterations in placentas from infants with evidence of intrauterine growth retardation, *Gruenwald* (1966) payed attention to the small, less branching villi observed with the light microscope. He stressed that the light-microscopic differences between chorionic villi from different places within the placental lobulus (subcotyledon) are important for the problem of sampling error. Phase-contrast microscopy of fresh placental tissue from SGA infants has shown lack of normal growth of chorionic villi and few syncytial sprouts (*Aladjem,* 1972). However, the relation to placental cotyledons was not considered.

The main bulk of dense chorionic villi is located within a circumferential area in the lobule (subcotyledon), which also has a thick juxtadecidual part. This probably explains the "homogeneous concept" of placental tissue suggested in phase-contrast and transmission electron-microscopic studies. The various types of chorionic villi may be related to placental arteries observed in angiographic studies. In the horizontal and inverted cotyledons seen on angiograms, the various types of villous tissue have probably changed place compared with their positions in the "normal" cotyledon. Transposition of the usual arrangement of villous tissue is certainly another source of the sampling error.

The variable morphology of chorionic villi within the cotyledon could have a physiologic explanation and be due to the blood flow in the IVS. The central part of the cotyledon is apparently hit by the initial jet from the spiral artery and the dense circumferential area by a more slowly returning blood flow. The thicker, less branching "central" villi may represent an area with fast flow. If this type has a lower degree of function or represents an immature type of chorionic villus, their predominant presence, even in the cotyledonary intermediate parts in the LBW placentas, is meaningful. The central type of chorionic villi correspond to the type characteristic for the first trimester. In the terminology of *Bleyl* and *Stefek* (1965) and of *Schumann* and *Wehler* (1971), the "youthful" chorionic villi are present in regions with high oxygen tension and nutrient content while maturation into the type characteristic for the dense part of the cotyledon is a reactive differentiation in response to decreasing oxygen tension in the maternal blood. The concept of immature chorionic villi in the center of the lobule is also supported by *Wigglesworth* (1969) and *Fox* (1964).

Whether this immaturity is a primary defect, involving both fetus and placenta, or is secondary to faulty implantation or impaired maternal nutrition cannot be decided. It can be noted that *Myers* and *Fujikura* (1968) found a reduction in the number of chorionic villi with absent fetal ciruclation but intact maternal circulation in the Rhesus monkey placenta. The growth of free, unattached chorionic villi is considered to be associated with the quantity of maternal blood (*Boyd* and *Hamilton,* 1967). This can explain the result of *Aherne* and *Dunnill* (1966), who found that the syncytial area of the placenta was reduced in the "small for date" syndrome. The results of *Laga* et al. (1972) point in the same direction. They found that the peripheral villous mass was considerably less in a lower socioeconomic group with children of low birth weight. The villous deficit was attributed to a decrease in number of villi rather than in the dimensions of individual villi. The main diameter of chorionic villi in the present study tallies with the finding by *Fujikura* et al. (1971). The chorionic villi thus seem to be reduced in number and height in SGA placentas.

The immature appearance of the chorionic villi and the syncytial surface might reflect an impairment of cellular growth of the villous tissie. *Winick* (1967) showed that cell division in the human placenta continues until 34-36 weeks of gestation. Further growth depends on cellular hypertrophy. Placentas from SGA children have been shown to contain fewer cells. The immature or growth-retarded appearance of the chorionic villi in the term SGA placentas can, in part, be explained by cellular hypoplasia having stopped growth at a preterm level. Accepting a maturation arrest theory does not give any information about the reason why the cells cease to divide. It is not possible to state whether the placental changes parallel the growth of the infant or reflect an impariment of the maternal vascular supply and thus represent secondarily an "insufficient" placenta. One of the SGA placentas did not have immature chorionic villi, a finding that might be explained by a genetically small-sized placenta. The infant, however, showed evidence of dysmaturity.

Angiographic studies (*Wigglesworth*, 1964), changes in spiral arteries (*Dixon* and *Robertson*, 1961), and Na-clearance studies (*Dixon* et al., 1963) indicate that uteroplacental blood flow is decreased in conditions associated with intrauterine growth retardation. Experimental evidence in animals also supports this (*Creasy* et al., 1972). Against this background it is temptying to explain the immature appearance of chorionic villi as caused by impairment of vascular supply.

b) Trophoblastic Layer and Syncytial Microvilli

The syncytial surface was granular due to the ubiquitous microvilli. The microvilli varied in height but were generally tall, slender, and branching. The branches often fused with each other. The tips were almost bulbous (Fig. 24). Compared with normal term placentas, the microvilli were more equal in height.

There was no apparent difference between the preterm and the term SGA placentas. No clear difference in the various areas of the cotyledon was found.

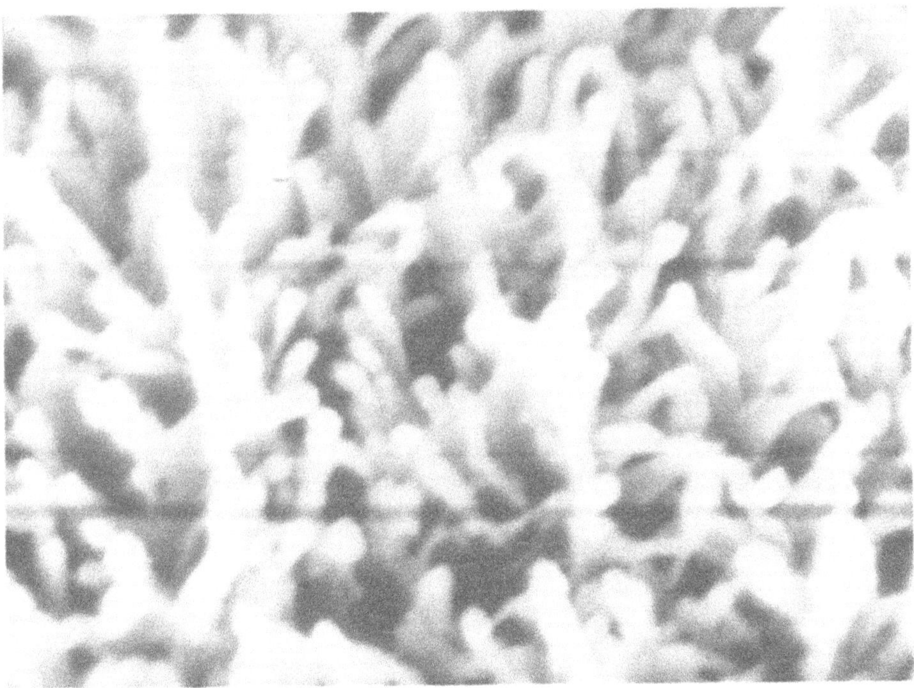

Fig. 24. Syncytial microvilli, long slender forms, in placenta from preterm SGA infant. Horizontal dark lines due to charging. SEM, x 23,000

The height and width of the microvilli were around 2.5 μ and 0.3 μ, respectively. The number of microvilli per square unit in all measured areas was 10–12 x 10^6 per mm^2.

The more luxuriant microvillous surface seen in SEM even at term in the SGA placentas corresponds to the appearance of normal villous tips and an earlier gestational age, and in that sense it represents an immature trait. The physiologic reason is not clear. The number and size of microvilli do not point to lowered activity. It could be a reactive change due to the smaller chorionic surface area in the SGA placenta, since a similar appearance can be found close to infarcts in mature placentas. The number of microvilli corresponds to the figures given by *Ikawa* (1959) and there seems to be no significant alteration in this respect during the third trimester. The SEM results point to a qualitative difference with a dominance of higher and cylindrical microvilli.

c) Syncytium

The description is restricted to the terminal villi. No definite differences were noted between premature AGA and SGA infants in tissue from central and intermediate areas

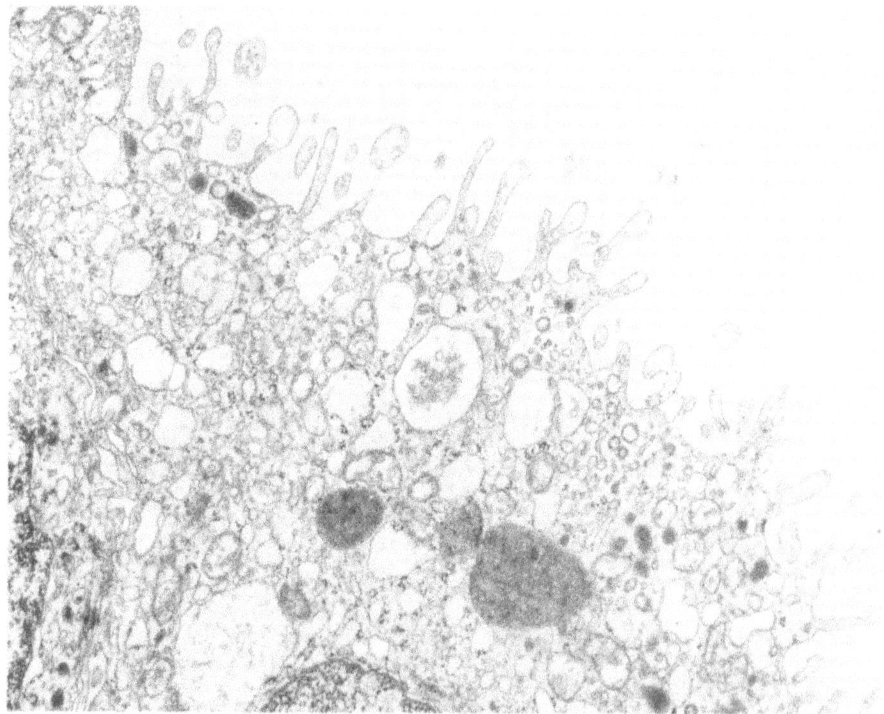

Fig. 25. Syncytial surface of distal chorionic villus with microvilli, dilated profiles of endoplasmatic reticulum, and osmiophilic droplets. Note microvilli attached to small syncytial crests. TEM, x 13,000

of the cotyledons. The microvilli of the syncytial trophoblast were well developed, usually tall and slender, and often they arose from promontories (Fig. 25). Branching and distension of the tips were common. In flat surface areas, the microvilli were shorter, thicker, and had more bulbous ends. The diameter was approximately 0.2 μ and the height was usually around 2 μ. Micropinocytotic vesicles were often present basally between the microvilli. The syncytial cytoplasm was rich in round or ellipsoid profiles of varying sizes. They were limited by a single membrane and contained granular or flocculent material with different densities. RNP granules were seen both free and attached to membranes of endoplasmatic reticulum. Dense droplets were few or moderate in number.

Mitochondria were ovoid or rod-shaped with lamellar cristae. They were diffusely distributed an numerous. Golgi complexes were infrequent. Glycogen particles were scattered throughout the syncytium. The nuclei were scattered and seldom formed clusters. The basal folded or microvillous part of the syncytium was usually in contact with the basal membrane.

The Langhans' cells were very few and never formed a complete layer. Their cytoplasm had low density. The mitochondria were more abundant and larger than in the syncytial trophoblast. On the other hand, the organelles were fewer. No mitoses were found.

Various changes in placental TEM ultrastructure in placentas from LBW infants have been reported. The descriptions are difficult to compare, since different definitions of LBW, dysmaturity, etc., have been used, and maternal complications have usually been involved. *Lister* (1968) found many blunted microvilli in TEM studies of placentas from infants with fetal malnutrition. Some of the placentas she studied were from mothers with diabetes and toxemia, which may have altered the structure. *MacLennan* et al. (1972) found occasional club-like microvilli and uneven surface projections in trophoblast cultured in 6% oxygen. Similar changes were observed in placental villi from a baby with signs of dysmaturity that was thought to be the result of hypoxia. They also noted profound vacuolation, thinning of the syncytiotrophoblast, and syncytial formation. Such changes were inconstant in the present material and were not related to SGA but rather to acute hypoxia such as after prolonged labor and even in delay in fixation of placental tissue. *Theuring* and *Kemnitz* (1974) studied seven placentas from small-for-date infants and reported thinnings of the syncytiotrophoblast and dilatations of the endoplasmatic reticulum. Similar findings have been seen in preeclampsia (*Franke* et al., 1971).

Lister (1963a, b) reported the ultrastructure of villi from the subchorial and basal parts of the placenta and, not surprisingly, found apparent differences. In the present study, no clear differences in the villi from the central and intermediate parts within a single cotyledon were found, not even between the different maturity groups. This can be explained by the fact that principally distal villi were studied, which seem to be similar in appearance, regardless of site.

Any attempt to describe internal syncytial structures such as multivesicular bodies, Langhans' cells, the basement membrane, Hofbauer cells, and fetal capillaries requires careful definition and selection of an area for comparable studies. The problem of placental sampling error is impossible to avoid in TEM when attempting to derive quantitative data, especially because the metabolic activity varies not only within the func-

46

tional units but probably also between various cotyledons (*Ramsey*, 1967). SEM has
an advantage in this respect since larger areas can be studied; however, it must be
stressed that the placental tissue studied was selected from normal subcotyledons
(lobule) as it appeared on the fresh cut surface. The results are only valid for such a
lobule. The angiographic studies indicate that cotyledons and subcotyledons do not
always have a regular appearance and probably reflect a great variability in chorionic
villous pattern.

d) Placental "Glycocalyx"

In ruthenium-stained sections, the syncytial surface had a distinct ruthenium-positive
layer, which also could be followed in the micropinocytotic vesicles opening onto the
surface (Fig. 26). There was an inner darker granular zone and an outer, more finely

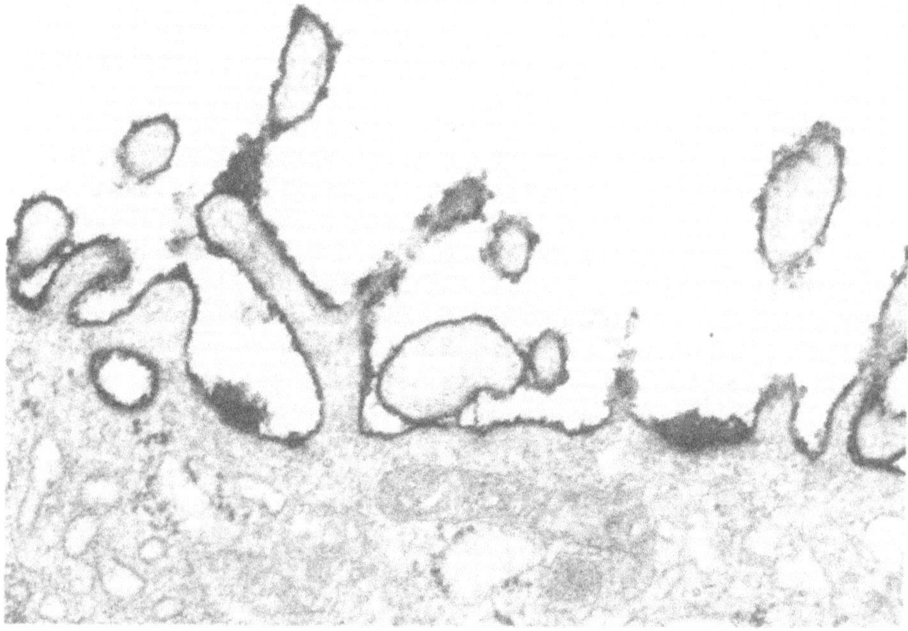

Fig. 26. Syncytium with distinct lining of ruthenium red from term SGA infant. Heavy
deposition *(arrows)* at the bases of microvilli and also in micropinocytotic vesicle.
TEM, x 55,000

granular, fading zone. In places, there were denser aggregates of the ruthenium-positive
material on the surface, especially at the tips of the microvilli and at their bases. The
thickness of the layer was approximately 200 Å and was more distinct than in placentas
from normal term pregnancies. In alveolated pits and micropinocytotic vesicles, which
sometimes had continuity with each other, the lining layer was thick (approximately

300 Å). The number of the ruthenium-labeled pits and vesicles differed between different areas of the syncytium. No apparent differences in number were noted between the various categories of placentas studied.

The micropinocytotic vesicles in the syncytium traced in the ruthenium red-stained sections closely resemble those that are involved in protein uptake in some cells, e.g., the proximal convoluted tubular epithelium of the kidney. A reduction in number could have been expected in the SGA placentas but was not found. It can be noted that by the ruthenium method, *Jollie* and *Triche* (1971) found no correlation between micropinocytotic activity and known transport rates across the rat visceral yolk-sac placenta.

It is difficult to interpret the significance of the denser ruthenium-positive layer on the syncytial surface in the LBW placentas, since several artifacts may be associated with this method. The method has been standardized and the more prominent lining layer in LBW is conceived as a real difference. Using ruthenium red, *Liebhart* (1974) also found a more intense staining reaction in immature placentas. The simplest explanation is that this finding reflects an immature trait since it is normally better developed in early pregnancy. *Martin* et al. (1974) used a battery of stains to demonstrate the the mucosubstance, which was identified as hyaluronic acid. With each of the techniques used, they found a variability in the intensity of staining in different regions along the syncytial surface, probably reflecting different functional zones, but there were only minor differences in placentas from early and term pregnancies. According to *Luft* (1966) substances binding ruthenium red are interpreted as representing acid mucopolysaccharides. It should also be noted that according to *Copley* and *Scheinthal* (1970) ruthenium red also stains fibrinogen and fibrin. Some studies indicate that the anionic side chains of acid mucopolysaccharides facilitate utilization and transfer of various ions and metabolites (*Goldstein*, 1969). It can be postulated that the better developed "glycocalyx" in the placentas from SGA infants then indicates a metabolic difference.

Apart from influencing structure measurements in SEM, this syncytial lining layer probably takes part in the function of the cell membrane, and thus one has to devise other methods to determine the distance that substances have to travel over cell membranes. The trophoblastic mucopolysaccharide layer also plays an important role by masking major histocompatibility differences between fetal and maternal tissues (*Currie* and *Bagshawe*, 1967).

It has been suggested (*Bradbury* et al., 1970) that the mucopolysaccharide layer acts through electrochemical repulsion. Its production is increased in response to histocompatibility (*Currie* and *Bagshawe*, 1967). The main role of the placental glycocalyx is, however, still unknown.

VII. Conclusions

The entity "low birth weight" with or without signs of intrauterine growth retardation is apparently a multifactorial condition for which no single explanation can be given. The causes could be on the maternal or on the fetal side, and they could also be at the

48

borderline in the uteroplacental unit. A "primary placental cause" is a very unusual event. Nevertheless, observation of placental changes will indirectly reveal other conditions that perhaps can be cured and eventually prevent fetal wastage.

In this review it has been pointed out that singleton LBW placentas have a high frequency of abnormal configuration, including placenta circumvallata, premature separation, abnormal cord insertion, infarction, and widespread subchorial thrombosis. Fresh infracts are frequent in toxemia and premature separation. Villitis is also an important cause of intrauterine growth retardation, but it is probably less frequent in communities with so-called high socioeconomic status.

By angiography, fewer cotyledons are found in extrachorial placentas, in placentas with a single umbilical artery and, to some extent, in placentas with marginal cord insertion, especially if the infant was small for gestational age. A large type of cotyledon with an abnormal vascular pattern, "seaweed," is noted in circumvallata placentas, in placentas with marginal velamentous cord insertion, and with a single umbilical artery, which in the investigated material is always associated with low birth weight. It is reasonable to believe that these placentas are implanted at a site with abnormal, "insufficient" spiral artery supply.

The central part of the cotyledon contains an "immature" type of chorionic villi seen with the scanning electron microscope. This type of chorionic villus was also present in the denser part of the cotyledon in placentas from SGA infants, in contrast to AGA infant placentas, which contain a "mature" type.

These changes probably indicate the presence of abnormal uterine vascular supply that, in most cases, is impaired. This, in turn, points to a mal-implanted ovum, possibly secondary to local uterine abnormality or perhaps uterine infection. This, then, places the emphasis on the uteroplacental unit and an impaired maternal blood supply as most important causes for low birth weight and intrauterine malnutrition. A current follow-up study by this author on the placentas from selected ante-natal risk patients with impaired uterine growth strongly confirms the over-representation of malformed, small placentas with peripheral cord insertions and an "insufficient" vascular pattern in a country where the socioeconomic status is optimal and villitis is uncommon.

Acknowledgment: I wish to express my warmest thanks to Professor Kurt Benirschke for stimulating me to write this article and also for critically reading the manuscript.

References

Ahrene, W., Dunnill, M.S.: Quantitative aspects of placental structure. J. Pathol. *91*, 123–139 (1966)

Aladjem, S., Facog, E.P., Fanaroff, A.: Placental score and neonatal outcome. A clinical and pathological study. Obstet. Gynecol. *39*, 591–602 (1972)

Altshuler, G., Russel, P., Ermocilla, R.: The placental pathology of small-for-gestational age infants. Am. J. Obstet. Gynecol. *121*, 351–359 (1975)

Altshuler, G.A., Russel, P.: The human placental villitides. A review of chronic intra-uterine infection. Curr. Top. Path. *60*, 63–112 (1975)

Arts, N.F.: Investigation on the vascular system of the placenta. Am. J. Obstet. Gynecol. *82*, 147–166 (1961)

Bacsich, P., Crawford, J.M.: On the probable genetic character of human placental types, with some remarks on the structure of placental cotyledons. J. Anat. *94*, 449 (1960)

Bacsich, P., Smout, C.F.V.: Some observations on foetal vessels of human placenta with account of corrosion technique. J. Anat. *72*, 358–364 (1938)

Barnes, A.C.: In discussion of: Cannell, D.E., Vernon, C.P.: Congenital heart disease and pregnancy. Am. J. Obstet. Gynecol. *85*, 749 (1963)

Bartolomew, R.A.: Criteria by which toxemia of pregnancy may be diagnosed from unlabeled formalin-fixed placentas. Am. J. Obstet. Gynecol. *82*, 277–290 (1961)

Battaglia, F.C., Woolever, C.A.: Fetal and neonatal complications associated with recurrent chorangiomas. Pediatrics *41*, 62–66 (1968)

Bazso, J. Le retard de croissance intra-uterine et ses causes. Gynecol. Prat. *17*, 293–303 (1966)

Benirschke, K., Brown, W.H.: A vascular anomaly of the umbilical cord. The absence of one umbilical artery in the umbilical cord of normal and abnormal fetuses. Obstet. Gynecol. *6*, 399–404 (1955)

Benirschke, K.: Major pathologic features of the placenta, cord and membranes. Birth Defects *1*, 52–63 (1965)

Benirschke, K., Driscoll, S.G.: The pathology of human placenta. Berlin, Heidelberg, New York: Springer 1967

Benirschke, K.: Placental causes of maldevelopment. In: Teratology, trends and application, pp. 148–164. Berlin, Heidelberg, New York: Springer 1975

Benson, R.C., Fujikura, T.: Circumvallate and circummarginate placenta. Obstet. Gynecol. *34*, 799–804 (1969)

Bergström, S.: Surface ultrastructure of the human amnion and chorion in early pregnancy. Obstet. Gynecol. *38*, 513–524 (1971)

Beyreiss, K., Graetz, H., Suss, K.J.: Pränatale Dystrophie bei Aplasie einer Nabelschnurarterie. Kinderärztl. Prax. *36*, 69–72 (1968)

Bieniarz, J., Maqueda, E., Caldeyro-Barcia, R.: Compression of aorta by the uterus in late human pregnancy. I. Variations between femoral and brachial pressure with changes from hypertension to hypotension. Am. J. Obstet. Gynecol. *95*, 795–808 (1966)

Billington, W.D.: Influence of immunological dissimilarity of mother and foetus on size of placenta in mice. Nature *202*, 317–318 (1964)

Bjerre, J., Östberg, G.: Infant mortality. Acta Paediat. Scand. *63*, 49–58 (1974)

Bøe, F.: Studies on vascularization of the human placenta. Acta Obstet. Gynecol. Scand. *32* [Suppl. 5], 1–92 (1953)

Borell, U., Fernström, I., Ohlsson, L., Wiqvist, N.: Influence of uterine contractions on the uteroplacental blood flow at term. Am. J. Obstet. Gynecol. *93*, 44–57 (1965)

Borell, U., Fernström, I., Westman, A.: Eine arteriographische Studie des Plazentarkreislaufs. Geburtshilfe Frauenheilkd. *18*, 1–9 (1958)

Bourne, G.L., Benirschke, K.: Absent umbilical artery. A review of 113 cases. Arch. Dis. Children *35*, 534–543 (1960)

Boyd, J.D., Hamilton, W.J.: Development and structure of the human placenta from the end of the 3rd month of gestation. Br. J. Obstet. Gynaecol. *74*, 161–226 (1967)

Boyd, J.D., Hamilton, W.J., Boyd, C.A.R.: The surface of the syncytium of the human chorionic villus. J. Anat. *102*, 553–563 (1968)

Bradbury, S., Billington, W.D., Kirby, D.R.S., Williams, E.A.: Histochemical chracterization of the surface mucoprotein of normal and abnormal human trophoblast. Histochem. J. *2*, 263–274 (1970)

Brody, S., Frenkel, D.A.: Marginal insertion of cord and premature labor. Am. J. Obstet. Gynecol. *65*, 1305–1312 (1953)

Brosens, J., Dixon, H.G.: The anatomy of the maternal side of the placenta. Br. J. Obstet. Gynaecol. *73*, 357–363 (1966)

Budlinger, H.: Plazentaveränderungen und ihre Beziehung zur Spättoxicose und perinatalen kindlichen Sterblichkeit. Fortschr. Geburtshilfe Gynäk. *17*, 86—110 (1964)

Bumm, E.: Zur Kenntnis der uteroplacentären Gefäße. Arch. Gynäk. *37*, 1—15 (1890)

Bumm, E.: Über die Entwicklung des mütterlichen Blutkreislaufes in der menschlichen Placenta.Arch. Gynäk. *43*, 181--195 (1893)

Busch, W.: Placenta bei der fetalen Mangelentwicklung. Makroskopie und Mikroskopie von 150 Placenten fetaler Mangelentwicklung. Arch. Gynäkol. *212*, 333—357 (1972)

Butler, N.R., Bonham, D.G.: Perinatal mortality. The first report of the British Perinatal Mortality Survey. Edinburgh: Livingstone 1958

Carter, J.E., Vellios, F., Huber, C.P.: Histologic classification and incidence of circulatory lesions of the human placenta, with review of the literature. Am. J. Clin. Pathol. *40*, 375—378 (1963)

Clifford, S.H.: Postmaturity with placental dysfunction. J. Pediatr. *44*, 1—13 (1954)

Cohen, A.L.: Critical point drying. In: Principles and techniques of scanning electron microscopy. Hayat, M.A. (ed.), pp. 44—112. New York: Van Nost and Reinold 1974

Copley, A.L., Scheinthal, B.M.: Nature of the endothelial layer as demonstrated by ruthenium red. Exp. Cell Res. *59*, 491—492 (1970)

Coulter, J.B.S., Scott, J.M.: Oedema of the umbilical cord and respiratory distress in the newborn. Br. J. Obstet. Gynecol. *82*, 453—459 (1975)

Crawford, J.M.: The foetal placental circulation. III. The anatomy of the cotyledons. Br. J. Obstet. Gynaecol. *63*, 542—546 (1956)

Crawford, J.: Vascular anatomy of the placenta. Am. J. Obstet. Gynecol. *84*, 1543—1567 (1962)

Creasy, R.K., Barrett, C.T., De Swiet, M., Kahanpää, K.V., Rudulph, A.M.: Experimental intrauterine growth retardation in the sheep. Am. J. Obstet. Gynecol. *112*, 566—573 (1972)

Currie, G.A., Bagshawe, K.D.: The masking of antigens on trophoblast and cancer cells. Lancet. *1967 I*, 708—710

De Costa, E.J., Gerbie, A.B., Andresen, R.H., Gallanis, T.C.: Placental tumours. Hemangiomas with special reference to an associated clinical syndrome. Obstet. Gynecol. *7*, 249-259 (1956)

Dixon, H.G., Robertson, W.B.: Vascular changes in the placental bed. Pathol. Microbiol. *24*, 622-629 (1961)

Dixon, H.G., Brownie, J.C.M., Davey, D.A.: Choriodecidual and myometrial blood flow. Lancet *1963 II*, 369—373

Dollmann, A.: The small-for-date infant and its placenta. A clinical-pathological study. In: Perinatal medicine, p. 288. Bern: Huber 1973

Echlin, P.: Applications to biological materials. In: The use of the scanning electron microscope. Hearle, J.W.S., Sparrow, J.T., Cross, P.M. (eds.), pp. 177—202. Oxford: Pergamon Pr. 1973

Enocksson, E.: Prognosis of low birth weight infants. A four year prospective study. Transact. Fourth European Contress of Perinatal Medicine, pp. 466—467. Stuttgart: Thieme 1975

Enocksson, E., Gyllenswärd, Å., Peterson, B.: Prosektiv studie av barn med låg födelsevikt. Abstr. Medicinsk Rikstämma (Stockholm) *29*, 361 (1972)

Faierman, E.: The significance of one umbilical artery. Arch. Dis. Children *35*, 285-288 (1960)

Fernström, I.: Arteriography of the uterine artery. Acta Radiol. [Suppl.] *122*, 1—128 (1955)

Fitzhardinge, P.M., Steven, E.M.: The small-for-date infant. II. Neurological and intellectual sequelae. Pediatrics *50*, 50—57 (1972)

Fox, H.: White infarcts of the placenta. Br. J. Obstet. Gynaecol. *70*, 980—991 (1963)

Fox, H.: The pattern of villous variability in the normal placenta. Br. J. Obstet. Gynaecol. *71*, 749–758 (1964)

Fox, H.: Pevillious fibrin deposition in the human placenta. Am. J. Obstet. Gynecol. *98*, 245–251 (1967)

Fox, H., Sen, D.K.: Placenta extrachorialis. A clinico-pathological study. Br. J. Obstet. Gynaecol. *79*, 32–35 (1972)

Franke, H., Gerl, D., Stössner, I.: Die Feinstruktur der Chorionzotten bei Spätgestose unterschiedlicher Schweregrade. Z. Geburtshilfe Gynaekol. *175*, 226–244 (1971)

Franken, H.: A contribution to clarification of structure and function of the placenta. Zbl. Gynäkol. *76*, 729–734 (1954)

Freese, V.E.: The fetal-maternal circulation of the placenta. Am. J. Obstet. Gynecol. *94*, 354–360 (1966)

Freese, V.E., Rauninger, K., Kaplan, H.: The fetal-maternal circulation of the placenta. II. An x-ray cinematografic study of pregnant rhesus monkey. Am. J. Obstet. Gyn Gynecol. *94*, 361–365 (1966)

Froehlich, L.A., Fujikura, T., Fisher, P.: Chorangiomas and their clinical implications. Obstet. Gynecol. *37*, 51–59 (1971)

Froehlich, L.A., Fujikura, T.: Follow-up of infants with single umbilical artery. Pediatrics *52*, 6–13 (1973)

Fujikura, T., Benson, R.C., Driscoll, S.G.: The bipartite placenta and its clinical features. Am. J. Obstet. Gynecol. *107*, 1013–1017 (1970)

Fujikura, T., Ezaki, K., Nishimura, H.: Chorionic villi and syncytial sprouts in spontaneous and induced abortions. Am. J. Obstet. Gynecol. *110*, 547–555 (1971)

Garrow, J.S., Hawes, J.F.: The relationship of the size and composition of the human placenta to its functional capacity. Br. J. Obstet. Gynaecol. *78*, 22–28 (1971)

Geller, H.-F.: Elektromikroskopische Befunde am Syncytium der menschlichen Plazenta. Geburtshilfe Frauenheilkd. *22*, 1234–1237 (1962)

Goldstein, M.A.: Anionic binding of ruthenium red in fish extraocular muscle. Z. Zellforsch. *102*, 459–465 (1969)

Grosser, O.: Frühentwicklung, Eihautbildung und Placentation des Menschen und der Säugetiere. München: Bergmann 1927

Gruenwald, P.: Abnormalities of placental vascularity in relation to intrauterine deprivation and retardation of fetal growth. Significance of avascular chorionic villi. N.Y. State J. Med. *61*, 1508–1513 (1961)

Gruenwald, P.: Chronic fetal distress and placental insufficiency. Biol. Neonate *5*, 215–265 (1963)

Gruenwald, P.: Examination of the placenta by the pathologist. Arch. Pathol. *77*, 41–46 (1964)

Gruenwald, P.: The lobular architecture of the human placenta. Johns Hopkin's Med. *119*, 172–190 (1966)

Gruenwald, P.: The supply line of the fetus. Definitions relating to fetal growth. In: The placenta and its maternal supply line. Gruenwald, P. (ed.). Lancaster: Med. Tech. Publ. 1975a

Gruenwald, P.: Fetal deprivation and placental pathology. Concepts and relationships. In: Perspectives in pediatric pathology, Vol. 2, pp. 101–149. Chicago: Year Bk Med. Publ. 1975b

Harnack, G.A. von, Bermuth, H. von: Mehrdimensionelle Reifediagnostik bei unter-gewichtigen Neugeborenen. Monatsschr. Kinderheilkd. *119*, 23–26 (1971)

Herbst, R., Multier, A.-M.: Inatsugi, Y.: Die räumliche Darstellung der menschlichen Chorinzotten mit dem JEOL-Raster-Elektronenmikroskop. Beitr. Elektronenmikr. Direktabbildung Oberflächen *1*, 297–302 (1968)

Herbst, R., Multier, A.-M., Hörman, G.: Elektronenoptische Untersuchungen an menschlichen Plazentazotten. Zbl. Gynäkol. *15*, 465–475 (1969)

Hertig, A.T., Sheldon, W.H.: An analysis of one thousand spontaneous abortions. Ann. Surg. *117*, 596–606 (1943)

Hibbard, B.M., Jeffcoate, T.N.A.: Abruptio placentae. J. Obstet. Gynecol. *27*, 155–167 (1966).

Hobbs, J.E., Price, C.N.: Placenta circumvallata. Am. J. Obstet. Gynecol. *45*, 39–45 (1940)

Hobel, C.J., Emmanoulides, G.C., Townsend, D.E., Ashiro, K.: Ligation of one umbilical artery in the fetal lamb. Experimental production of fetal malnutrition. Obstet. Gynecol. *36*, 582–588 (1970)

Hunt, A.B.: Discussion of a paper by Paalman and Van der Veer. Am. J. Obstet. Gynecol. *65*, 497 (1953)

Ikawa, A.: Observation on the epithelium of human chorionic villi with the electron microscope. Acta Obstet. Gynecol. Jpn. *6*, 220–234 (1959)

Ivermark, B., Sandstedt, B.: Svepelectronmicroscopi av placenta. Documenta KVA *1*, 34–37 (1971)

Jollie, W.P., Triche, T.J.: Ruthenium labeling of micropinocytotic activity in the rat visceral yolk-sac placenta. J. Ultrastruct. Res. *35*, 541–553 (1971)

Kastschenko, N.: Das menschliche Chorionepithel und dessen Rolle bei der Histogenese der Placenta. Arch. Anat. Phys. Lpz. 451–480 (1885)

Kaufmann, P., Stegner, H.E.: Über die funktionelle Differenzierung des Zottensyncytiums in der menschlichen Placenta. Z. Zellforsch. *135*, 361–382 (1972)

Kloosterman, G.J., Huidekoper, B.L.: The significance of the placenta in "obstetrical mortality." Gynaecologia *138*, 529–550 (1954)

Koeningsberger, M.R.: Judgement of fetal age. I. Neurological evaluation. Pediatr. Clin. North Am. *13*, 823–833 (1966)

Krohn, K., Ivemark, B.I., Salo, K.: A microangiographic study of fetal arterial vasculature in the human placenta in uncomplicated pregnancy. Acta Obstet. Gynecol. Scand. *49*, 205–214 (1970)

Krone, H.A.: Die Bedeutung der Eibettstörungen für die Entstehung menschlicher Mißbildungen. Stuttgart: Fischer 1961

Krone, H.A., Jopp, H., Scheller, W.: Die Bedeutung anamnestischer Befunde für verschiedene Formen des Nabelschnuransatzes. Z. Geburtshilfe Perinatal. *163*, 205–213 (1965)

Laga, E.M., Driscoll, S.G., Munro, H.N.: Comparison of placentas from two socioeconomic groups. I. Morphometry. Pediatrics *50*, 24–32 (1972)

Le Marec, B., Kerisit, J., De Villartay, A., Ferrand, B., Toulouse, R., Senecal, J.: L'artère ombilicale unique. Etude de 31 cas. J. Gynecol. Obst. Biol. Reprod. *1*, 825–841 (1972)

Lemtis, H.: Über die Architektonik des Zottengefäßeapparates der menschlichen Plazenta. Anat. Anz. *102*, 106–133 (1955)

Liebhart, M.: Polysaccharide surface coat (glycocalyx) of human placental villi. Pathol. Eur. *9*, 3–5 (1974)

Lister, U.M.: Ultrastructure of the human mature placenta. I. The maternal surface. Br. J. Obstet. Gynaecol. *70*, 373–386 (1963a)

Lister, U.M.: Ultrastructure of the human mature placenta. II. The foetal side. Br. J. Obstet. Gynaecol. *70*, 766–776 (1963b)

Lister, U.M.: Placental ultrastructure in foetal malnutrition. In: International Symposium on foeto-placental unit, p. 2. Excerpta Med. Found. 1968

Little, A.: Aplasia of the umbilical artery. Bull. Sloane Hosp. Wom. *4*, 127–131 (1958)

Little, W.A.: Placental infarction. Obstet. Gynecol. *15*, 109–130 (1960a)

Little, W.A.: The significance of placental foetal weight ratios. Am. J. Obstet. Gynecol. *79*, 134–137 (1960b)

Longo, L.D.: Disorder of Placentas. Transfer. In: Pathophysiology of Gestation, Vol. 2, pp. 1–76. Assali, N.S. (ed.). New York: Academic Press 1972

Lubchenko, L.O., Hansman, C., Dressler, M., Boyd, E.: Intrauterine growth as estimated from live-born birth weight data at 24 to 42 weeks of gestation. Pediatrics *32*, 793–800 (1963)

Ludwig, H.: Surface structure of the human term placenta and of the uterine wall post partum in the screen scan electron microscope. Am. J. Obstet. Gynecol. *111*, 328–344 (1971)

Ludwig, H., Metzger, H.: The human female reproductive tract. A scanning electron microscopic atlas. Berlin, Heidelberg, New York: Springer 1976

Luft, J.H.: Fine structure of capillary and endocapillary layer as revealed by Ruthenium red. Fed. Proc. *25*, 1773–1783 (1966)

MacLennan, A.H., Sharp, F., Shaw-Dunn, J.: The ultrastructure of human trophoblast in spontaneous and induced hypoxia using a system of organ culture. Br. J. Obstet. Gynaecol. *79*, 113–121 (1972)

Marais, W.D.: Human decidual spiral arterial studies. Part I. Br. J. Obstet. Gynaecol. *69*, 1-12 (1962a)

Marais, W.D.: Human decidual spiral arterial studies. Part IV. Br. J. Obstet. Gynaecol. *69*, 234–238 (1962b)

Marais, W.D.: Human decidual spiral arterial studies. Part V. Br. J. Obstet. Gynaecol. *69*, 944–955 (1962c)

Marais, W.D.: Human decidual spiral arterial studies. Part VI. Postmortem circulation studies on an in situ placenta. S. Afr. Med. J. *36*, 678–681 (1962d)

Marchetti, A.A.: A consideration of certain types of benign tumors of the placenta. Surg. Gynecol. Obstet. *68*, 733–743 (1939)

Martin, B.J., Spicer, S.S., Smythe, N.M.: Cytochemical studies of the maternal surface of the syncytiotrophoblast of human early and term placenta. Anat. Rec. *178*, 769–786 (1974)

McKeown, T., Record, R.G.: The influence of placental size on fetal growth in man, with special reference to multiple pregnancy. J. Endocrinol. *9*, 418–426 (1953)

Monie, I.W.: Velamentous insertion of cord in early pregnancy. Am. J. Obstet. Gynecol. *93*, 276–281 (1965)

Morgan, J.: Circumvallata placenta. Br. J. Obstet. Gynaec. *62*, 899–900 (1955)

Myers, R., Fujikura, T.: Placental changes after experimental abruptio placentae and vessel ligation of rhesus monkey placenta. Am. J. Obstet. Gynecol. *100*, 946–951 (1968)

Naftolin, F., Khudr, G., Benirschke, K.: The syndrome of chronic abruptio placentae, hydrorrhea and circumvallate placenta. Am. J. Obstet. Gynecol. *116*, 347–350 (1973)

Okudaira, Y., Hashimoto, T., Hamanaka, N., Yoshinare, S.: Electron microscope study on the trophoblastic cell column of human placenta. J. Electron Microsc. *20*, 93–106 (1971)

Ounsted, M., Ounsted, C.: Rate of intrauterine growth. Nature *220*, 599–600 (1968)

Panigel, M.: Placental perfusion experiments. Am. J. Obstet. Gynecol. *84*, 1664–1683 (1962)

Pinkerton, J.H.M.: Placenta circumvallata. Its aetiology and clinical significance. Br. J. Obstet. Gynaec. *63*, 743–747 (1956)

Potter, E.L., Davies, M.E.: Perinatal mortality. Am. J. Obstet. Gynecol. *105*, 335–348 (1969)

Ramsey, E.M., Martin, C.B., Donner, M.W.: Fetal and maternal placental circulation. Am. J. Obstet. Gynecol. *98*, 419–423 (1967)

Reichwein, D., Vogel, M.: Formen und Häufigkeit maternoplazentarer Durchblutungsstörungen bei Neugeborenen unterschiedlicher Gewichts- und Reifeklassen. Z. Geburtshilfe Perinatol. *176*, 364–378 (1972)

Reynolds, S.R.M.: Formation of fetal cotyledons in the hemochorial placenta. Am. J. Obstet. Gynecol. *94*, 425–439 (1966)

54

Romney, S.L., Reid, D.E.: Observations on the fetal aspects of placental circulation.
Am. J. Obstet. Gynecol. *61*, 83–98 (1951)

Rosso, P., Winick, M.: Intrauterine growth retardation. A new systematic approach
based on clinical and biological characteristics of this condition. J. Perinat. Med.
2, 147–160 (1974)

Rumboltz, W., McGogan, L.S.: Placental insufficiency and the small undernourished
full-term infant. J. Obstet. Gynecol. *1*, 294–301 (1953)

Sandstedt, B.: Studies on the human placenta with special reference to low birth weight.
Thesis, Karolinska Institutet (Stockholm) 1974

Saint-Anne Dargassier, S.: Le nouveau-né à terme, aspect neurologique. Biol. Neonat.
4, 174–200 (1962)

Schordania, J.: Der architektonische Aufbau der Gefäße der menschlichen Nachgeburt
und ihre Beziehung zur Entwicklung der Frucht. Arch. Chir. Gynäkol. *135*,
568–598 (1929)

Schuhmann, R., Wehler, V.: Histologische Unterschiede an Plazentazotten innerhalb
der materno-fetalen Strömungseinheit. Arch. Gynäkol. *210*, 425–439 (1971)

Scott, J.S.: Placenta extrachorialis (placenta marginata and placenta circumvallata).
Br. J. Obstet. Gynaec. *67*, 904–918 (1960)

Scott, J.M., Usher, R.: Fetal malnutrition: Its incidence, causes and effects. Am. J.
Obstet. Gynecol. *94*, 951–963 (1966)

Scott, J.M., Jordan, J.M.: Placental insufficiency and the small-for-dates baby.
Am. J. Obstet. Gynecol. *113*, 823–832 (1972)

Sexton, L.I., Hertig, A.T., Duncan, E.R., Kellog, F.S., Patterson, W.S.: Premature
separation of the normally implanted placenta. Am. J. Obstet. Gynecol. *59*,
13–24 (1950)

Shanklin, D.R.: The human placenta. A clinico-pathologic study. J. Obstet. Gynecol.
11, 129–138 (1958)

Shanklin, D.R., Sotelo-Avila, C.: The pathogenesis and significance of placenta extrachorialis. Lab. Invest. *15*, 1111 (1966)

Shanklin, D.R.: The influence of placental lesions on the newborn infant. In:
Symposium on the small-for-date infant. Pediatric Clin. North Am. *17*, 25–42
(1970)

Sjöstedt, S., Englesson, G., Roth, G.: Dysmaturity. Arch. Dis. Child. *33*, 123–130
(1958)

Smart, P.J.G.: Some observations on the vascular morphology of the foetal side of the
human placenta. Br. J. Obstet. Gynaec. *69*, 929–933 (1962)

Söderling, B.: Pseudoprematurity. Acta Pediatr. Scand. *42*, 520–525 (1953)

Spanner, R.: Mütterlicher und kindlicher Kreislauf der menschlichen Placenta und
seine Strombahnen. Z. Anat. Entwicklungsgesch. *105*, 163–242 (1935)

Steigrad, K.: Über die Beziehung von Plazentarinfarkten zur Schwangerschaftsnephro-
pathie. Gynaecologia *134*, 273–321 (1952)

Stieve, H.: Die Entwicklung und der Bau der menschlichen Plazenta. II. Zotten,
Zottenraumgitter und Gefäße in der zweiten Hälfte der Schwangerschaft.
Z. Mikrosk. Anat. Forsch. *50*, 1–120 (1941a)

Stieve, H.: Das Zottenraumgitter der riefen menschlichen Plazenta. Z. Geburtshilfe
Perinatol. *122*, 289–316 (1941b)

Strauss, F.: Bau und Funktion der menschlichen Plazenta. Fortschr. Geburtshilfe
Gynäkol. *17*, 3–11 (1964)

Strong, J.J., Corney, G.: The placenta in twin pregnancy. Oxford: Pergamon Press
1967

Theuring, F., Kemnitz, P.: Elektronenmikroskopische Plazentabefunde bei fetaler intra-
uteriner Wachstumsretardierung. Zbl. Allg. Pathol. *118*, 82–89 (1974)

Thomas, J.: Die gestörte Vascularisation der menschlichen Plazenta und ihre Auswirkung
auf die Frucht. Geburtshilfe Frauenheilkd. *19*, 801–811 (1959)

Thomas, J.: Untersuchungsergebnisse über die Aplasie einer Nabelarterie unter besonderer Berücksichtigung der Zwillingsschwangerschaft. Geburtshilfe Frauenheilkd. *21*, 984–992 (1961)

Torpin, R., Hart, B.F.: Placenta bilobata. Am. J. Obstet. Gynecol. *1*, 38–49 (1941)

Usher, R., McLean, F., Scott, K.E.: Judgement of foetal age. II. Clinical significance of gestational age on objective method for its assessment. Pediatr. Clin. North Am. *13*, 835–862 (1966)

Wallenburg, H.C.S., Hutchinson, D.L., Schuler, H.M., Stolte, L.A., Janssens, J.: The pathogenesis of placental infarction. II. An experimental study in the rhesus monkey placenta. Am. J. Obstet. Gynecol. *116*, 841–846 (1973)

Walton, A., Hammond, J.: The maternal effects on growth and conformation in Shire horse-Shetland pony crosses. Proc. R. Soc. Lond. (Biol.) *125*, 311–335 (1938)

Warburton, D., Naylor, A.F.: The effect of parity on placental weight and birth weight: an immunological phenomenon. A report of the collaborative study of cerebral palsy. Am. J. Hum. Genet. *23*, 41–54 (1971)

Widmaier, G.: Zur Ultrastruktur der menschlichen Plazentazotten. Arch. Gynäkol. *207*, 513–527 (1969)

Wigglesworth, J.S.: Morphological variations in the insufficient placenta. Br. J. Obstet. Gynaecol. *71*, 871–874 (1964)

Wigglesworth, J.S.: Vascular anatomy of the human placenta and its significance for placental pathology. Br. J. Obstet. Gynaecol. *76*, 979–989 (1969)

Wilkin, P.: Contribution à l'étude de la circulation placentaire d'origine foetale. Gynécol. Obstét. *53*, 239–262 (1954)

Wilkin, P.: Pathologie der Plazenta. Paris: Masson 1965

Williams, J.W.: Placenta circumvallata. Am. J. Obstet. Gynecol. *13*, 1–16 (1927)

Wilson, M.G.: Placental abnormalities and fetal disease. Am. J. Dis. Child. *108*, 154–163 (1964)

Winick, M.: Cellular growth of human placenta. III. Intrauterine growth failure. J. of Pediatr. *71*, 390–395 (1967)

Wulf, K.H., Becker, V.: Die morphologischen und funktionellen Grundlagen der Plazentainsuffizienz. Arch. Gynaecol. *219*, 368–369 (1975)

Wynn, R.M.: Cytotrophoblastic specializations: An ultrastructural study of the human placenta. Am. J. Obstet. Gynecol. *114*, 339–353 (1972)

Wynn, R.M.: Fine structure of the placenta. In: The Placenta and its Maternal Supply Line. Gruenwald, P. (ed.), pp. 56–79. Lancaster: MTP. 1975

Yoshida, Y.: Ultrastructure and secretory function of the syncytial trophoblast of human placenta in early pregnancy. Exp. Cell Res. *34*, 305–317 (1961)

Younoszai, M.K., Haworth, J.C.: Placental dimensions and relations in preterm, term, and growth-retarded infants. Am. J. Obstet. Gynecol. *103*, 267–271 (1969)

Zeek, P.M., Assali, N.S.: The formation, regression and differential diagnosis of true infarcts of the placenta. J. Obstet. Gynecol. *64*, 1191–1201 (1952)

Placental Insufficiency

Histomorphologic Diagnosis and Classification

W.-W. HÖPKER and BEATE OHLENDORF

I. General Aspects 58
II. Disorders of Maturation and Circulation 59

  1. Placentation Disorders 59
  2. Circulation Disorders 66

III. Clinical Syndromes 72

  1. Placental Insufficiency 72
  2. Fetal Underweight, Disorders of Gestation Period 74
  3. Hemolytic Disease of Newborns 77
  4. Maternal Diabetes Mellitus 77
  5. EPH Gestosis 77

References 80

Systematic and more-or-less detailed instructions regarding the morphologic diagnosis of placental disorders have been published by several authors (*Hörmann*, 1958; *Becker*, 1962; *Gruenwald*, 1964; *Döring* and *Kloos*, 1964; *Benirschke* and *Driscoll*, 1967). The functional concepts backing each of these diagnostic interpretations have been considerably modified and supplemented in the following years (*Strauss*, 1967). Some of the more recent reviews and compilations (*Boyd* and *Hamilton*, 1970; *Becker*, 1971; *Flenker*, 1974; *Becker*, 1977) have given but little room to a new concept of differentiation and interpretation that was developed and presented by the team of *Kloos* and *Vogel* (*Kloos* and *Vogel*, 1968; *Vogel*, 1968; *Kloos* and *Vogel*, 1974). Their ideas have subsequently found admission into several international publications, with slight modifications to terminology. Increased knowledge has been gained in the field of morphogenesis and physiology of placental perfusion (*Schuhmann* et al., 1977; *Schiebler*, 1977). The wide range of physiologic variations in placental differentiation suggests and even demands a new interpretation of histologic findings (*Becker*, 1977).

In our presentation the nomenclature proposed by *Kloos* and *Vogel* (1974) is adopted as far as possible; their classification was modified and extended in some essential aspects. This terminology, used in our working group for several years (*Ohlendorf*, 1977), was found adequate for exact morphologic classification of placental insufficiency and related disorders.

I. General Aspects

Morphologic diagnostics of the placenta should always include functional criteria (*Becker*, 1977). The clinician is asked to provide data about duration of pregnancy, body weight, and length of the fetus. The so-called placentofetal ratio (placenta weight : fetus weight) is an important parameter in the assessment of maturation disorders associated in some way with retarded or arrested development. Macroscopic inspection has to ascertain disturbed implantation or circulatory disorders and document the relative proportions of the areas involved.

Specimens must be sampled not only from areas of obvious pathologic change, but also from apparently healthy tissue. The specimens should exemplify a large cross section of the organ to permit adequate anatomic identification of each histologic slide, i.e., to determine its origin from the chorionic plate, base, or "placenton" (= placento-maternal unit). As a rule, a selective excision of five specimens is sufficient.

The four histologic criteria of placental maturation (*Becker*, 1963) may also serve as appropriate criteria of differentiation:
  1) Reduction of diameter with consecutive extension of surface in chorionic villi;
  2) Substitution of villous stroma by proliferating capillaries, formation of sinusoids;
  3) Formation of nuclear bridges between the resorptive nodules of different villi;
     these external fortifying structures are the result of intervillous stroma reduction;
  4) Hardening of arterial walls with fibrous stiffening of perivascular spaces.

When subdivised according to functional aspects, morphologic findings may be dynamically interpreted (*Schuhmann* and *Wehler*, 1971): The placenta is subdivided into 60–80 placentons or placentomaternal units, each supplied by its own spiral artery from the maternal decidua. A placentomaternal unit stretches from the chorionic plate to the basal attachment area. Its central structures are rather loose, villi in this area being less differentiated than in peripheral parts. Therefore, a horizontal section will show apparently immature areas alternating with mature parts. A similar discordance of differentiation can be found in vertical sections: subchorionic areas show more advanced maturation than those near the basis.

Histologic assessment must begin with an exact delineation of stages of placental maturity (*Becker*, 1963). The wide range of physiologic variations has to be correlated with actual macroscopic and microscopic findings from more than one placentomaternal unit if possible. This procedure of sampling and assessment will prevent misinterpretation (e.g., diagnosing embryonic villi together with a subnormal placentofetal ratio in the case of a mature infant at full term). No histologic finding, taken by itself and out of context, will permit relevant interpretation of the situation in the respective organ: we need additional data about the site from which it was taken and the area covered.

II. Disorders of Maturation and Circulation

1. Placentation Disorders (Table 1)

The term "placentation disorders" is reserved for the impairment or severe disturbance of epithelial, stromal, and vascular development during which these placental tissues are also affected to different degrees (*Becker*, 1969; *Kaufmann*, 1971). Each of these structural compartments can be either arrested or retarded in its normal development. Acceleration or dissociation are observed as well as paraplasia or malformation. The placenta responds to primary changes (disorders of implantation or primary disorders of placentation) by either compensatory or inflammatory and regressive reaction.

Kloos and *Vogel* (1974) have defined placentation disorders as either primary or secondary. *Persistence of embryonic villi* (Fig. 1) is caused by the arrest of stromal and vascular development during the first trimester. Vascularity of villi is insufficient; the trophoblast has merely one layer without villous bridges; and intervillous spaces

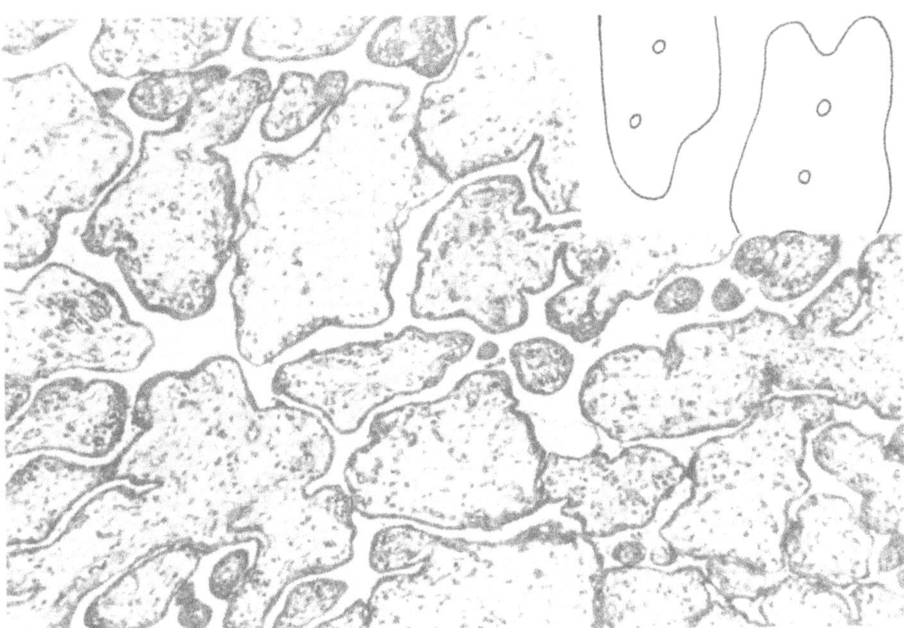

Fig. 1. Persisting embryonic villi, trophoblast without villous bridges; primordial embryonic connective tissue, Hofbauer cells (H & E, x 95). Insert: Schema

are wide, Hofbauer cells, abundant. *Arrested ramification* (Fig. 2) is characterized by more advanced differentiation. Plump, enlarged villi are rich in histiocytes, but vascularity is poor. *Discordant retardation* (Fig. 3) shows voluminous villi with padlike processes and highly cellular stroma. Capillarity is reduced, sinusoidal differentiation of vessels, lacking. The trophoblast shows partly monolayered, partly multilayered structures and distinct signs of regression with pyknosis and reduction of nuclear diameters.

Table 1. Placentation disorders (after *Kloos* and *Vogel*, 1974, modified and augmented)

			Formal Pathogenesis			Time	
			Epithelium	Stroma	Vessels	Trimester	PFR
Primary Disorders of Placentation	Arrest	Persistence of embryonic villi (Fig. 1)	F	AR	AR	I	↑↑↑↑
		Arrested ramification (Fig. 2)	AR	AR	AR	I	
		Discordant retardation (Fig. 3)	AR	F	AR	I	
	Retardation	Concordant retardation type A (Fig. 4)	R	R	R	II	↑↑↑
		Concordant retardation type B (Fig. 5)					
	Dissociation	Centro-peripheral discontinued vascularity (Fig. 6)	central R periph. AC	central R periph. AC	central R periph. AC	II	↑↑
		Intercalary defective rami-fication (Fig. 7)	AC	AC	AC	II–III	
	Paraplasia	Chorangiomatosis (Fig. 8)	R	F	F	II	↑
Secondary Disorders of Placentation	Compensation	Angiomatosis type A (Fig. 9)	S	S	AC	II–III	
		Angiomatosis type B (Fig. 10)	S	S		II–III	↕
	Reaction	Obliterating angiopathy (Fig. 11)	S	S	O	II–III (I ?)	

Abbreviations: AC = acceleration; AR = arrest; F = faulty differentiation; O = obliteration; R = retardation; S = synchronous development; PFR = placentofetal ratio

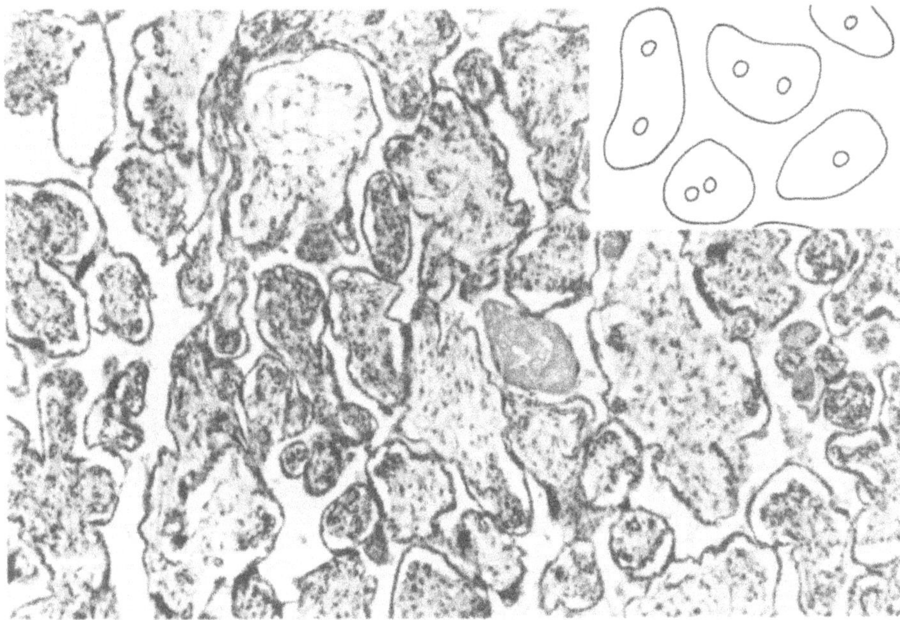

Fig. 2. Arrested ramification: plump villi, abundance of histiocytes, Hofbauer cells, wide meshwork of villous stroma. (H & E, x 95)

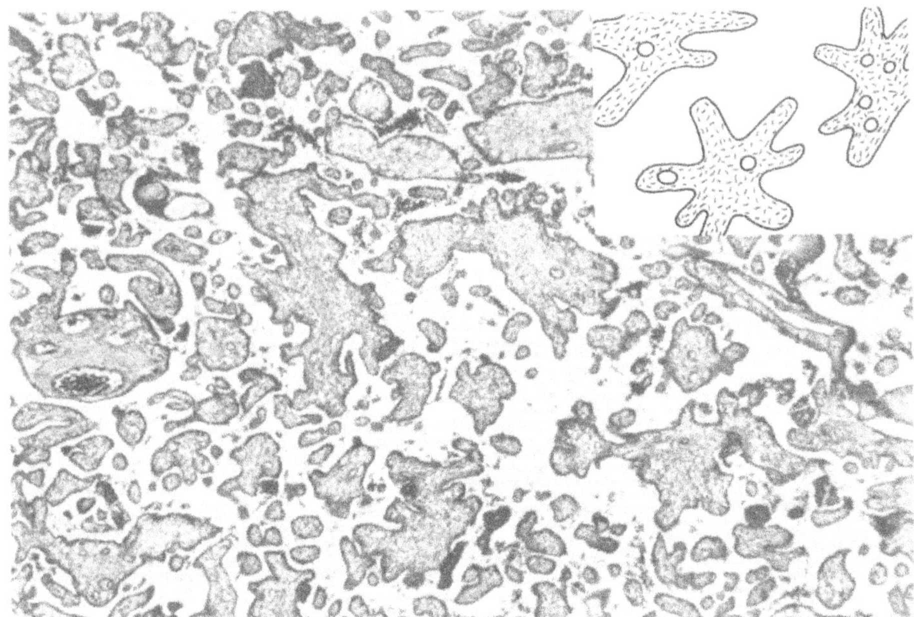

Fig. 3. Discordant retardation: voluminous villi with padlike processes, highly cellular stroma, reduced capillarity, failing sinusoidal differentiation. (H & E, x 38)

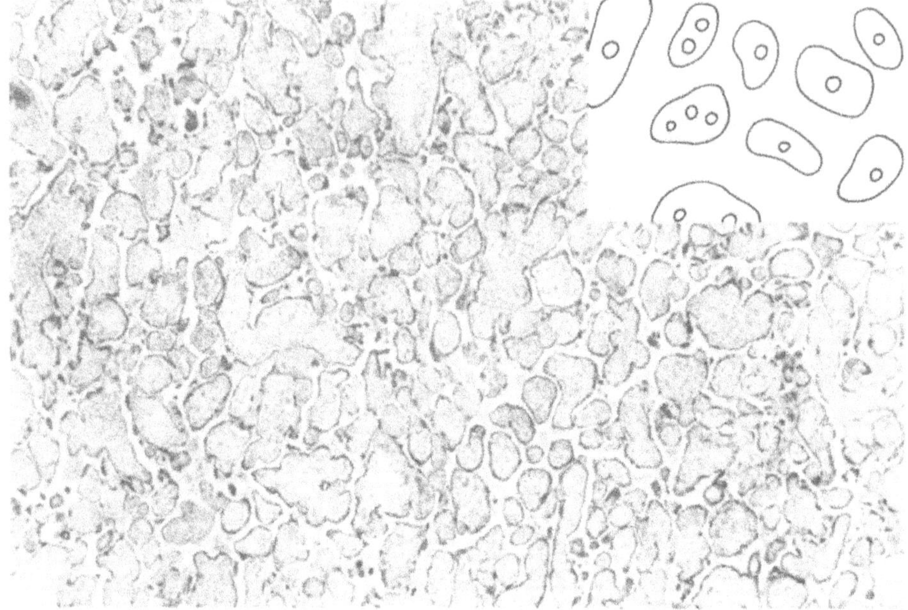

Fig. 4. Concordant retardation/type A: uniform, plump villi, poor fibrillar differentiation and reticular structure of stroma. (H & E, x 38)

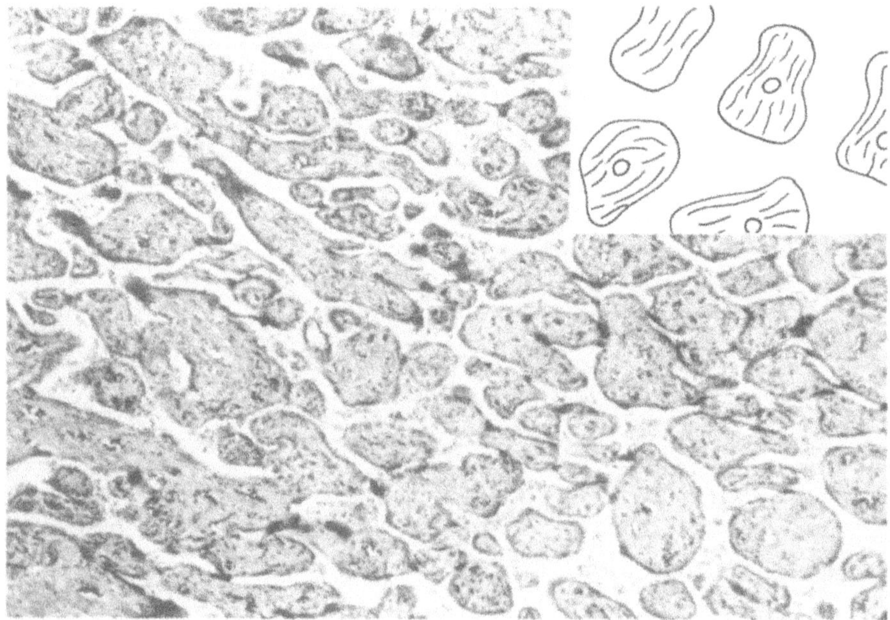

Fig. 5. Concordant retardation/type B: uniform, plump villi, abundant histiocytes and fibroblasts, and precollagenous fibrillar differentiation. (H & E, x 95)

Phenomena of c o n c o r d a n t r e t a r d a t i o n are manifested during the second trimester. The histologic picture is dominated by regular, coarse villi with poor fibrillar differentiation and reticular structure of stroma. The trophoblast is mostly monolayered and vascularity of villi is poor in central as well as in peripheral parts. There is a *type A* (without fibrillar differentiation of the villous stroma, Fig. 4) and a *type B* (abundance of precollagenous fibers and increased number of histiocytes and fibroblasts, Fig. 5).

Dissociative disorders of the development during the 2nd and 3rd trimester may lead to *centroperipheral discontinuity of vascularization* (Fig. 6). Histologically, ramification is apparently regular, the number of arteries and veins in the trunci is normal,

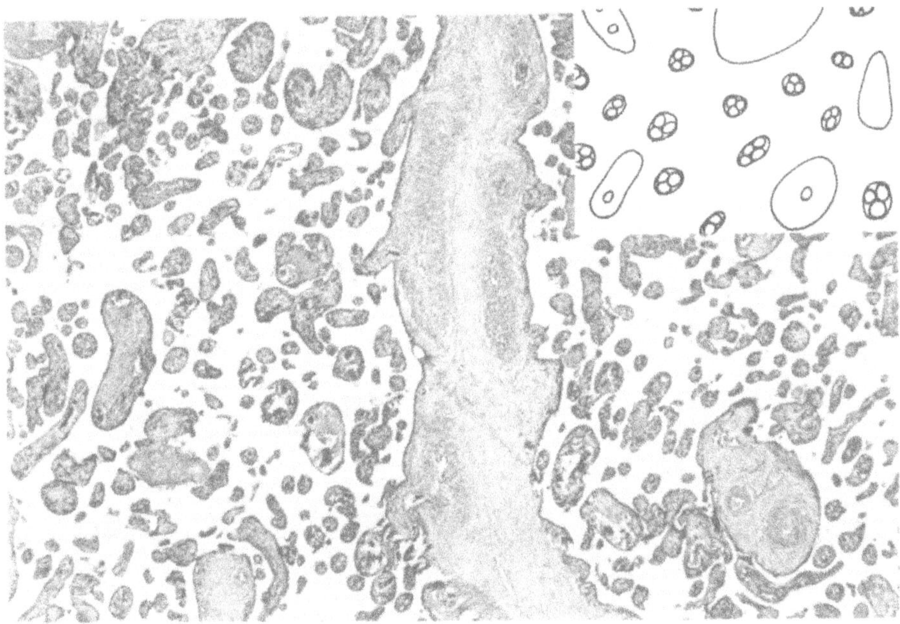

Fig. 6. Discontinued centroperipheral vascularity: regular ramification, normal number of arteries and veins in the truncus. Poor vascularity of large and medium-sized rami, regular vascularity of smaller rami. (H & E, x 38)

but the fibrous "cuffs" are insufficient. Large and medium-sized branches are poorly vascularized, whereas smaller villous branchings show a sufficient number of well-differentiated vessels. In contrast, *intercalary defective ramification* (Fig. 7) is characterized by complete absence of large and medium rami and by a reduced number of peripheral villi. Moreover, the terminal diameter of villi is severely reduced.

A pattern of paraplastic change is seen in the rare picture of *chorangiomatosis* (Fig. 8). Reticular stroma of varying cellularity shows a proliferation of narrow (type A) or sinusoidal (type B) vessels. Trophoblast development is retarded, its structure, monolayered.

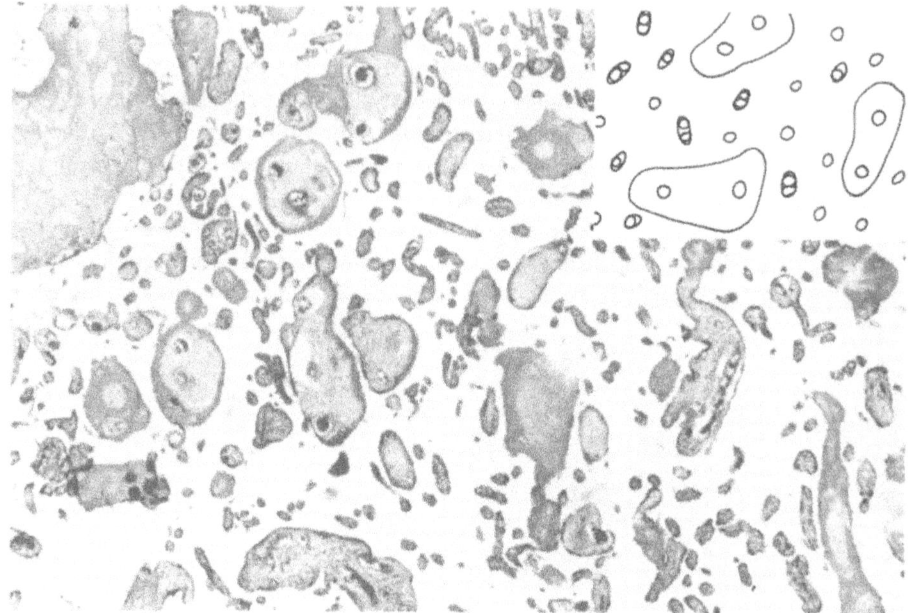

Fig. 7. Intercalary defective ramification: absence of large and medium-sized rami, small number of peripheral rami, strongly reduced diameter of terminal villi. (H & E, x 95)

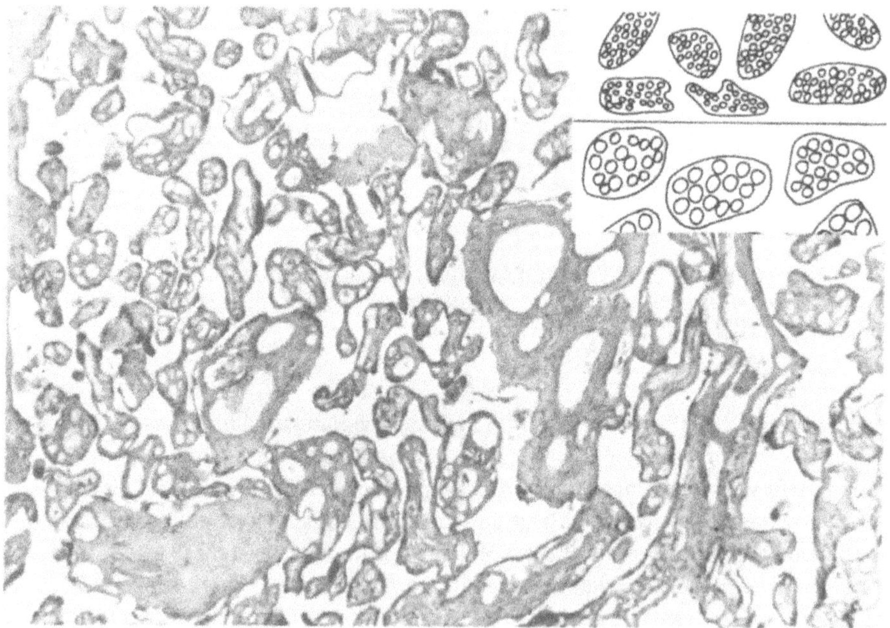

Fig. 8. Chorangiomatosis: plump villi, reticular stroma of varying cellularity, capillary hyperplasia, proliferation of narrow (type A) or sinusoidal (type B) vessels. (H & E, x 95)

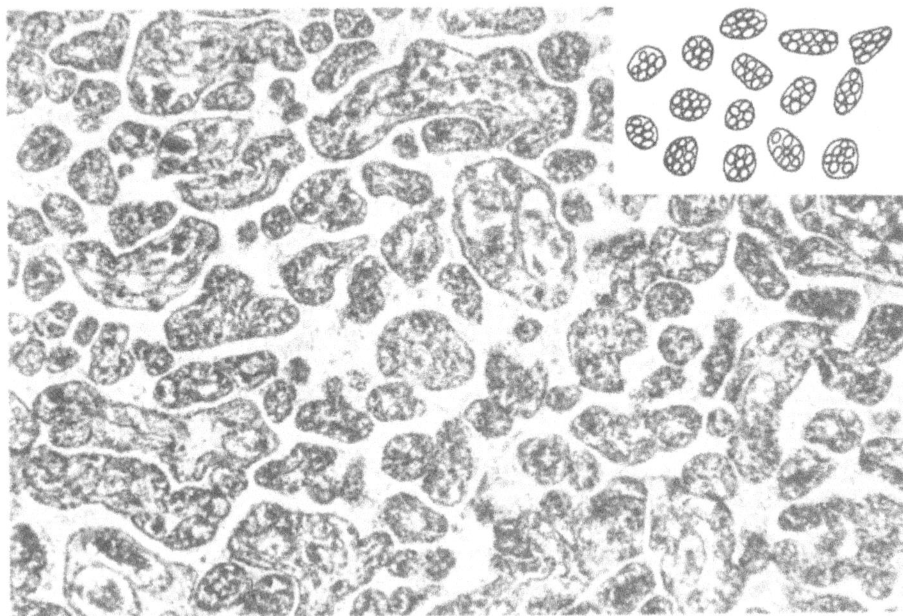

Fig. 9. Angiomatosis/type A: regular mesenchymal and epithelial differentiation, focally excessive vascularity in peripheral villi. (H & E, x 95)

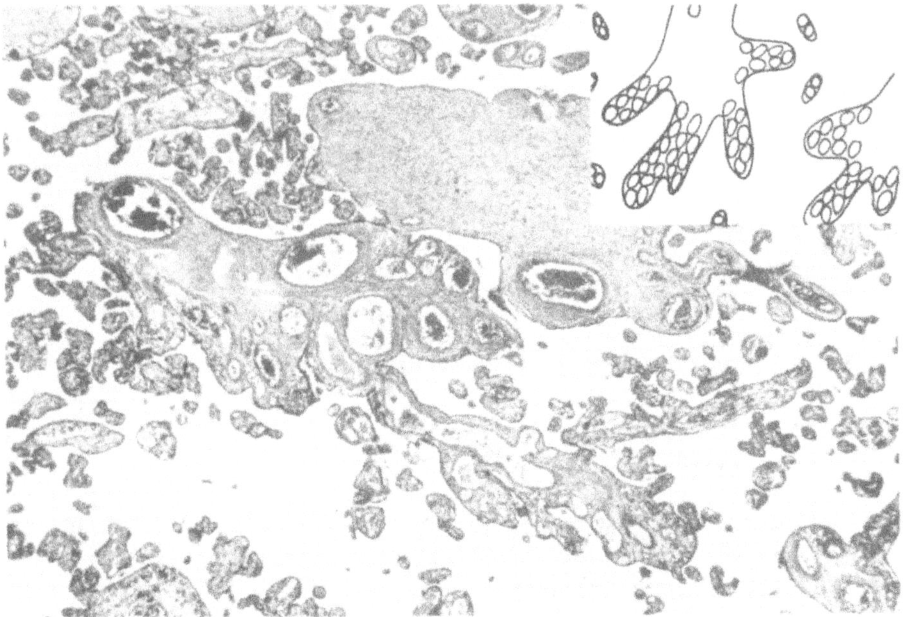

Fig. 10. Angiomatosis/type B: regular epithelial and mesenchymal differentiation, focally angiomatous hyperplasia of paravascular truncus blastema. (H & E, x 38)

66

This picture must be clearly separated from that of *angiomatosis*, which is interpreted as an acceleration of the vascular system in terms of compensatory reaction. Histologically, mesenchymal and epithelial formations of regular differentiation are found besides focal excessive vascularity in peripheral villi (type A, Fig. 9). Type B (Fig. 10) is characterized by angiomatous hyperplasia of the paravascular truncus blastema.

The classification of *obliterating angiopathy* presents an unsolved problem. In agreement with *Becker* (1977) we would recognize an independent disease pattern rather than a mere supravital or postvital phenomenon (*Becker* and *Dolling*, 1965; *Peceny*, 1972; *Reichwein* and *Vogel*, 1972; *Bender* and *Werner*, 1974). The histologic picture (Fig. 11) shows villi of apparently correct development and ramification, but with a severe stenosis or occlusion of vessels with dense, broad fibrous cuffs.

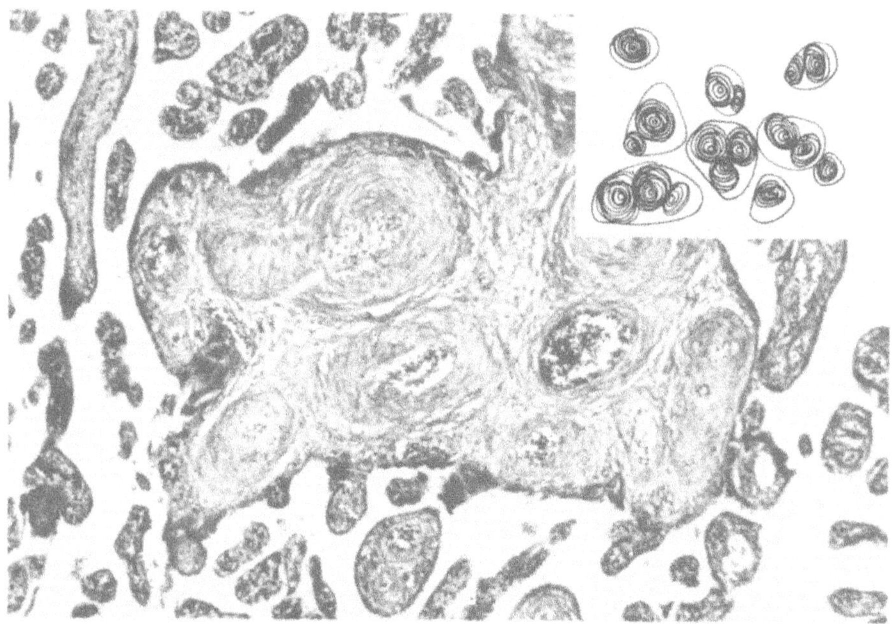

Fig. 11. Obliterating angiopathy: villi developed and ramified according to age; vessels surrounded by dense, fibrous cuffs with partial stricture of lumen. (H & E, x 95)

2. Circulation Disorders (Table 2)

Except for the very rare picture of the anemic or white infarct (*Fox*, 1963), all circulatory disorders of the placenta are of uterine, i.e., maternal origin. Size, shape, and borders of unsupplied areas correlate to the actual cause of the disturbance (*Kloos* and *Vogel*, 1974): correct interpretation requires an adequate understanding of the functional subdivision into placentomaternal units of placental supply, the above-mentioned placentons (*Moll* and *Künzel*, 1974).

Table 2. Circulation disorders of the placenta (terminology adapted from *Kloos* and *Vogel*, 1974; *Becker*, 1977)

Name of lesion	Size	Localization	Pathophysiologic features	Morphology
Deposits of microfibrin (Fig. 12)	Microscopic dimensions	Ubiquitous (relevant for diagnosis: intermediate)	Fluent transition to normal features. Factors: flow-through rate of inter-villous area and villi, pH values increase during EPH gestosis	Disseminated minifocal precipitation of fibrin at surface of villi and be-tween them (bridge formation)
Gridlike infarction (Fig. 13)	A few mm	Intermediate	Involved are the "watershed" areas of fetomaternal flow units	Small foci of villous adhesion with fibrin deposits between villi
Focal collapse of villi (Fig. 14)	1 cm ϕ	Basal	Functional occlusion of decidual spiral artery. Disturbed circulation in one fetomaternal unit	Collapsed intervillous area with marginal hyperemia, stromal bleeding, necrosis, organization. Placentation disorder: compensation
Placental infarction hemorrhagic (red) (Fig. 15)	Mostly 2 cm ϕ	Basal to subchorionic	Deficiency of several maternofetal units	Intervillous and stromal bleeding, necrosis of villi, insudatles of fibrin, ghost villi, mosaic pattern, organization
anemic (white)	Dependent on vascular involvement	Intermediate, subchorionic	Occlusion of one placental vessel, functional terminal artery (e.g., in placentitis	Coagulation necrosis, organization, vascular process (e.g., inflammation)
Intervillous hemorrhage/aneurysm (Fig. 16)	1 cm ϕ	Subchorionic, intermediate	Intervillous anomaly, bleeding from decidual or villous vessel, one feto-maternal unit is involved	Villus-displacing hemorrhage. Villous adhesions in the vicinity; marginal hyperemia
Intervillous thrombosis (Fig. 17)				Villus-displacing thrombus; capsule-like merging of villi
Subchorionic pseudo-infarction (Fig. 18)	1 cm ϕ	Subchorionic	Functional narrowing of intervillous spaces by fibrinous deposits (dead-water-area); physiologic process	Reticular precipitation of fibrin-including villi; frequent regressive changes (e.g., calcification)

68

Microdeposits of fibrin (Fig. 12) as well as *subchorionic pseudoinfarction* (Fig. 13) may be seen as physiologic phenomena to a certain degree. The amount of precipitated fibrin correlates with certain diseases of the mother, in particular with EPH gestosis and diabetes mellitus. The frequency of precipitates increases toward the chorion, showing a marked preponderance between placentons. This phenomenon is called the "last field" * in German and "watershed infarct" in Angloamerican terminology. — A similar pattern appears in the *"gridlike"* infarction (Fig. 14) and in the *focal collapse of villi* (Fig. 15).

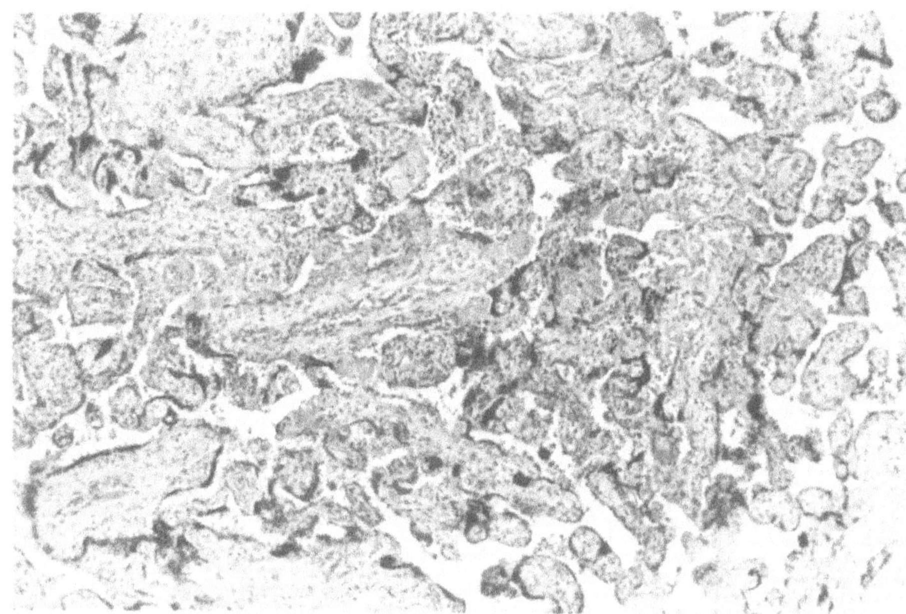

Fig. 12. Microdeposits of fibrin: minimal foci of fibrin precipitation forming intervillous bridges in the vicinity of trophoblast buds. (H & E, x 95)

Hemorrhagic placental infarction (Fig. 16) is provoked by occlusion or obliteration of one or several spiral arteries (*Carter* et al., 1963; *Wallenburg* et al., 1973). The disturbance involves one or several of the fetomaternal circulatory units. The definition of different varieties of placental infarction corresponds to the functional units of the organ. *Intervillous aneurysma* (Fig. 17) and *intervillous thrombosis* (Fig. 18) are always limited to a single placenton; they even pass through similar stages of organization.

Correct histologic differentiation of diverse circulatory disorders of the placenta requires adequate documentation of macroscopic findings in each case. Unsupplied areas may show either regressive alterations or phenomena of organization, according

---

* The metaphor is taken from the last and hence worst-supplied field when water is pumped up a steep slope

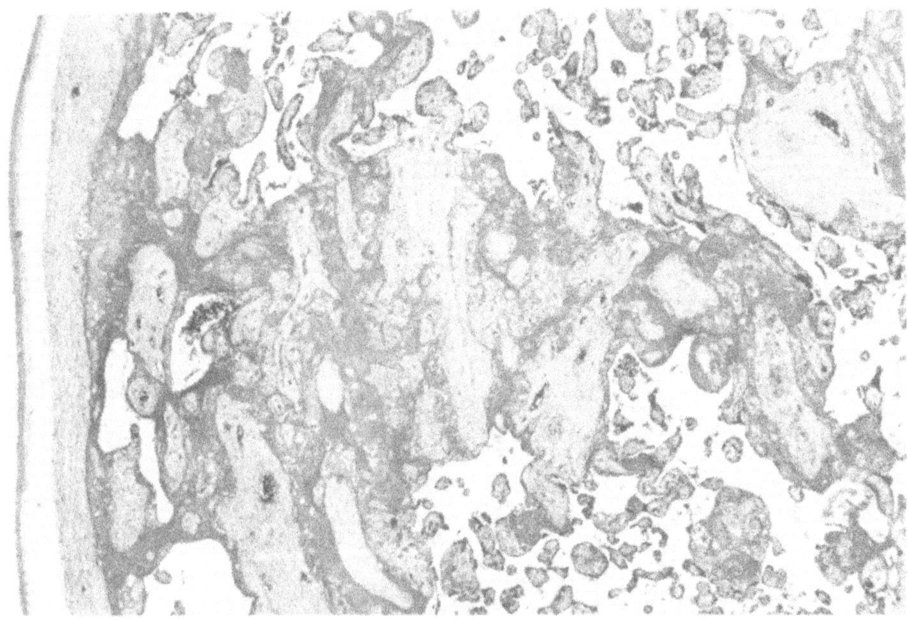

Fig. 13. Subchorionic pseudoinfarction: subchorionic fibrin-precipitation involving the villi. (H & E, x 38)

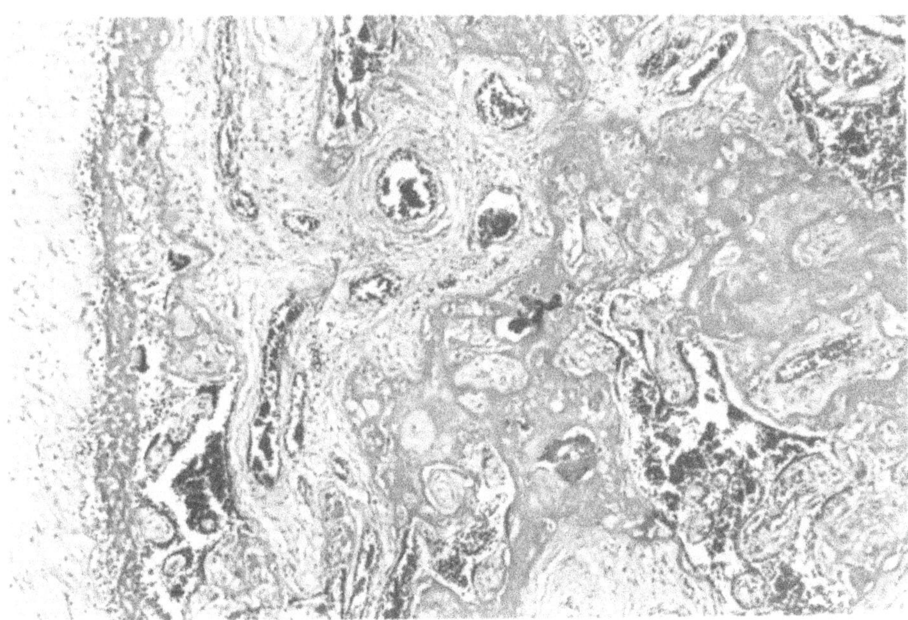

Fig. 14. Gridlike infarction: minimal foci of villous adhesion with netlike fibrin deposits in intervillous spaces. (H & E, x 95)

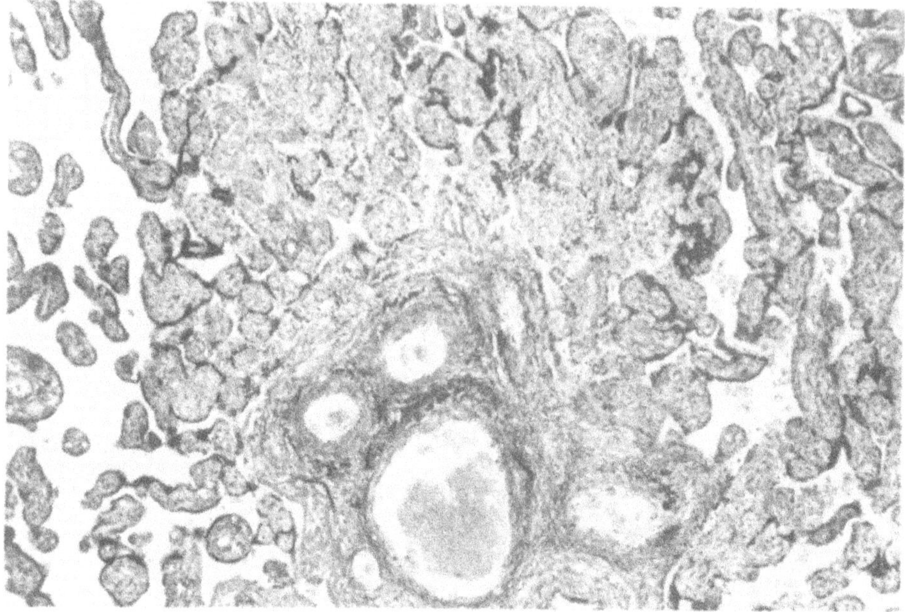

Fig. 15. Focal collapse of villi: collapsed intervillum with closely packed villi, marginal hyperemia. (H & E, x 95)

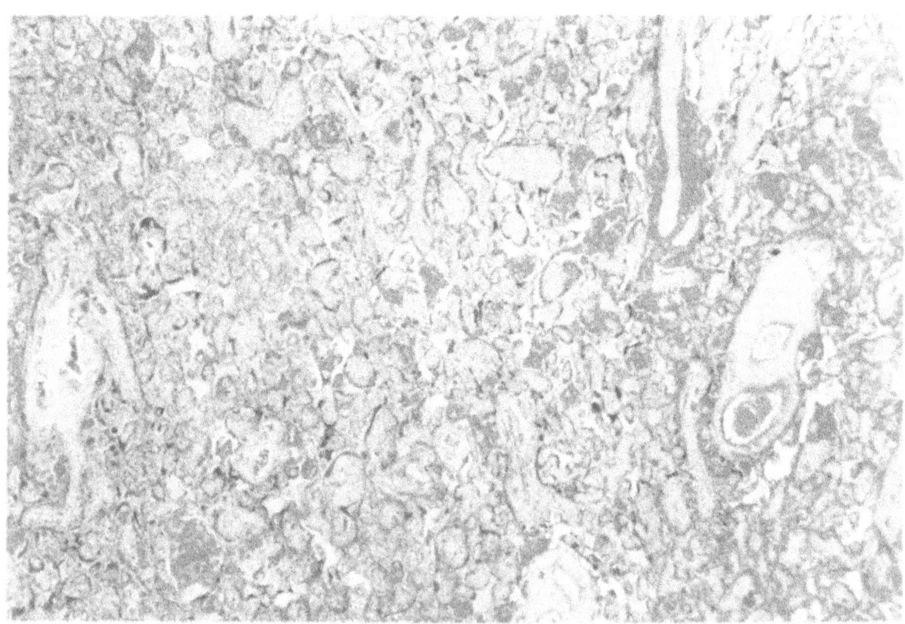

Fig. 16. Placental infarction, macroscopically extending over the whole depth of the organ. Fresh and older hemorrhages into the villous and intervillous stroma. Netlike fibrin precipitations. Poorly staining necrotic villi, "ghost villi." (H & E, x 38)

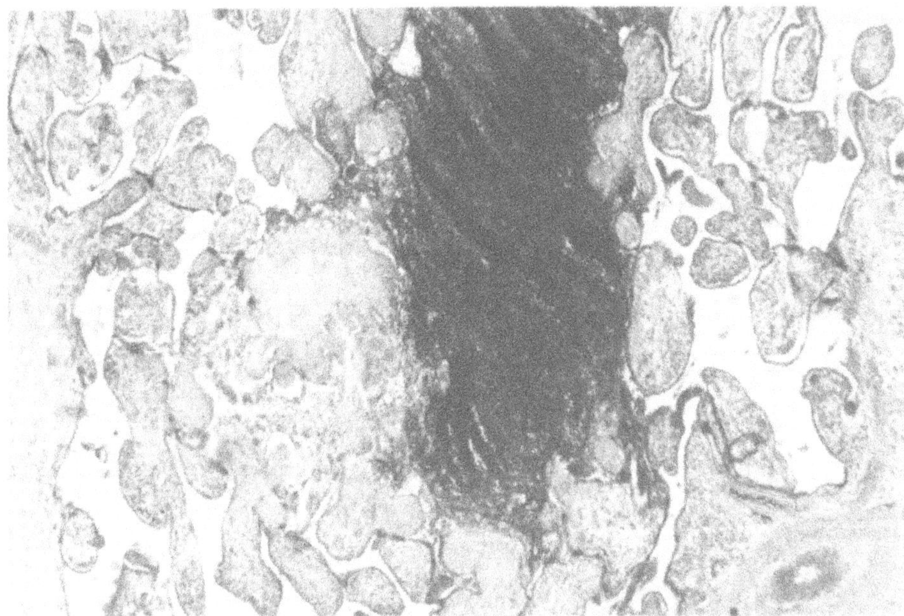

Fig. 17. Intervillous hemorrhage or aneurysm: villus-displacing hematoma with conglutination of neighboring areas by a fine network of fibrin. (H & E, x 47,5)

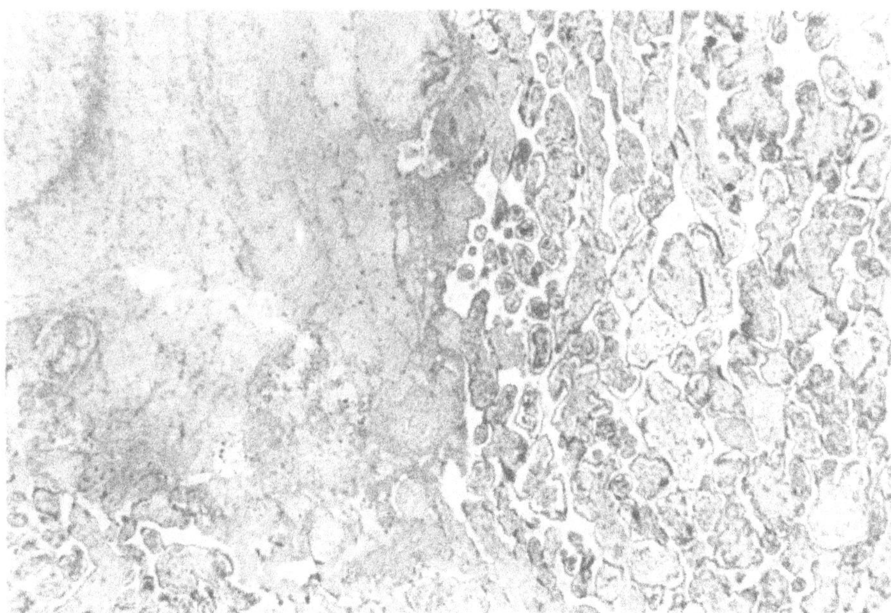

Fig. 18. Intervillous thrombosis: intervillous hemorrhage, partly coagulated, with marginal organization of varying duration. (H & E, x 38)

72

to their respective history. Changes vary from obliterating angiopathy, to r e c a n a l-
i z e d t h r o m b i (Fig. 19), and, eventually, extensive calcification and secondary
disorders of placentation in the vicinity. A placenta that shows disturbed circulation
has suffered, as a rule, previous disturbances of development.

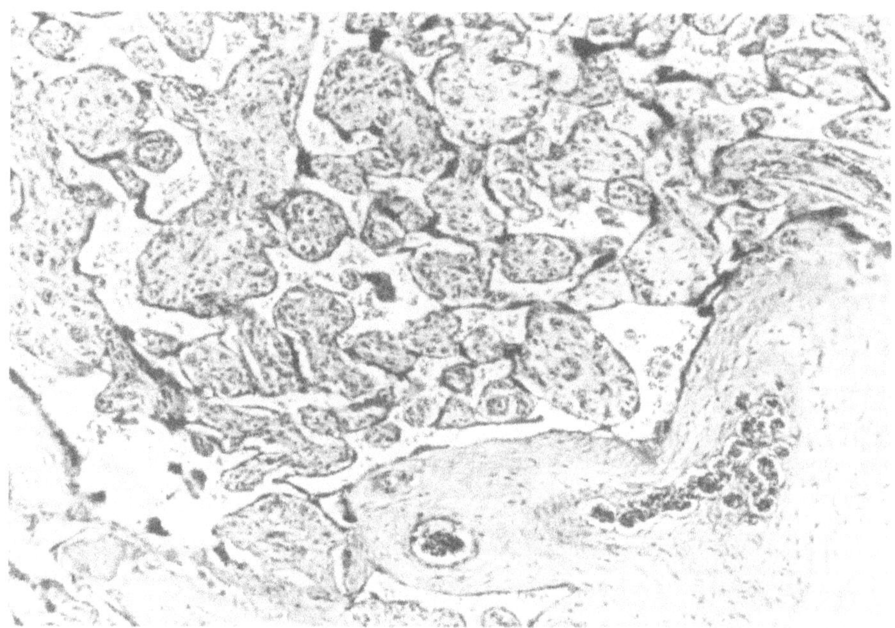

Fig. 19. Recanalized thrombus: "angiomatous" or "cavernous" lumen of large truncal
vessel. (H & E, x 95)

III. Clinical Syndromes

Any morphologic interpretation of clinical findings, even a tentative evaluation of the
function of a placenta, will require accurate classification among the disorders affect-
ing placentation and circulation.

1. Placental Insufficiency (Table 3)

The inability of the placenta to maintain adequate fetomaternal exchange is called
placental insufficiency (*Becker*, 1972). The possible causes are:
  1) Disturbance of the intervillous blood flow, provoked by maternal factors localized
in decidua or uterus;

Table 3. Placental insufficiency in the proper sense (acute or chronic) and in a broader sense (preterm detachment, intrauterine fetal death)

Name of disturbance	Definition	Pathogenesis	Placentofetal ratio	Morphology
Placental insufficiency acute	Respiratory insufficiency with or without abruptio totalis/ partialis	1. Acute disturbance of decidual perfusion → circulatory disorder of placenta 2. Disturbed placentation with or without circulatory disorder	Uncharacteristic	1. mature villi 2. disturbed placentation: dissociation retardation hyperplasia 3. disturbed circulation
chronic	First nutritional or hormonal, later (factultative) respiratory insufficiency	1. Chronic disturbance of decidual perfusion → disturbed placentation → disturbed placental circulation 2. Frequent in hemolytic disease of newborns, diabetes mellitus, EPH gestosis	According to basic disease	1. mature villi 2. disturbed placentation: arrest retardation dissociation 3. disturbed circulation (infarction placenta) 4. obliterating angiopathy
Premature separation	Always retroplacental hematoma, circulatory disorder	1. Disturbed implantation → placentation 2. Additional factors: → hydramnion, multiple pregnancy (mechanical, hormonal factors) → changes in spiral artery, → decidual necrosis → disturbed circulation (EPH-gestosis)	Uncharacteristic	1. mature villi 2. disturbed circulation: collapse of villi intervillous bleeding infarction 3. disturbed implantation 4. disturbed placentation
Fetal death in utero	Latent placental insufficiency, acute or chronic	1. Disturbed implantation placentation 2. Circulatory disorder	Uncharacteristic	1. signs of retention in the stroma: condensation, swelling; in vessels: swelling, proliferation (obliteration), fibrinous insudation; in chorion: increase of nuclear nodules, necrosis, morphallaxis 2. disturbed implantation and placentation

2) Faulty differentiation of the membranes of metabolic exchange (disorders of placentation in the proper sense);

3) Insufficiency of specific placental functions (impairment of active transport or hormone production).

Acute placental insufficiency (*Hibbard* and *Jeffcoate*, 1966) arises from impaired decidual perfusion and can be compared to respiratory insufficiency (*Kubli*, 1968). *Chronic placental insufficiency* is interpreted, as a rule, in terms of nutritional or hormonal, later even of possibly respiratory insufficiency. The placentofetal ratio as well as the morphologic findings are determined by the basic disease of the mother and by the duration of pregnancy. Quite a number of cases clinically manifesting placental insufficiency yield no relevant morphologic findings; disorders of uterine attachment or decidual differentiation (mostly of vascular nature) should be discussed in this context.

2. Fetal Underweight, Disorders of Gestation Period (Table 4)

It seems necessary to distinguish the terms *premature birth* (prematurity) (*Becker*, 1961; *Reichwein* and *Vogel*, 1972), *fetal dystrophy* (*Thomas*, 1959), and *fetal hypotrophy* (*Scott* and *Usher*, 1966; *Schuhmann*, 1969; *v. Harnack* and *v. Bermuth*, 1971; *Busch*, 1972; *Scott* and *Jordan*, 1972; *Dollmann*, 1973; *Rosso* and *Winick*, 1974; *Altshuler* et al., 1975; *Vogel*, 1977). Placental prematurity is probably provoked by an insufficient supply to the implantation area and latent oxygen deficiency. The result is acceleration of placental maturation and, eventually, generalized insufficiency of the placenta at the end of pregnancy. The corresponding histologic findings show maturitas praecox (*Becker*, 1960) with characteristic dissociation phenomena (*Kloos* and *Vogel*, 1974). A reverse mechanism is discussed for the pathogenesis of the placenta in retarded delivery. A large cardiac minute-volume of the mother may provide excessive oxygen supply to the area of implantation, but fail to give the necessary stimulus for placental differentiation. The histologic picture of the organ shows retarded villi.

Pre-existing primary disorders of placentation, with circulatory disorders during the 3rd trimester, characterize the placenta in fetal dystrophy. The actual cause is seen in subacute placental insufficiency, the effects of which are manifested in the fetus. The role of the decidual or implantation area of the placenta has been underestimated until now (*Becker*, 1977). During the 1st and 2nd trimester this area may give rise to increased placental growth or to hyperplasia associated with retarded maturation. In accordance with the actual functional value of the respective implantation area, acceleration begins during the 4th or 5th month. Consequences vary, resulting in either the harmonious type of fetal hypotrophy (placental nanism) or the disharmonious type with normal length but reduced weight of the fetus. Histology reveals concordant retardation, often associated with intercalary defects of ramification.

Table 4. Placenta-derived fetal disorders. Symptoms in the neonate for which explanation is sought in the placenta

	Definition	Pathogenesis	Plazentofetal ratio	Morphology
Prematurity of birth (placentogenic causes)	Gestation period reduced to less than 36 weeks	1. Small cardiac minute-volume of the mother, $\downarrow\downarrow$ or corresponding uterine factor: → insufficient supply to the site of implantation → latent O_2-deficiency 2. Acceleration, prematurity of placenta, global insufficiency; Symptoms: low placental weight, prematurtiy of villi, premature detachment of placenta		1. mature villi 2. disturbed placentation: dissociation (maturitas praecox)
Fetal dystrophy (placentogenic causes)	Subacute placental insufficiency; stage I: absence of vernix caseosa; stage II: meconium in amniotic fluid; stage III: thick fluid, discolored skin	Primary disorders of placentation commonly are superimposed by circulatory disorders (late gestosis, retarded birth)	Uncharacteristic	1. mature villi 2. disturbed placentation: retardation 3. circulation disorders
Fetal hypotrophy (placentogenic causes)	Chronic placental insufficiency — "small for date" children; body w. under 10th percentile; harmonious: placental nanism; disharmonious: normal length, reduced weight	Insufficient blood supply to the uterus → undersized decidual area compensatory mechanisms: 1. increased growth → hyperplasia concordant retardation 2. Accelerated placental maturation; critical phase: 4th month: harmonious type; 5th month: disharmonious type	Uncharacteristic	1. disturbed implantation 2. disturbed placentation: retardation, dissociation 3. mature villi 4. circulation disorders espec. gridlike infarcts)
Retarded birth (placentogenic causes)	Prolonged gestation period, over 40 weeks	1. Large cardiac minute-volume of the mother, $\uparrow\uparrow$ or corresponding uterine factor → oversupply to the site of implantation → abundant O_2 supply 2. No stimulus for differentiation → retardation		1. mature villi 2. disturbed placentation: retardation, compensation 3. regressive changes (calcification, fibrosis, pseudo-infarction, "maturitas retardata")

Table 5. Correlated pathology of hemolytic disease of newborns, diabetes mellitus, and EPH gestosis

	Definition	Pathogenesis	Placentofetal ratio	Morphology
Hemolytic disease of newborns (Fig. 20)	Infant hemolysis caused by blood group incompatibility of mother and child	Placenta-inherent maternal antibodies hemo-antigens of the child (Rh-, ABO-system), action dependent on: 1. timing (=mode of placental disorders, compensation) and 2. 2. intensity: extension of the placental area involved)	$\uparrow\uparrow\uparrow\uparrow$	1. mature villi 2. disturbed placentation: arrest, retardation 3. erythroblasts
Diabetes mellitus (Figs. 21 and 22)	Diabetes mellitus of the mother at time of conception	Changes depend on: 1. duration of diabetes mellitus; 2. metabolic guidance during pregnancy; 3. additional complications in the mother. True stromal and vascular proliferation in the placenta. Vascular changes in the uterus.	According to compensation $\updownarrow\updownarrow$	1. mature villi 2. disturbed placentation: arrest, dissociation, compensation, obliteration 3. disturbed circulation
EPH Gestosis (Figs. 22 and 23)	Edema, proteinuria, hypertension	Insufficiency of decidual circulation, pre-dominant respiratory insufficiency of placenta: 1. basic disease (e.g., diabetes mellitus, hypertension) 2. vascular dysfunction: primary: uterine vessels, spiral artries; secondary: wall ischemia (twins, hydrops; etc.)	Uncharacter-istic	1. mature villi 2. disturbed placentation arrest, dissociation, compensation, obliteration 3. intervillous fibrin deposits 4. circulation disorders, mainly gridlike infarction

3. Hemolytic Disease of Newborns (Table 5)

The incidence of the hemolytic disease of newborns (Fig. 20) was considerably reduced with recent therapeutic achievements. In these cases the placentofetal ratio shows a characteristic increase. Histologic features are the disturbed maturation with arrest or retardation of villi, changes which probably take place during the 1st or 2nd trimester. Evidence of erythroblasts in the fetal blood (in histology or placental sections) at the end of the gestation period is an additional helpful finding (*Becker* and *Bleyl,* 1961; *Kloos* and *Vogel,* 1974).

4. Maternal Diabetes Mellitus (Table 5)

Morphologic changes of the placenta in maternal diabetes (Figs. 21 and 22) may vary in intensity and especially duration. If the disease has preceded the actual pregnancy by a long time, circulatory disorders provoked by decidual vascular changes will predominate; if the maternal diabetes has escaped clinical guidance or stabilization, placental changes will arise from placentation disorders. Arrest of development and retarded maturation are associated with genuine stromal or vascular proliferation (*Vogel,* 1967; *Emmrich* and *Gödel,* 1972; *Emmrich* and *Müller,* 1974; *Kloos* and *Vogel,* 1974).

5. EPH Gestosis (Table 5)

EPH gestosis (*e*dema, *p*roteinuria, and *h*ypertension) is as a rule caused by the combined effects of disturbed placentation plus secondary vascular disturbance of circulation, resulting from the basic disease (Figs. 22 and 23). The clinical picture in most cases shows respiratory placental insufficiency. Histology reveals a significant increase of disseminated intervillous fibrin precipitation (*Kloos* and *Vogel,* 1974). This pattern characterizes the actual circulatory status of the uteroplacental unit (*Frank,* 1967; *Franke* et al., 1971).

In clinically manifested placental insufficiency, histomorphologic changes as presented in Tables 1–5, are found in approximately two-thirds of all organs investigated. In most of the other cases clinical evidence is not matched by any, or by merely an insufficient morphologic counterpart. Therefore, the list of symptoms in our tables always begins with the evidence of mature, well-differentiated villi. Moreover, histologic changes in *one and the same* placenta may show a very wide range of variations.

Fig. 21. Stillborn infant (autopsy no. 1086/75), 8th month, of 38-year-old tripara with diabetes mellitus. Other two children living. Extensive fresh infarction of the placenta. Several large foci reaching from the basal to the covering plate are macroscopically visible. The majority of villi show incomplete and partly discordant maturation. (H & E, x 38)

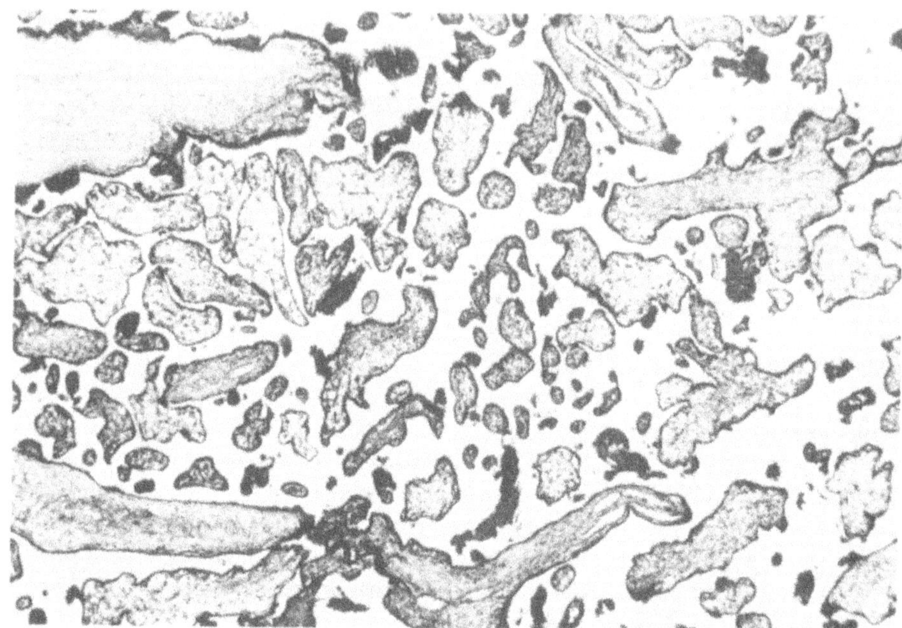

Fig. 20. Stillborn infant (autopsy no. 91/77), 8th month of pregnancy, of 38-year-old tripara. Other children both living. Severe fetal and placental hydrops in Rh-erythroblastosis. Persisting embryonic villi, intercalary defective ramification. (H & E, x 38)

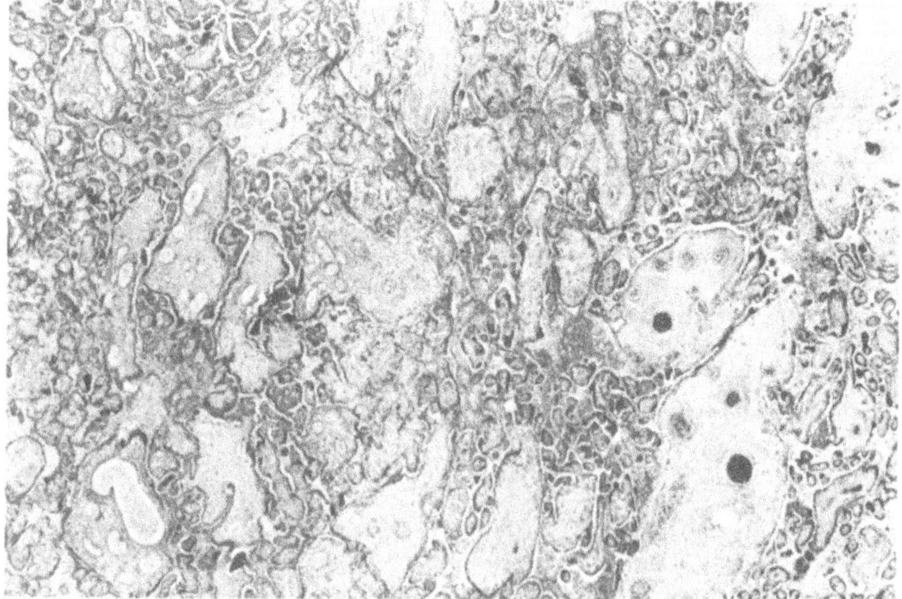

Fig. 21. (Legend see page 77)

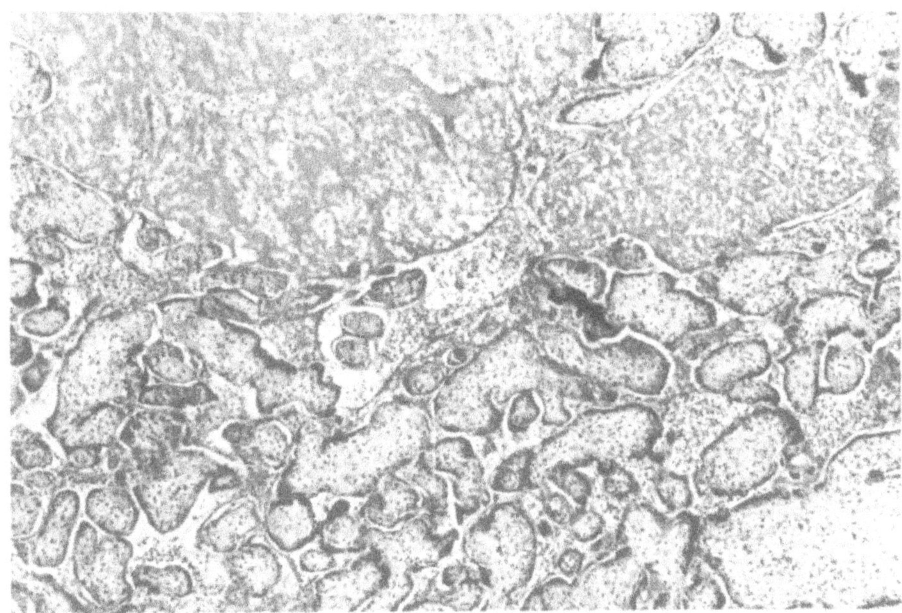

Fig. 22. Stillborn infant (autopsy no. 2/75), 9th month. Pre-eclampsia of mother with diabetes mellitus. Discordantly retarded villi with villus-displacing intervillous thrombosis. (H & E, x 38)

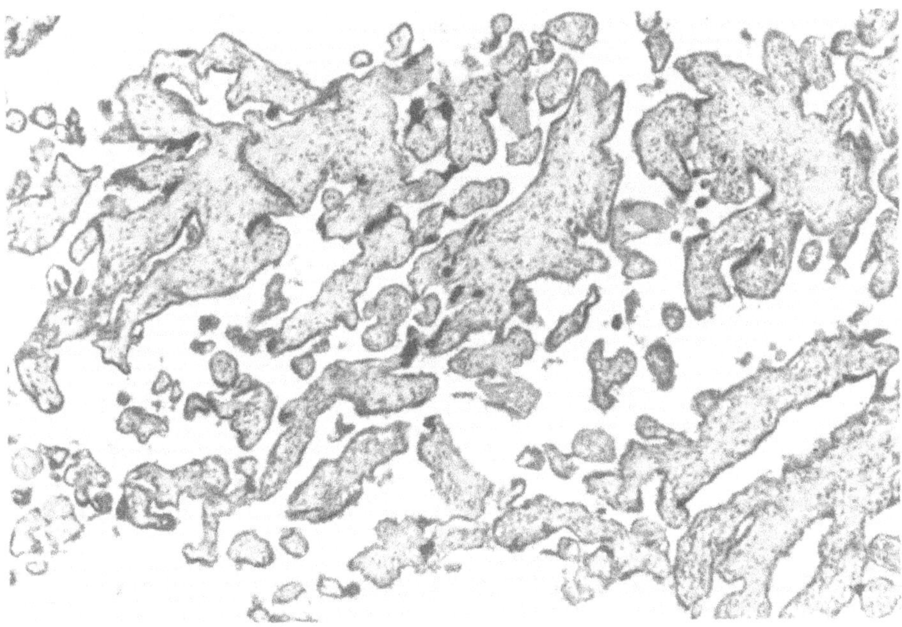

Fig. 23. Stillborn infant (autopsy no. 161/75), 8th month, cervical insufficiency in early pregnancy. A 25-year-old dipara, first pregnancy ended by abortion. At present EPH gestosis. Discordant retardation. (H & E, x 95)

References

Altshuler, G., Ermocilla, R., Russel, P.: The placental pathology of small for gestational age infants. Am. J. Obstet. Gynecol. *121*, 351–359 (1975)

Becker, V.: Über Maturitas praecox placentae. Verh. Dtsch. Ges. Pathol. *44*, 256–260 (1960)

Becker, V.: Plazentare Ursachen von Früh- und Totgeburten. Dtsch. Med. Wschr. *90*, 1060–1062 (1961)

Becker, V.: Funktionelle Morphologie der Plazenta. Arch. Gynaekol. *198*, 3–28 (1962)

Becker, V.: Funktionelle Morphologie der Plazenta. Verh. Dtsch. Ges. Gynaekol. *34*, 3–28 (1963)

Becker, V.: Die Plazenta bei der Geburt. Fortschr. Med. *87*, 132–134 (1969)

Becker, V.: Die Chronopathologie der Plazenta. Dtsch. Med. Wschr. *96*, 1845–1849 (1971)

Becker, V.: Pathologisch-anatomische Aspekte zur Plazentainsuffizienz. Z. Geburtshilfe Perinatol. *176*, 349–355 (1972)

Becker, V.: Neue Erkenntnisse über die Orthologie und Pathologie der Plazenta. Beiheft Z. Geburtshilfe Perinatol. *8*, 26–44 (1977)

Becker, V., Bleyl, U.: Plazentarzotte bei Schwangerschaftstoxikose und fetaler Erythroblastose im fluoreszenzmikroskopischen Bilde. Virchows Arch.[Pathol. Anat.] *334*, 516–527 (1961)

Becker, V., Dolling, D.: Gefäßverschlüsse in der Plazenta von Totgeborenen. Virchows Arch. [Pathol. Anat.] *338*, 305–314 (1965)

Bender, H.G., Werner, Ch.: Zur Endangiitis obliterans der Plazenta-Gefäße. Verh. Dtsch. Ges. Pathol. *58*, 499 (1974)

Benirschke, K., Driscoll, S.G.: The pathology of the human placenta. In: Handb. spez. path. Anat. Histol. Bd. VII/5 Placenta. Uehlinger, E. (ed.), pp. 96–568. Berlin, Heidelberg, New York: Springer 1967

Boyd, J.D., Hamilton, W.J.: The human placenta. Cambridge: Hefter & Sous 1970

Carter, J.E., Vellios, F., Huber, C.P.: Histologic classification and incidence of circulatory lesions of the human placenta, with review of the literature. Am J. Clin. Pathol. *40*, 375–378 (1963)

Dollmann, A.: The small-for-date infant and its placenta: a clinical-pathological study. In: Perinatal medicine. Bern: Huber 1973

Döring, W., Kloos, K.: Morphologische Routinediagnostik der Plazenta. Münch. Med. Wschr. *106*, 1849–1855 (1964)

Emmrich, P., Gödel, E.: Morphologie der Placenta bei mütterlichem Diabetes mellitus. Zentralbl. Allg. Pathol. *116*, 56–63 (1972)

Emmrich, P., Müller, G.: Größe der Chorionzotten in der Plazenta bei mütterlichem Diabetes mellitus. Zentralbl. Allg. Pathol. *118*, 504–509 (1974)

Flenker, H.: Orthologie und Pathologie der menschlichen Plazenta. 2. Pathologie der Plazenta. Fortschr. Med. *92*, 381–386 (1974)

Fox, H.: White infarcts of the placenta. J. Obstet. Gynecol. Br. Cwlth. *70*, 980–991 (1963)

Frank, G.: Histologische Befunde bei Gestoseplacenten. Verh. Dtsch. Ges. Pathol. *51*, 381–385 (1967)

Franke, H., Gerl, D., Stössner, I.: Die Feinstruktur der Chorionzotten bei Spätgestose unterschiedlicher Schweregrade. Z. Geburtshilfe Gynaekol. *175*, 226–244 (1971)

Gruenwald, P.: Examination of the placenta by the pathologist. Arch. Pathol. *77*, 41–46 (1964)

v. Harnack, G.A., v. Bermuth, H.: Mehrdimensionale Reifediagnostik bei untergewichtigen Neugeborenen. Mschr. Kinderheilkd. *119*, 23–26 (1971)

Hibbard, B.M., Jeffcoate, T.N.A.: Abruptio placentae. J. Obstet. Gynecol. *27*, 155–167 (1966)

Hörmann, G.: Zur Systematik einer Pathologie der menschlichen Plazenta. Arch. Gynaekol. *191*, 297–344 (1958)

Kaufmann, P.: Die Entwicklung der menschlichen Plazenta. Geburtshilfe Frauenheilkd. *175*, 263–277 (1971)

Kloos, K., Vogel, M.: Placentationsstörungen. Histologische Untersuchungen über Placentareifeströungen am Routinematerial. Virchows Arch. [Pathol. Anat.] *343*, 245–257 (1968)

Kloos, K., Vogel, M.: Pathologie der Perinatalperiode. Stuttgart: Thieme 1974

Kubli, F.: Die chronische Plazentainsuffizienz. Gynaekologe *1*, 53–60 (1968)

Moll, W., Künzel, W.: Deter uteroplazentare Kreislauf. Z. Geburtshilfe Perinatol. *178*, 1–18 (1974)

Ohlendorf, B.: Zur Systematik der Plazentationsstörungen. Diss. Münster 1977

Peceny, J.: Die Plazenta bei Totgeborenen. Zentralbl. Allg. Pathol. *115*, 600–606 (1972)

Reichwein, D., Vogel, M.: Formen und Häufigkeit maternoplazentarer Durchblutungsstörungen bei Neugeborenen unterschiedlicher Gewichts- und Reifeklassen. Z. Geburtshilfe Perinatol. *176*, 364–378 (1972)

Rosso, P., Winick, M.: Intrauterine growth retardation. A new systematic approach based on clinical and biological characteristics of this condition. J. Perinat. Med. *2*, 147–160 (1974)

Scott, J.M., Jordan, J.M.: Placental insufficiency and the small-for-date baby. Am. J. Obstet. Gynecol. *113*, 823–832 (1972)

Scott, J.M., Usher, R.: Fetal malnutrition: its incidence, causes and effects. Am. J. Obstet. Gynecol. *94*, 951–963 (1966)

Schuhmann, R.: Hypotrophes reifes Kind an Termin aus placentarer Ursache (sog. placentarer Zwerg). Beitr. pathol. Anat. *138*, 426–435 (1969)

Schuhmann, R., Borst, R., Geier, G., Kraus, H.: Über die Plazentone der reifen menschlichen Plazenta. In: Neue Erkenntnisse über die Orthologie und Pathologie der Plazenta. Beiheft Z. Geburtshilfe Perinatol. *8*, 13–25 (1977)

Schuhmann, R.: Wehler, V.: Histologische Unterschiede an Plazentazotten innerhalb der materno-fetalen Strömungseinheit. Arch. Gynaekol. *210*, 425–439 (1971)

Schiebler, T.H.: Zur funktionellen Morphologie der reifen menschlichen Plazenta. In: Neue Erkenntnisse über die Orthologie und Pathologie der Plazenta. Beiheft Z. Geburtshilfe Perinatol. *8*, 1–12 (1977)

Strauss, F.: Die normale Anatomie der menschlichen Plazenta. In: Handb. der spez. pathol. Anat. Histol., Bd. VII/5 Placenta. Uehlinger, E. (ed.), pp. 1–96. Berlin, Heidelberg, New York: Springer 1967

Thomas, J.: Die gestörte Vaskularisation der menschlichen Plazenta und ihre Auswirkungen auf die Frucht. Geburtshilfe Frauenheilkd. *19*, 801–811 (1959)

Vogel, M.: Plakopathia diabetica. Entwicklungsstörungen der Placenta bei Diabetes mellitus der Mutter. Virchows Arch. [Pathol. Anat.] *343*, 51–63 (1967)

Vogel, M.: Epikritische und prognostische Plazentadiagnostik. Münch. Med. Wschr. *110*, 1182–1187 (1968)

Vogel, M.: Morphologische Plazentabefunde bei fetaler Hypo- und Hypertrophie. In: Neue Erkenntnisse über die Orthologie und Pathologie der Plazenta. Beiheft Z. Geburtshilfe Perinatol. *8*, 45–52 (1977)

Wallenburg, H.C.S., Hutchinson, D.L., Schuler, H.M., Stolte, L.A., Janssens, J.: The pathogenesis of placental infarction. II. An experimental study in the rhesus monkey placenta. Am. J. Obstet. Gynecol. *116*, 841–846 (1973)

Interactions Between Maternal and Fetal/Neonatal Lymphocytes*

LARS B. OLDING

I. Introduction 83
II. Immunologic Basis for Maternal and Fetal/Neonatal Cell Interactions . . 84

   1. Immunocompetence of the Pregnant Individual 84
   2. Immunocompetence of the Fetus 86
   3. Permeability of the Placental Barrier to Leukocytes 88

III. Interactions Between Human Maternal and Cord Blood Lymphocytes . . . 89

   1. Lymphocytes from Newborn Abrogate the Proliferation of Lympho-
      cytes from Mothers and Other Adults 89
   2. Only Newborns' Lymphocytes with an Intact DNA Synthesis Suppress
      Mitosis 91
   3. Lymphocytes from Newborns Do Not Kill Maternal Lymphocytes . . . 91
   4. Nonlymphoid Fetal Cells Are Not Able to Suppress the Proliferation of
      Maternal Lymphocytes 93
   5. Suppressor T Lymphocytes Are Present in the Newborn Baby 94
   6. Evidence that the Abrogation of Maternal Lymphocyte Proliferation is
      Mediated by a Soluble Small-Molecular-Weight suppressive Substance(s)
      Released by Activated Lymphocytes from Newborns 94

IV. Conclusions 97

References 99

I. Introduction

One of the most fascinating and challenging phenomena in immunology is the successful grafting of the fetus onto the uterus and the maintenance of fetus and placenta
throughout gestation. The fetus inherits genetic material from its father and, accordingly, should be recognized as alien, "non-self," by the mother's immunocompetent
cells and subsequently rejected. Obviously, rejection does not occur in the vast majority of pregnancies. Still, we have learned from several investigations that maternal
immunocompetent cells are able to react against fetal antigens both in vitro and in

* The research was supported by grants from the National Foundation March of Dimes,
No. 1–364, the Swedish Cancer Society, Expressen's Prenatal Research Fund (Stockholm),
Magnus Bergvall's Foundation (Stockholm), and U.S. Public Health Service grant AI-07007.
This is publication number 1331 from the Department of Immunopathology, Scripps
Clinic and Research Foundation, La Jolla, California 92037.

vivo (reviewed by *Beer* and *Billingham,* 1971; *Edwards* et al., 1975). It also seems as if disparity between maternal and fetal histocompatibility antigens favor, to some extent, the invasiveness of the trophoblast and the size of the placenta (*James,* 1965; *Billington,* 1965; *Beer* and *Billingham,* 1971). Even though factors regulating the successful outcome of the pregnancy are still unknown in many ways, the advancements in immunology and endocrinology during the last decade have enabled us to discern some of the events that occur in the complicated interplay between mother and fetus.

Attention has been paid to such factors as the modulation of the maternal immune reactions by gestational hormones, and the expression of alloantigens on the surface of the trophoblast (the "frontier" cell involved in implantation of the fertilized ovum). Changes in the composition of immunocompetent cells in the maternal blood during pregnancy have been recognized. The experiments by *Hellström* et al. (1969), which suggested that a factor in the serum of pregnant mice (presumably antifetal antibody) could block the cell-mediated killing of fetal tissue cells by maternal lymphoid cells in vitro (and thereby promote a state of immunologic enhancement) have sparked large efforts to find similar immunosuppressive soluble substances in the human maternal serum or plasma. The main emphasis has focused on alloantibodies to paternal antigens, immune complexes, and substances specifically related to pregnancy and the fetus, like α-fetoprotein and "pregnancy-zone protein." It is beyond the scope of this paper to review these investigations inasmuch as they have already been comprehensively reviewed (*Beer* and *Billingham,* 1971; Ciba Found. Symp., 1972; *Edwards* et al., 1975).

This communication will focus on *one* aspect of the immunologic interplay between mother and fetus, namely, interactions between maternal and fetal lymphoid cells.

This paper will describe in detail recently published investigations of the author and his colleagues (*Olding* and *Oldstone,* 1974, 1976; *Olding* et al., 1974, 1977) as well as current ongoing work. Comparison of these findings with investigations reported by other workers will be made. The first part of this review will provide background data related to these investigations, including (1) immunocompetence of pregnant women, (2) antigenicity of the early embryo and immunocompetence of the fetus, and (3) permeability of the placenta for lymphoid cells.

II. Immunologic Basis for Maternal and Fetal/Neonatal Cell Interactions

1. Immunocompetence of the Pregnant Individual

During recent years, several reports about the physiologic state of lymphoid cells during pregnancy have been published. They have been comprehensively reviewed by *Howe* (1975). Recent experiments indicate that the T and B-cell compartments of lymphocytes in the peripheral blood and lymphoid organs of animals shift during pregnancy. Thus, *Howe* (1975) showed that during pregnancy, T cells decrease in the peripheral blood of mice and B cells increase correspondingly. Further, an increased number of lymphocytes are trapped in lymph nodes, especially those draining the uterus. *Howe's* investigation suggested that soluble substances in the fetal tissues, presumably alloantibodies directed against paternal antigens, increased the homing of T lymphocytes toward the lymph nodes. It is at present unclear whether similar mechanisms operate in man. Recently it was found that there is a relative decrease of T cells in the blood of pregnant women in the first but not in the last trimester of pregnancy (*Strelkauskas* et al., 1975)

Investigations of the influence of hormones on the immune response during pregnancy have been reviewed by *Edwards* et al. (1975), and will not be discussed further in this paper. It might be mentioned, however, that investigators generally agree that human placental lactogen (HPL) and human chorionic gonadotrophin (HCG) are able to suppress mixed lymphocyte reactions (MLR) (*Contractor* and *Davies*, 1973).

The reactivity of lymphocytes from pregnant women has been investigated extensively. The use of mitogens such as phytohemagglutinin (PHA) to stimulate them has given divergent results: PHA was reported to depress (*Purtilo* et al., 1972), and to have no effect (*Harrison*, 1972) on the activity of lymphocytes from pregnant as compared with nonpregnant women. Enhanced reactivity to PHA has also been reported (*Carr* and *Stites*, 1972).

Specific, cell-mediated immunity against neonatal (fetal) lymphocytes by maternal lymphocytes has also been tested by several workers. Thus, MLR, which is generally believed to be the in vitro correlate of the recognition phase of the cellular immune response to allografts in vivo, has been used to test the specific maternal reactivity to paternal antigens on the surface of fetal lymphocytes. Using the one-way MLR, *Ceppelini* et al. (1971) found that lymphocytes from mothers and their newborn babies displayed decreased mutual reactivity. However, whereas the mother's lymphocytes also showed a decreased reactivity toward lymphocytes from the father and from unrelated adults, the reactivity of the baby's lymphocytes toward lymphocytes of the father and unrelated adults did not differ significantly from that between unrelated nonpregnant adults. In contrast, *Carr* et al. (1974), who studied the kinetics of the MLR between maternal and neonatal lymphocytes in man, found no reduction in the reactivity of the mother's lymphocytes against those of her baby.

After *Hellström* et al. (1969) found an immunosuppressive factor in sera from pregnant mice, investigations turned toward finding a similar substance in the plasma or serum of pregnant women. These experiments studying the MLR between unrelated adult lymphocytes have revealed that such substances – presumably alloantibodies to paternal antigens on fetal cells – which are able to block MLR (*Leventhal* et al., 1970; *Kasakura*, 1971; *Revillard* et al., 1973; *Robert* et al., 1973; and others) exist.

In addition, deposits of immunoglobulin, mainly IgG, have been detected on the trophoblastic basement membrane of the placenta (*McCormick* et al., 1971). Eluates of the IgG in the trophoblast basement membrane suppress the in vitro reaction of unrelated lymphocytes to tuberculin and PHA and to alien lymphocytes in MLR, according to an investigation by *Faulk* et al. (1974). These investigators suggested that these placental immunoglobulin deposits represented maternal blocking antibody to a trophoblast antigen, which has not yet been characterized. The IgG in the trophoblast basement membrane may originate from circulating antigen-antibody complexes (immune complexes) regularly found in the serum of pregnant women (*Masson* et al., 1977). It is tempting to speculate that such immune complexes block the cell-mediated immunity by the pregnant woman against her fetus, as has been suggested by experiments by *Tamerius* et al. (1975).

The ability of human maternal lymphocytes to produce cell-mediated (antibody-independent) lympholysis of fetal cells has been tested in vitro by cytotoxicity assays using ^{51}Cr-labeled target cells. Apparently maternal lymphoid cells do not induce spontaneous cytotoxicity (*Bonnard* and *Lemos*, 1972; *Olding* et al., 1974). Even after attempts to amplify the sensitivity of the cytotoxicity assay, by maximal prestimulation of the effector (killer) cells against the target cells in MLR and by sensitization of the target cells by pretreatment with PHA, cell-mediated lysis of the neonatal lymphocytes occurred only occasionally (*Bonnard* and *Lemos*, 1972) or never (*Olding* et al., 1974).

So far the importance of killer cells derived from so-called K cells (*Perlmann* et al., 1972), which are dependent on specific antitarget cell antibodies for their cytolytic activity, has not been established in human pregnancy. The same is true for killing by macrophages.

2. Immunocompetence of the Fetus

Interest in the antigenicity and immunogenicity of fetal tissues has been focused primarily on the trophoblast. This is understandable, because this cell invades the endometrium during implantation and is accordingly the first fetal cell to be exposed to maternal immunocompetent cells. In addition, the trophoblast constitutes the ultimate placental barrier between the fetal and maternal circulation throughout pregnancy.

Experiments investigating the expression of major and minor histocompatibility antigens in the pre- and postimplantation trophoblast have recently been reviewed (*Edidin*, 1972; *Johnson,* 1975; *Faulk* et al., 1975) and will not be treated further. It should be mentioned, however, that the evidence indicating that the trophoblast carries transplantation antigens (such as H-2 in mice and HL-A in man) or blood group substances is still uncertain. According to some investigations, the HL-A antigens on cultured human trophoblasts are expressed as early as the 12th week of gestation (*Loke* et al., 1971; *Bodmer*, 1972), although they are less dense on trophoblasts than on fetal skin (*Loke,*, 1975). However, it has been questioned whether the cultures contained trophoblasts exclusively or whether nontrophoblastic cells could have contributed significantly to the amount of detected HL-A antigens (see workshop report referred by *Johnson,* 1974). Moreover, *Faulk* and *Temple* (1977), using immunofluorescent and antibody-peroxidase techniques, were unable to find any evidence of HL-A or β_2 microglobulin (closely associated with HL-A) on the trophoblastic cells covering the chorionic villi of 6- and 13-week, and full term placentas. In contrast, the stromal and endothelial cells inside the villi displayed both HL-A and β_2 microglobulin.

A recent report by *Searle* et al. (1976) merits consideration in this context. They found that in mice, H-2 antigens are present on the preimplantation trophectoderm in the blastocyst but that they disappear during implantation. It is unknown whether a similar mechanism operates in the human blastocyst.

There seems to be general agreement that transplantation antigens are present on nontrophoblastic cells in the early human embryo. Quantitative assays have revealed that HL-A antigens in different human fetal tissues are very similar, relative to weight, to those of corresponding adult tissues (*Pellegrino* et al., 1970).

The question as to whether blood group antigens are present on the human trophoblast is still controversial. Using a modern and sensitive immunoferritin labeling technique, *Loke* and *Ballard* (1973) found a small amount of blood group A substances on the surface of human trophoblasts, while *Goto* et al. (1976), using a similar method, did not.

It has been suggested that HL-A or blood group antigens on the surface of a trophoblast, if present, are masked by mucoproteins rich in sialic acid that are present in the periphery (glycocalyx) of the trophoblast (*Kirby* et al., 1964; *Bradbury* et al., 1965). Removal of these mucoproteins by neuraminidase increases the immunogenicity of the trophoblasts (*Currie* et al., 1968). It was suggested recently that the surface alloantigens of fetal lymphocytes are likewise masked by mucoprotein rich in sialic acid (*Tiilikainen* et al., 1974).

It is far beyond the scope of this paper to discuss all investigations on the ability of the fetus to mount immune responses that have been published. Comprehensive reviews by *Beer* and *Billingham* (1971), by a Ciba Foundation Symposium report (1972), and by *Edwards* et al. (1975) are recommended. In this context it need only be mentioned that human fetal lymphocytes, able to recognize foreign cell antigens in MLR, have been observed in the liver as early as the 10th week of gestation, i.e., before the thymus has developed fully, whereas response to mitogen (PHA) has been found in the 13th week of gestation (*Carr* et al., 1973). MLR-reactive lymphocytes can be found in the thymus as early as the 12th week of gestation (*Hayward* and *Soothill,* 1972). PHA-induced cytotoxicity against xenogeneic target cells (chicken erythrocytes) in vitro has been demonstrated during the 14th week of gestation (*Stites* et al., 1972). However, there seems to be a dichotomy between induced proliferation and cytotoxicity of human fetal lymphoid cells. Thus, whereas PHA can stimulate the proliferation of the fetal thymus cells, the cells are not cytotoxic in vitro. The reverse occurs in fetal bone marrow. On the other hand, lymphocytes in fetal peripheral blood, like those of the adult, are able to both proliferate and exhibit cytotoxicity when stimulated with PHA (*Stites* et al., 1972).

It is well known that the human fetus is able to mount a significant humoral response involving IgM and at least trace amounts of IgD and IgE. This ability has been valuable in detecting congenital infections contracted in utero (*Alford* et al., 1968).

In contrast, most laboratory animals studied show decreased ability to mount humoral responses during the neonatal period. This has been attributed to a normally occurring intrinsic deficiency or to the immaturity of different kinds of leukocytes in the newborn animal. Mice were usually used in these experiments. Newborn mice have functionally mature macrophages (*Fidler* et al., 1972) and B cells that can differentiate to antibody-producing plasma cells after appropriate stimulation (*Spear* and *Edelman,* 1974; *Mosier* et al., 1974). This has been borne out in experiments using T-cell independent (e.g., bacterial) antigens to induce an antibody response. In contrast, the "helper" T function, i.e., the ability of T cells to cooperate with B cells and macrophages in inducing specific antibody responses, does not seem to operate until several weeks after birth (*Spear* and *Edelman,* 1974; *Mosier* et al., 1974). This has been shown in experiments using T-cell dependent antigens like sheep red blood cells. Moreover, a suppressive action that suppresses the antibody response not only in the newborn mice but also in adult animals (*Mosier* and *Johnson,* 1975) seems to be associated with the newborn animal's T lymphocytes.

3. Permeability of the Placental Barrier to Leukocytes

It has become increasingly clear in the last few years that the human placental barrier, i.e., the barrier between the fetal capillaries in the chorionic villi and the maternal circulation in the intervillous space, is to some extent permeable to leukocytes. The literature on this topic has been reviewed by *Benirschke* and *Sullivan* (1968), *Benirschke* (1971), and *Adinolfi* (1975).

Briefly, the transfer of leukocytes both from fetus to mother and from mother to fetus has been tested. It is well documented that fetal leukocytes can travel from the fetal to the maternal circulation, as was convincingly shown by *Walknowska* et al. (1969). They searched for mitogen-stimulated, dividing fetal lymphocytes with a Y chromosome in the blood of pregnant women carrying male fetuses. The peripheral blood of 19 out of 21 pregnant women contained dividing lymphocytes of male sex. The incidence of fetal lymphocytes amounted to 0.14–0.8% (corresponding to 10–20 ml of fetal whole blood). Fetal leukocytes were observed in the maternal circulation as early as the 14th week of gestation. *Schröder* and *de la Chapelle* (1972) found similar results using the interphase fluorescent Y body as an indicator for male fetal lymphocytes in the maternal blood.

The passage of leukocytes from mother to fetus has also been investigated, but with conflicting results. Large-scale investigations of cord blood lymphocytes from male newborns, comprising altogether 231 newborns and 25,880 metaphase cells, revealed only three cells with a 46-XX karyotype, i.e., only 0.01% maternal cells could be induced to divide by mitogen (*Turner* et al., 1966; *Angell* and *Adinolfi,* 1969; *Olding,* 1972; *Adinolfi* and *Gorvette,* 1974). Recent investigations (*Olding* et al., 1974), however, have clearly shown that the presence of lymphocytes from newborn babies prevents maternal lymphocytes from dividing, which means that maternal cells may remain undetected in the cord blood by the chromosome marker technique used. Furthermore, some human perinatal deaths have presumably occurred by graft-versus-host (GvH) reactions caused by spontaneous transplacental passage of maternal lymphocytes into the fetal circulation (*Billingham* and *Silvers,* 1971) or by intrauterine blood transfusions given to fetuses of Rh-sensitized mothers (*Parkman* et al., 1974). *Beer* et al. (1972) and *Beer* and *Billingham* (1973) reproduced these clinical results in a series of elegant experiments on rats. The bone marrow of inbred female rats was destroyed by cyclophosphamide, and then reconstituted with bone marrow graft from F_1 hybrids carrying heterologous paternal antigens. The females thus carrying chimeric bone marrow cells were mated with syngeneic males. More than 50% of the offspring suffered postnatal runt disease, which suggested that chimeric cells from the mother had been transferred across the placenta to the fetus, where they mounted GvH reactions and runt disease.

In summary, human maternal cells interact with fetal lymphoid cells, as is evident from the following observations: (1) No obvious tolerant state seems to exist between mother and fetus, (2) the human fetus is able to express early antigenicity and immunogenicity, (3) the fetal lymphocytes are able to mount humoral responses, and display even in early intrauterine life mature cellular immune reactions in vitro, such as immune recognition in MLR, reactivity to mitogens like PHA, and cytotoxicity against alien cells, (4) leukocytes travel through the placenta, not only from fetus to mother but possibly also in the opposite direction, enabling cell-to-cell contact between maternal and fetal immunocompetent cells.

III. Interactions Between Human Maternal and Cord Blood Lymphocytes

1. Lymphocytes from Newborns Abrogate the Proliferation of Lymphocytes from Mothers and Other Adults

Initially we studied the interactions in vitro between lymphocytes from recently delivered mothers or nonpregnant adult women and lymphocytes from the cord blood of newborn babies (*Olding* et al., 1974; *Olding* and *Oldstone*, 1974). Mononuclear leukocytes from mothers delivered less than 1 h before or from nonpregnant adult women were co-cultured (1:1) with mononuclear leukocytes from the cord blood of newborn babies. The cord blood was sampled immediately after the baby was born but before the placenta was expulsed. The lymphocytes in the blood were enriched by Ficoll-Hypaque gradient centrifugation as described by *Mendelsohn* et al. (1971).

In our first experiments we mixed living cells from newborns and from their mothers. To separate dividing lymphocytes of the baby from those of the mother in co-culture, we used cord blood of male babies and employed the sex chromosomes as markers for the two compartments of cells. The sex chromosomes were visualized by fluorescence after the fixed cells were stained with quinacrine dihydrochloride (*Olding* et al., 1974). The specific fluorescence of the Y chromosome served as a marker for the dividing baby cells (Fig. 1), and the 46-XX cells as markers for the female (maternal) cells. Lymphocytes from mother-and-baby pairs were co-cultured for 5–6 days to allow mutual allogeneic stimulation with blastoid formation and ensuing division, i.e., with two-way MLR. Co-cultures containing PHA were run in parallel for three days and subsequently harvested, because the MLR often did not provide a sufficient number of dividing cells for an adequate chromosome investigation. PHA-P (Difco) was used in a final concentration of 50 μg/ml, which gave a similar mitogenic response both in the babys' and the maternal lymphocytes (*Olding* et al., 1974). In all experiments, RPMI-1640 medium with 20% fetal calf serum, L-glutamine, and antibiotics was used, and the cultures were incubated in 5% CO_2 in air and at 37°C.

The results of these experiments are shown in Table 1. In all experiments in which newborns' lymphocytes were mixed with lymphocytes from either the natural mother

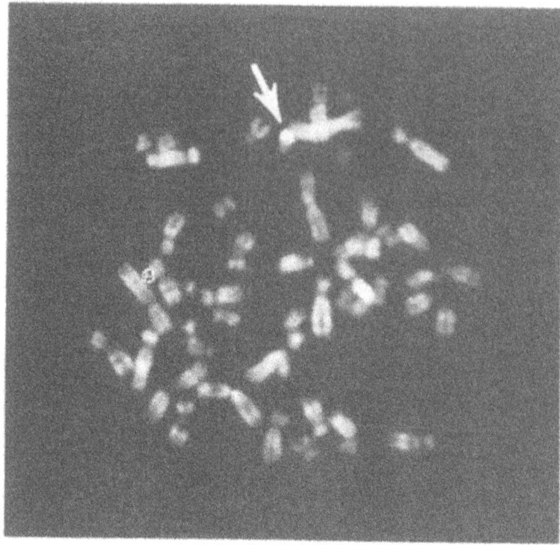

Fig. 1. Metaphase cell of male baby origin in co-culture of maternal and cord blood lymphocytes. The chromosomes are made visible by fluorescent chromosome technique (see text). The typical fluorescent pattern of the Y chromosome is shown in the picture (*arrow*). x 1000

Table 1. Abrogation of mitosis of lymphocytes from mothers and other adults by lymphocytes from newborns [a]

Mixed culture (1:1) Male	female	No. of cases	PHA[b]	% Metaphase cells having a Y chromosome
Newborn +	natural mother	18	+	97 (88−100)
Newborn +	natural mother	6	0	96 (90−100)
Newborn +	alien mother	3	+	91 (90−93)
Newborn +	nonpregnant	1	+	88
Newborn +	nonpregnant	1	0	92
Adult +	nonpregnant	2	+	53 (53−54)
Adult +	nonpregnant	1	0	60

[a] $1-2 \times 10^6$ mononuclear leukocytes from cord blood of newborn infants and from adults were enriched by Ficoll-Hypaque gradient centrifugation and co-cultured in RPMI-1640 medium with 20% fetal calf serum. After 60−72 h, dividing cells were arrested in metaphase by colchicine. Chromosomes were prepared and stained with quinacrine-dihydrochloride and subsequently screened in a fluorescent microscope (*Olding* et al., 1974).

[b] +, 50 μg PHA-P(Difco)/ml of medium; 0, no PHA added

or alien mothers, dividing cells from the baby predominated, amounting to 88%−100%. Dividing baby cells also predominated (88%−92%) in co-cultures comprising lymphocytes from nonpregnant women. In contrast, the distribution of dividing male and female cells was almost the same when lymphocytes from adult males were co-cultured with lymphocytes from adult females. This indicated that the strong predominance of dividing cells from the newborns in co-culture with adult females had nothing to do with the fact that the cells were male and perhaps able to express suppressing activity linked to the Y chromosome. The baby cell mitoses prevailing in the co-cultures depended largely on a suppression of the maternal lymphocytes, and to a much lesser degree, on an enhanced stimulation of the baby cells. Thus, we found on the average a 13-fold suppression of the maternal cells as compared to a twofold stimulation of the newborns' cells (*Olding* and *Oldstone*, 1976). In other experiments we showed that lymphocytes from one baby did not suppress the division of lymphocytes from another baby (*Olding* and *Oldstone*, 1976). An interpretation of this phenomenon might be that newborns' lymphocytes lack the receptor for a substance they release that mediates the suppressive effect.

2. Only Newborns' Lymphocytes with an Intact DNA Synthesis Suppress Mitosis

In recent experiments we tried to determine whether the suppression exerted by newborns' cord blood lymphocytes requires cells actively synthesizing DNA, or whether the suppression can operate merely by means of antigens expressed by the baby's lymphocytes. Lymphocytes from newborns were irradiated and subsequently mixed (1:1) with living maternal lymphocytes in one-way MLR in the presence or absence of mitogen (Table 2). With the chromosome technique, dividing cells from the baby could not be detected in any of the co-cultures.

The maternal lymphoid cells were stimulated to varying degrees, judging from their uptake of ^{3}H-thymidine. Thus, the maternal lymphocytes responded to the alloantigens displayed by the inactivated cord lymphocytes in a manner similar to a regular one-way MLR between alien cells. The details of these investigations have been published elsewhere (*Olding* et al., 1977).

3. Lymphocytes from Newborns Do Not Kill Maternal Lymphocytes

In a separate series of experiments it was shown that the suppression of mitosis in maternal cells by the newborn babies is not linked to any significant killing of the maternal cells. Neither does it seem that maternal lymphocytes kill lymphocytes from the baby. This was deduced from cytotoxicity assays designed as previously reported (*Olding* et al., 1974). Briefly, mononuclear leukocytes derived from the cord blood of newborns and from venous blood of recently delivered mothers were used interchangeably as effector (killer) cells or target cells. The release of ^{51}Cr from labeled target cells exposed to effector cells was compared to the spontaneous release from control cells. Different kinds of sera (fetal calf, autologous maternal or baby, or maternal + baby) were used in different experiments. The ratio of effector to target cells varied between 25:1 and 100:1.

In none of these experiments was there any significant lysis of either maternal or baby lymphocytes judging from their release of ^{51}Cr (*Olding* et al., 1974). In other experiments the sensitivity of the cytotoxicity assay was further amplified by presensitizing the effector cells to the target cells in two-way MLR and by sensitizing the target cells with PHA. The results are shown in Table 3.

Table 2. Inability of irradiated lymphocytes from newborns to suppress mitogen- (PHA) or allogen- (MLR)induced proliferation of mothers' lymphocytes [a]

Case no.	PHA[b]	Culture time (days)	Uptake of ^{3}H-thymidine (c.p.m. x 10^{-3} ± SEM)			Stimulation of mothers' lymphocytes[f]
			Mother [c]	Newborn [d]	Mother + newborn (1:1) [e]	
1	+	3	34.1 ± 3.3	2.5 ± 0.5	30.6 ± 0.8	1.8
2	+	3	48.7 ± 3.6	2.1 ± 0.3	45.4 ± 3.4	1.9
3	+	3	73.8 ± 14.0	3.5 ± 0.5	78.2 ± 10.1	2.1
4	+	3	97.9 ± 11.3	3.5 ± 0.4	92.2 ± 5.5	1.9
5	0	6	1.7 ± 0.4	0.6 ± 0.3	7.9 ± 3.6	9.0
6	0	6	3.5 ± 0.3	0.4 ± 0.01	21.6 ± 1.7	12.2
7	0	6	6.7 ± 1.4	0.1 ± 0.06	25.1 ± 4.3	3.7
8	0	6	1.9 ± 0.1	0.3 ± 0.1	14.9 ± 1.4	14.9
9	0	6	6.7 ± 1.4	0.7 ± 0.3	72.1 ± 7.7	10.7

[a] Enriched mononuclear leukocytes (see footnote, Table 1) from the cord blood of newborn male babies and from vein blood of their mothers were suspended in RPMI-1640 medium with 10% human pooled AB serum, placed in Microtiter plate wells and incubated in 5% CO_2 in air at 37°C 4 h before harvest. The cells in each well were labeled with ^{3}H-thymidine.

[b] +, PHA-P (Difco) 50 μg/ml of medium; 0, no PHA added.

[c] 2 x 10^5 cells (in triplicate).

[d] 2 x 10^5 cells (in triplicate) irradiated with 6000 rad.

[e] 1 x 10^5 maternal cells + 1 x 10^5 irradiated baby cells (in triplicate). No dividing baby cells were found in the co-cultures judging from chromosome assays.

[f] c.p.m. of maternal cells in co-culture/c.p.m. of maternal cells in single cultures.

Table 3. Absence of significant cell-mediated lysis among maternal lymphocytes co-cultured with lymphocytes of newborns[a]

Experiment no.	Effector cells	^{51}Cr-labeled target cells (PHA-sens.)	Ratio effector/ target	Specific ^{51}Cr release (6 h) %[b]
1	Newborn	Mother	100:1	0.5
2	Newborn	Mother	40:1	−5.5
3	Mother	Newborn	40:1	−1.7
4	Newborn + mother	Mother	25:1	1.4
5	Newborn + mother	Mother	25:1	0.2
6	Newborn + mother	Mother	25:1	−2.9
7	Newborn + mother	Newborn	50:1	−1.7
8	Newborn + mother	Newborn	25:1	−2.5

[a] As for enrichment of mononuclear leukocytes, labeling with ^{51}Cr, and measuring of released isotope − see *Olding* et al. (1974). Lymphocytes from pairs of mother and her own baby were used in all experiments. In experiments 4−8 effector lymphocytes were presensitized in vitro against the target cells by co-culture (1:1) for 3 days in RPMI-1640 medium with 20% fetal calf serum and with 50 μg PHA-P/ml of medium before being tested against maternal or newborn target cells. The latter were sensitized with PHA-P for 3 days in culture before being used in the cytotoxicity assay.

[b] Calculations of ^{51}Cr release were based on the following formula [^{51}Cr in culture fluid/total ^{51}Cr in culture (cells + fluid)] x 100. Before calculating the specific release, the spontaneous release in co-cultures of labeled and unlabeled autologous target cells was subtracted from the experimental value.

Not even in these highly sensitive assays were significant numbers of maternal or cord blood lymphocytes killed. Other workers have found similar results, although a significant killing of baby's lymphocytes by maternal lymphocytes has infrequently been reported (*Bonnard* and *Lemos*, 1972). Hence, if killing occurs, it is limited in extent. Our cytotoxicity assays strongly indicate that the predominance of dividing lymphocytes of the newborn co-cultured with maternal lymphocytes was not due to selective killing of maternal cells by the newborn's cells.

4. Nonlymphoid Fetal Cells Are Not Able to Suppress the Proliferation of Maternal Lymphocytes

In another series of experiments, we tried to determine whether the ability of cord blood lymphocytes to abrogate proliferation of maternal lymphocytes was restricted to fetal mononuclear leukocytes or whether other kinds of fetal cells could also exert this effect. Accordingly, fibroblasts derived from different fetal organs such as bone marrow and spleen, as well as amniotic cells from the placenta, were co-cultured with maternal lymphocytes as described (*Olding* and *Oldstone*, 1976). Amniotic cells were collected from full-term placentas, and laboratory cell lines of fibroblasts were used. The maternal lymphocytes were seeded on semiconfluent monolayers of fetal cells, and mitogen was added to stimulate proliferation of the maternal cells. The experiments have so far not shown that fetal cells other than lymphocytes have the ability to abrogate mitosis of maternal mitogen-induced lymphocytes (Table 4). Similarly, there was no indication that a rapidly growing lymphoid cell line can produce the same suppressive effect. This was evident from our experiments using co-cultures of maternal lymphocytes and lymphoblastoid thymus (T) cell lines of male sex (Molt-4, CCRF-HSB-4).

Table 4. Analysis of fetal, newborn, or other human cells that abrogate mitosis of maternal lymphocytes[a]

Cells tested	Inhibition of maternal lymphocytes
Fetal spleen fibroblasts	No
Fetal bone marrow fibroblasts	No
Amnion cells	No[b]
Lymphoblastoid T-cell lines (Molt-4, CCRF-HSB-2)	No
Newborns' T lymphocytes	Yes[b]

[a] For experimental design and details — see *Olding* and *Oldstone* (1976).

[b] Cells sampled from natural mothers.

5. Suppressor T Lymphocytes Are Present in the Newborn Baby

In the next step of our investigation we separated thymus-derived (T) and bone marrow-derived (B) lymphocytes, as well as monocytes from the newborns' cord blood, and tested these compartments of cells separately against maternal lymphocytes (*Olding* and *Oldstone*, 1976). In order to enrich T- and B-cell populations we used different rosetting techniques (E-AET, EAC 1423) followed by separation on a Ficoll-Hypaque gradient. Monocytes were enriched by means of glass adherence. The baby cell populations thus enriched were co-cultured with maternal lymphocytes and stimulated with T- and B-cell mitogens, using the same chromosome assay as in our previous experiments.

A summary of these results, published elsewhere (*Olding* and *Oldstone*, 1976), are shown in Table 5. Whereas enriched T lymphocytes from the newborns' cord blood strongly suppressed the maternal lymphocytes (78%–100%), the newborns' B lymphocytes did not. Neither did monocytes from the cord blood suppress proliferation of the maternal lymphocytes.

6. Evidence That the Abrogation of Maternal Lymphocyte Proliferation is Mediated by a Soluble Small-Molecular-Weight Suppressive Substance(s) Released by Activated Lymphocytes from Newborns

We used the next series of experiments to elucidate whether cell-to-cell contact was necessary for suppression or whether a soluble substance(s) released by the cord blood

Table 5. T-lymphocyte dependence of the mitotic inhibition exerted by lymphocytes from newborn babies[a]

Male newborns' cells	Co-cultured with	No. of cases	Mitogen	% Metaphase cells of baby origin (with a Y chromosome)
T lymphocytes	Maternal (crude) lymphocytes	8	PHA[b]	93 (78–100)
B lymphocytes	Maternal (crude) lymphocytes	4	PWM[c]	34 (15–59)
Monocytes	Maternal (crude) lymphocytes	2	PHA	3 (0–6)

[a] Enriched mononuclear leukocytes (see footnote, Table 1) were separated in T, B, and monocyte cell populations by means of rosetting with E-AET and EAC 1423 cells followed by gradient centrifugation, and by glass adherence (*Olding* and *Oldstone*, 1976). Co-culture (1:1 in RPMI-1640 medium with 20% fetal calf serum). For chromosome preparations – see footnote of Table 1 and *Olding* et al. (1974).

[b] 50 μg (Difco)/ml of medium.

[c] Pokeweed mitogen, PWM, 50 μg/ml of medium

lymphocytes could bring about the same effect. For that purpose we modified the Marbrook-Diener culture system (*Marbrook*, 1967), principally as described by *Feldman* and *Basten (1972)*. Briefly, the outer chamber contained a small glass vial with a bottom diameter of 25 mm. The inner chamber consisted of a glass tube measuring 12 mm in diameter, which was inserted into the outer chamber (vial). The lower opening of the tube was sealed off by a cell-impermeable membrane. We used a Nuclepore (0.4 μ size, General Electric Co.) or a dialysis membrane (Union Carbide Corp.). The baby's lymphocytes rested on the membrane in the inner chamber while lymphocytes from mothers or other adults were placed on the bottom of the vial. Four x 10^6 baby's lymphocytes were suspended in 1 ml of growth medium; 8 x 10^6 maternal cells were suspended in 4 ml of the medium. RPMI-1640 medium supplied with 10% human pooled AB serum, L-glutamine, and antibiotics served as growth medium for both populations of cells. Equal amounts of PHA-P (50 μg/ml) were added to both populations of cells, and the cultures were incubated for 60–72 h in 5% CO_2 in air and at 37°C. Four hours before harvest the lymphocytes in both chambers were checked for viability and subsequently transferred to Microtitre round-bottom wells (1 x 10^5 cells per well) and labeled with [^{3}H]-thymidine. After incubating for 5 more hours, the cells were harvested with a microculture harvesting device on glass fiber filters that were dried, and the radioactivity was subsequently measured by a scintillation spectrometer.

Table 6 shows typical results that emerged from experiments using a dialysis membrane. Similar results were obtained using Nuclepore membranes. A detailed report of the experiments has been published elsewhere (*Olding* et al., 1977). It is obvious that the baby's cord lymphocytes released a soluble substance or substances that significantly suppressed the proliferation of mitogen-stimulated maternal lymphocytes by 40%–

71%. Control experiments using lymphocytes from nonpregnant adult women in the outer chamber and lymphocytes from either unrelated nonpregnant women or from unrelated adult males in the inner chamber did not exhibit suppression.

Table 6. Effect of exposing maternal lymphocytes to dialyzable product(s) released by mitogen-stimulated mononuclear leukocytes from newborns[a]

Case no.	Lymphocytes from	Exposed to dialyzable leukocyte product(s) from	Uptake of ^{3}H-thymidine c.p.m. x 10^{-3} $\pm$ SEM	% Suppression
1	Mother	None	154.8 $\pm$ 7.5	
		Newborn	93.3 $\pm$ 3.3	40
2	Mother	None	156.7 $\pm$ 3.9	
		Newborn	80.1 $\pm$ 2.7	47
3	Mother	None	148.6 $\pm$ 19.1	
		Newborn	42.1 $\pm$ 0.5	71
4	Nonpregnant female	None	95.6 $\pm$ 0.9	
		Unrelated nonpregnant female	115.9 $\pm$ 1.4	0
5	Nonpregnant female	None	126.6 $\pm$ 15.5	0
		Unrelated adult male	152.2 $\pm$ 1.9	0
6	Newborn	None	265.1 $\pm$ 9.4	
		Unrelated newborn	267.2 $\pm$ 4.9	0

[a] 4×10^6 lymphocytes in 1 ml of growth medium (RPMI-1640 with 10% human pooled AB serum and 50 μg PHA-P per ml) in an inner chamber separated from 8×10^6 lymphocytes in 4 ml of growth medium in an outer chamber by a dialysis membrane were incubated for 3 days in 37°C and 5% CO_2. 4 h before harvest the cells were transferred to round-bottom Microtitre wells (1×10^5 cells per well in triplicate) and labeled with 1 μCi ^{3}H-TdR per well. The Table shows some typical results. Other experiments gave similar results.

In addition, our experiments have shown that mitogen-stimulated lymphocytes from one baby do not inhibit the division of lymphocytes from another baby.

These experiments clearly indicate that mitogen-stimulated lymphocytes from the cord blood release a dialyzable small molecule(s) able to suppress the proliferation of adult mitogen-induced lymphocytes. Because this substance can pass through a dialysis membrane, one can estimate that the molecular weight is less than 20,000.

Investigations designed to identify this substance(s) and its physical properties are in progress in our laboratory.

IV. Conclusions

Our observation that lymphocytes from human newborns are able to abrogate the proliferation of lymphocytes from the natural mother, from alien mothers, and even from unrelated nonpregnant women has not been reported previously. However, investigations using animal models have indicated that the newborn offers an adverse environment for inducing immune responses. For example, *Dixon* and *Weigle* (1956, 1959) found that antigen-primed lymph node cells combined with specific antigen (bovine serum albumin) adoptively transferred from adult rabbits into newborn homologous rabbits induced no antibody responses. (The same was true for a bacterial antigen derived from *Shigella paradysenteriae*, provided that the adult donors were exposed to the antigen less than three days before the cell transfer.) In contrast, the same procedure induced a significant response in X-irradiated adult recipients. In retrospect, these experiments tally with the concept that immunosuppressive cells and/or immunosuppressive substance(s) are present in the newborn.

Our experiments clearly indicate that the mitogenic suppression exerted by lymphocytes from human newborns is a selective function of suppressor T lymphocytes. The term "suppressor" is used here in a broad sense, and encompasses the capacity of T cells to suppress not only an immune response mounted by B cells but also the functions of another T cell population, such as proliferation (*Gershon* et al., 1974; *Folch* and *Waksman,* 1974; *Rich* and *Rich,* 1975; *Wallis* et al., 1976) or cytotoxicity toward allogeneic cells (*Peavy* and *Pierce,* 1974).

Our observation that the healthy human newborn harbors suppressor T cells has recently been confirmed by other authors using a similar fluorescent chromosome technique in co-cultures of maternal and newborns' lymphocytes (*Gille* et al., 1977). In addition, direct evidence for such cells in newborn animals has only recently been presented. For example, T cells from newborn mice able to inhibit antibody responses (*Mosier* and *Johnson,* 1975) or cellular immune reactions in MLR (*Wallis* et al., 1976) have been reported.

It has not yet been demonstrated that the mitogenic suppression exhibited by human baby T cells in vitro also operates in vivo, which seems to be true for mice (*Skowron-Cenrzak* and *Ptak,* 1976). The investigators showed that in F_1 hybride mice, local GvH reactions elicited by parental spleen lymphocytes were abrogated by lymphoid cells from mouse fetuses or newborns but not from adult animals. The investigation also revealed that the suppressor T lymphocytes were responsible for the abrogation.

Although suppressor T cells in healthy human newborns have not been previously reported, such cells have been implicated in human immunodeficiencies. The work was pioneered by *Waldmann* et al. (1974), who showed that suppressor T cells, which abrogate the Ig synthesis of normal human B lymphocytes, can cause common variable hypogammaglobulinemia. Subsequently, *Siegal* et al. (1976) found that leukocytes from hypogammaglobulinemic patients were able to suppress the differentiation of B cells from unrelated normal individuals. *Stobo* et al. (1976) found evidence for suppressor T cell function in patients with fungal infections. Recently, suppressor cell activity, along with dysfunction of T and B lymphocytes, was found in a three-month-old infant who suffered from malabsorption and recurrent infections (*Hansson* et al.,

1976). One may speculate that the immunosuppressive activity was caused by suppressor T-cell activity remaining from the neonatal period.

The literature on suppressor T cells has expanded rapidly in the last few years, after *Gershon* and *Kondo* (1970) first suggested that T cells were linked to the specific suppression of an immune response. Since comprehensive reviews on suppressor T cells have recently been published (*Möller,* 1975), this matter will not be reviewed in detail here. It might be mentioned, however, that investigators generally agree that suppressive activity can be provoked specifically by antigens (*Feldmann,* 1974; and others) or nonspecifically by T-cell mitogens like con A and PHA (*Dutton,* 1975), or by allogeneic cells (*Gershon* et al., 1972). The exact mechanisms by which the suppression is induced remains controversial. Several authors have focused their attention on suppressive molecular substances released by T suppressor cells (*Tada* et al., 1975). Others think that the suppressor activity might be associated with subclasses of T cells that may emerge during maturation, from immature precursor (T_1) cells to antigen-primed differentiated (T_2) cells (*Mosier* and *Cantor,* 1971).

The concept that suppression and stimulation are linked to different subclasses of T cells has gained further support in elegant experiments carried out on mice by *Cantor* and *Boyse* (1975a, b), *Jandinski* et al. (1976) and *Cantor* et al. (1976). Briefly, they used ongeneic lines of C57B1/6(B6) mice that differed with respect to the alleles present in the so-called Ly gene locus. They could separate classes of T cells by the surface antigens controlled by this locus (Ly 1, Ly 2, and Ly 3 antigens). About 50% of the Ly-positive T cells had both Ly 1, 2, and 3 antigens, whereas 33% had only Ly 1 and 5—10% Ly 2 and 3 antigens. Furthermore, the subclass bearing Ly 123 antigens appeared early in neonatal life, while the Ly 1 and Ly 23 subclasses developed later. The different T-cell clones could be isolated by treating the cells with antisera specific to the.Ly antigens, together with complement. The functions of both populations could therefore be studied separately. It was shown that Ly 1 T cells exhibit helper but not killer activity, while Ly 2, 3 T cells display both suppressor and cytotoxic activity. It is likely that similar subclasses of T cells with different functions also operate in man. Such subclasses carrying receptors for different immunologlobulins have been described by *Moretta* et al. (1976, 1977), and recently *Oldstone* et al. (1977) found evidence that the suppressor T-cell activity in the human newborn is restricted to lymphocytes carrying Fc receptors for IgG. This observation raises the interesting question whether the fetal suppressor T cells are triggered by immune complexes regularily found in human pregnancies (*Masson* et al., 1977)

Our data suggest that the mitogenic suppression of maternal and other adult lymphocytes are caused by a small dialyzable molecule (or molecules) released by stimulated lymphocytes from newborns (and presumably also from fetuses).

So far, the substance(s) seems to be specific for the lymphocytes of newborns: PHA-stimulated lymphocytes from adults did not suppress proliferation of lymphocytes from other adults. This bbservation rules out suppression by immunosuppressive, nondialyzable substances like immunoglobulins, α-fetoprotein (*Murgita* and *Tomasi,* 1975a, b; *Dattwyler* et al., 1975), and "pregnancy-zone protein" (*Stigbrand* et al., 1976). However, because this work is in its infancy, it is likely that other suppressive substances, dialyzable and nondialyzable, will be found. Of interest in this context is a recent report by *Murgita* et al. (1977) that suppressor T cells can be induced in spleen cells of mice by α-fetoprotein.

T lymphocytes and the small suppressive molecules they produce might exert their immunosuppressive effects in different ways. Thus, fetal lymphocytes might modulate the maternal cellular immune response locally, against the (fetal) trophoblasts on the chorionic villi of the placenta. This effect might be exerted either by fetal lymphocytes that travel through the barrier, or by the release of suppressive soluble substance(s) by fetal lymphocytes circulating in the capillaries in the chorionic villi. In the latter case, the substance(s) might diffuse through the thin barrier separating the fetal capillaries and the maternal blood in the intervillous space of the placenta. This barrier is only 2–5 microns thick (*Aherne* et al., 1966). Such a mechanism might help protect the (fetal) trophoblast layer in the placenta against immune rejection by maternal lymphocytes. It is also conceivable that maternal lymphocytes, which are eventually transferred through the placental barrier, might be effectively prohibited from mounting any immune responses in the fetus.

Finally, one may speculate that the described mitogenic inhibition by baby lymphocytes may help protect the fetus against latent or "dormant" viruses living in maternal leukocytes that are transferred across the placenta to the fetus. Viruses belonging to the herpesvirus group are especially able to remain in the host cells in a latent state after the primary infection, but can be re-activated and eventually produce disease under certain conditions. Such conditions include, for example, pregnancy, organ transplantation, massive blood transfusions, and malignancy (reviewed by *Weller*, 1971a, b). Allogeneic reactions between leukocytes carrying the latent virus and allogeneic recipient cells might be an important factor in reactivating the virus during these situations. In experiments using mouse models, it has recently been shown that allogeneic reaction with ensuing lymphoblast formation and mitosis is important for virus activation (*Hirsch*, et al., 1972, 1973; *Olding* et al., 1975). It is feasible that fetal lymphocytes might prevent activation of viruses in the placenta by suppressing mitosis of maternal leukocytes carrying viruses in a latent stage.

Acknowledgments: The author thanks Drs. Michael B.A. Oldstone, Kurt Benirschke, and Hans Wigzell for reviewing the manuscript; Agnetha Olofsson for her technical laboratory assistance; Maureen Shumate for editorial assistance; and Sally Hendrix for typing the manuscript.

References

Adinolfi, M., Gorvette, D.P.: The transfer of lymphocytes through the human placenta. In: Proceedings. 1st Int. Congr. Immunol. in Obstetrics and Gynaecology (Padua). Amsterdam: Excerpta Med. Intern. Congress Series No. 327, pp. 177–182, 1974

Adinolfi, M.: The human placenta as a filter for cells and plasma proteins. In: Immunobiology of trophoblast. Edwards, R.G., Howe, C.W., Johnson, M.H. (eds.). Cambridge: Cambridge University Press 1975

Aherne, W., Dunnill, M.S.: Morphometry of the human placenta. Br. Med. Bull. *22*, 5–8 (1966)

Alford, C.A., Blankenship, W.J., Straumfjord, J.V., Cassady, G.: In: Intrauterine infections. Bergsma, D. (ed.), pp. 5–19. New York: National Foundation 1968

Angell, L., Adinolfi, M.: cited by: Adinolfi, M., Wood, C.: Ontogenesis of immuno-globulins and components of complements in man. In: Immunology and development. Adinolfi, M. (ed.), pp. 27–32. London: Spastic Int. Med. Publ. 1969

Beer, A.E., Billingham, R.E.: Immunobiology of mammalian reproduction. In: Advances in Immunology. Dixon, F.J., Kunkel, H.G. (eds.). New York, London: Academic Press 1971

Beer, A.E., Billingham, R.E., Yang, S.L.: Maternal induced transplantation, immunity, tolerance and runt disease in rats. J. Exp. Med. *135*, 808–826 (1972)

Beer, A.E., Billingham, R.-E.: Maternally acquired runt disease. Science *179*, 240–243 (1973)

Benirschke, K., Sullivan, M.M.: The human placenta in relationship to the development of chimerism. In: The foeto-placental unit. Proceedings of an Internation Symposium. Milan: Excerpta Med. Int. Congr. Series No. 183, pp. 37–44, 1968

Benirschke, K.: Chimerism, mosaicism and hybrids. In: Human Genetics. Proceedings Fourth International Congress Human Genetics (Paris), pp. 212–231. Amsterdam: Excerpta Med. Found. 1971

Billingham, R., Silvers, W.: The Immunobiology of Tissue Transplantation. New Jersey: Prentice-Hall Englewood Cliffs 1971

Billington, W.D.: The invasiveness of transplanted mouse trophoblast and the influence of immunological factors. J. Reprod. Fert. *10*, 343–352 (1965)

Bodmer, W.F.: Evolutionary significance of the HL-A system. Nature *237*, 139–140 (1972)

Bonnard, G.D., Lemos, L.: The cellular immunity of mother versus child at delivery: sensitization in unidirectional mixed lymphocyte culture and subsequent ^{51}Cr-release cytotoxicity test. Transplant. Proc. *4*, 177–179 (1972)

Bradbury, S., Billington, W.D., Kirby, D.R.S.: A histochemical and electron micro-scopical study of the fibrinoid of the mouse placenta. J. R. Microsc. Soc. *84*, 199–206 (1965)

Cantor, H., Boyse, E.A.: Functional subclasses of T lymphocytes bearing different Ly antigens. I. The generation of functionally distinct T-cell subclasses is a differentiative process independent of antigen. J. Exp. Med. *141*, 1376–1389 (1975a)

Cantor, H., Boyse, E.A.: Functional subclasses of T lymphocytes bearing different Ly antigens. II. Cooperation between subclasses of Ly$^+$ cells in the generation of killer activity. J. Exp. Med. *143*, 1390–1399 (1975b)

Cantor, H., Shen, F.W., Boyse, E.A.: Separation of helper T cells from suppressor T cells expressing different Ly components. II. Activation by antigen: after immunization antigen-specific suppressor and helper activities are mediated by distinct T-cell subclasses. J. Exp. Med. *143*, 1391–1401 (1976)

Carr, M.C., Stites, D.P.: Reactivity of maternal lymphocytes to phytohaemagglutinin. Lancet *1972 I*, 1073

Carr, M.C., Stites, D.P., Fudenberg, H.H.: Dissociation of responses to phytohemagglutinine and adult allogeneic lymphocytes in human foetal lymphoid tissues. Nature New Biol. *241*, 279–281 (1973)

Carr, M.C., Stites, D.P., Fudenberg, H.H.: Cellular immune aspects of the human fetal-maternal relationship. III. Mixed lymphocyte reactivity between related maternal and cord blood lymphocytes. Cell. Immunol. *11*, 332–341 (1974)

Ceppellini, R., Bonnard, G.D., Coppo, F., Miggiano, V.C.: Mixed leukocyte cultures and HL-A antigens. I. Reactivity of young fetuses, newborns, and mothers at delivery. Transplant. Proc. *3*, 58–70 (1971)

Ciba Foundation Symposium: Ontogeny of acquired immunity. Amsterdam, London, New York: Elsevier-Excerpta Medica-North-Holland Associated Scientific Publishers 1972

Contractor, S.F., Davies, H.: Effect of human chorionic somatomammotrophin and HCG on phytohemagglutinin-induced lymphocyte transformation. Nature New Biol. *243*, 284–286 (1973)

Currie, G., Van Doorninck, W., Bagshawe, K.: Effect of neuroaminidase on the immunogenicity of early mouse trophoblast. Nature *219*, 191–192 (1968)

Dattwyler, R.J., Murgita, R.A., Tomasi, T.B.: The binding of alpha-feto-protein to murine T cells. Nature *256*, 656–657 (1975)

Dixon, F.J., Weigle, W.O.: The nature of the immunologic inadequacy of neonatal rabbits as revealed by cell transfer studies. J. Exp. Med. *105*, 75–83 (1956)

Dixon, F.J., Weigle, O.: The nature of the immunologic inadequacy of neonatal rabbits. II. Antibody formation by neonatal splenic cells transferred to adult recipients. J. Exp. Med. *110*, 139–146 (1959)

Dutton, R.: Suppressor T cells. Transplant. Rev. *26*, 39–55 (1975)

Edidin, M.: Histocompatibility genes, transplantation antigens, and pregnancy. In: Transplantation Antigens, Markers of Biological Individuality. Kahan, B.D., Reisfeld, R.A. (eds.). New York: Academic Press 1972

Edwards, R.G., Howe, C.W.S., Johnson, M.H. (eds.): Immunobiology of Trophoblast. Cambridge: Cambridge University Press 1975

Faulk, P.W., Jeannet, M., Creighton, W.D., Carbonara, A.: Immunological studies of the human placenta. Characterization of immunoglobulins on the trophoblastic basement membranes. J. Clin. Invest. *54*, 1011–1019 (1974)

Faulk, W.P., Trenchew, P., Dorling, J., Holborow, J.: Antigens on postimplantation placentae. In: Immunobiology of Trophoblast. Edwards, R.G., Howe, C.W.S., Johnson, M.H. (eds.). Cambridge: Cambridge University Press 1975

Faulk, W.P., Temple, A.: Distribution of β_2 microglobulin in HLA in chorionic villi of human placentae. Nature *262*, 799–802 (1977)

Feldmann, M.: T cell suppression in vitro. II. Nature of specific suppressive factor. Eur. J. Immunol. *4*, 660–666 (1974)

Feldmann, M., Basten, A.: Cell interaction in the immune response in vitro. III. Specific collaboration across a cell impermeable membrane. J. Exp. Med. *136*, 49–62 (1972)

Fidler, J.M., Chiscon, M.O., Golub, E.S.: Functional development of the interacting cells in the immune response. II. Development of immunocompetence to heterologous erythrocytes in vitro. J. Immunol. *109*, 136–140 (1972)

Folch, H., Waksman, B.H.: The splenic suppressor cell. II. Suppression of the mixed lymphocyte reaction by thymus dependent adherent cells. J. Immunol. *113*, 140–144 (1974)

Gershon, R.K., Cohen, P., Hencin, R., Liebhaber, S.A.: Suppressor T cells. J. Immunol. *108*, 586–590 (1972)

Gershon, R.K., Kondo, K.: Cell interactions in the production of tolerance: The role of thymic lymphocytes. Immunology *18*, 723–737 (1970)

Gershon, R.K., Lance, E.M., Kondo, G.: Immuno-regulatory role of spleen localizing thymocytes. J. Immunol. *112*, 546–554 (1974)

Gille, J., Williams, J.H., Hoffman, C.P.: The feto-maternal lymphocyte interaction in preeclampsia and in uncomplicated pregnancy. Europ. J. Obstet. Gynec. Reprod. Biol. *7/4*, 227–238 (1977)

Goto, S., Hishino, M., Tomoda, Y., Ishizuka, N.: Immunoelectron microscopy of the human chorionic villus in search of blood group A and B antigens. Lab. Invest. *35*, 530–536 (1976)

Hansson, L.Å., Lindholm, L., Carlsson, B., Fasth, A., Fällström, S.P., Wadsworth, C., Vährendh, G.: Suppressor cell activity in a male infant with T- and B-lymphocyte dysfunction treated with thymosin. Scand. J. Immunol. *5*, 1227–1231 (1976)

Harrison, G.P.: Immunocompetence of maternal lymphocytes. Lancet *1972 II*, 1319–1320

Hayward, A.R., Soothill, J.F.: Reaction to antigen by human foetal thymus lymphocytes. In: Ciba Foundation Symposium: Ontogeny of Acquired Immunity. pp. 261–268. Amsterdam, London, New York: Elsevier-Excerpta Medical North Holland, Associated Scientific Publishers 1972

Hellström, K.E., Hellström, I., Brawn, J.: Abrogation of cellular immunity to antigenically foreign mouse embryonic cells by a serum factor. Nature *224*, 914–915 (1969)

Hirsch, M.S., Phillips, S.M., Solnik, C., Black, P.H., Schwartz, R.S., Carpenter, C.B.: Activation of leukemia viruses by graft versus host and mixed lymphocyte reactions in vitro. Proc. Natl. Acad. Sci. US *69*, 1069–1072 (1972)

Hirsch, M.S., Ellis, D.A., Black, P.H., Monaco, A.P., Wood, S.: Leukemia virus activation during homograft rejection. Science *180*, 500 (1973)

Howe, C.: Lymphocyte physiology during pregnancy: in vivo and in vitro studies. In: Immunobiology of Trophoblast, pp. 131–146. Cambridge: Cambridge University Press 1975

James, D.A.: Effects of antigenic dissimilarity between mother and foetus on placental size in mice. Nature *205*, 613–614 (1965)

Jandinski, J., Cantor, H., Tadakuma, T., Peavy, D.L., Pierce, C.W.: Separation of helper T cells from suppressor T cells expressing different Ly components. I. Polyclonal activation: suppressor and helper activities are inherent properties of distinct T cell subclasses. J. Exp. Med. *143*, 1382–1390 (1976)

Johnson, M.H. (ref.): Foeto-maternal interactions (Workshop report). In: Progress in Immunology II. Vol. II, p. 400. Brent, L., Holborow, J. (eds.). Amsterdam, Oxford, New York: North Holland and American Elsevier 1974

Johnson, M.H.: Antigens of the pre-implantation trophoblast. In: Immunobiology of trophoblast. Edwards, R.G., Howe, C.W.S., Johnson, M.H. (eds.), pp. 87–112. Cambridge: Cambridge University Press 1975

Kasakura, S.J.: A factor in maternal plasma that suppresses the reactivity of mixed leukocyte cultures. J. Immunol. *107*, 1296–1301 (1971)

Kirby, D.R.S., Billington, W.D., Bradbury, S., Goldstein, D.: Antigen barrier of the mouse placenta. Nature *204*, 548–549 (1964)

Leventhal, B.G., Buell, D.N., Yankee, R., Rogentine, G.N., Terasaki, P.: The mixed leukocyte response. Effect of maternal plasma. In: Proceedings of the Fifth Leukocyte Culture Conference, pp. 473–485. New York: Academic Press 1970

Loke, Y.W., Joysey, V.C., Borland, R.: HL-A antigens on human trophoblast cells. Nature *232*, 403–405 (1971)

Loke, Y.W., Ballard, A.C.: Blood group A antigens on the human trophoblast cells. Nature *245*, 329–330 (1973)

Loke, Y.W. (Discussion): In: Immunobiology of trophoblast. Edwards, R.-G., Howe, C.W.S., Johnson, M.H. (eds.), p. 101. Cambridge: Cambridge University Press 1975

Marbrook, J.: Primary immune response in cultres of spleen cells. Lancet *1967 II*, 1279–1281

Masson, P.L., Delire, M., Cambiaso, C.L.: Circulating immune complexes in normal human pregnancy. Nature *266*, 542–543 (1977)

McCormick, J.N., Faulk, W.P., Fox, H., Fudenberg, H.H.: Immunohistological and elution studies of the human placenta. J. Exp. Med. *133*, 1–18 (1971)

Mendelsohn, J., Skinner, A., Kornfeld, S.J.: The rapid induction by phytohemagglutinin of increased α-aminoisobuturic acid uptake by lymphocytes. J. Clin. Invest. *50*, 818–826 (1971)

Möller, G. (ed.): Suppressor T lymphocytes. Transplant. Rev. *26*, 1–205 (1975)

Moretta, L., Ferrarini, M., Mingari, M.C., Moretta, A., Webb, S.: Subpopulations of human T cells identified by receptors for immunoglobulins and mitogen responsiveness. J. Immunol. *117*, 2171–2176 (1976)

Moretta, L., Webb, S.R., Grossi, C.E., Lydyard, P.M., Cooper, M.: Functional analysis of two human T-cell subpopulations: Help and suppression of B-cell responses by T cells bearing receptors for IgM or IgG. J. Exp. Med. *146*, 184–200 (1977)

Mosier, D., Cantor, H.: Functional maturation of mouse thymic lymphocytes. Eur. J. Immunol. *1*, 459–461 (1971)

Mosier, D.E., Johnson, B.M., Paul, W.E., McMaster, P.R.B.: Cellular requirements for the primary in vitro antibody response to DNP-Ficoll. J. Exp. Med. *139*, 1354–1360 (1974)

Mosier, D.E., Johnson, B.M.: Ontogeny of mouse lymphocyte function. II. Development of the ability to produce antibody is modulated by T lymphocytes. J. Exp. Med. *141*, 216–226 (1975)

Murgita, R.A., Tomasi, T.B.: Suppression of the immune response by α-fetoprotein. I. The effect of mouse α-fetoprotein on the primary and secondary antibody response. J. Exp. Med. *141*, 269–286 (1975a)

Murgita, R.A., Tomasi, T.B.: Suppression of the immune response by α-fetoprotein. II. The effect of mouse α-fetoprotein on mixed lymphocyte reactivity and mitogen-induced lymphocyte transformation. J. Exp. Med. *141*, 440–452 (1975b)

Murgita, R.A., Goidl., E.A., Kontiainen, S., Wigzell, H.: α-fetoprotein induces suppresor T cells in vitro. Nature *267*, 257–259 (1977)

Olding, L.: The possibility of materno-foetal transfer of lymphocytes in man. Acta Paed. Scand. *61*, 73–75 (1972)

Olding, L.B., Oldstone, M.B.A.: Lymphocytes from human newborns abrogate mitosis of their mother's lymphocytes. Nature *249*, 161–162 (1974)

Olding, L.B., Benirschke, K., Oldstone, M.B.A.: Inhibition of mitosis of lymphocytes from human adults by lymphocytes from human newborns. Clin. Immunol. Immunopathol. *3*, 79–89 (1974)

Olding, L.B., Jensen, F.C., Oldstone, M.B.A.: Pathogenesis of cytomegalo-virus infection. I. Activation of virus from bone marrow-derived lymphocytes by in vitro allogeneic reaction. J. Exp. Med. *141*, 561–572 (1975)

Olding, L.B., Oldstone, M.B.A.: Thymus-derived peripheral lymphocytes from human newborns inhibit division of their mother's lymphocytes. J. Immunol. *116*, 682–686 (1976)

Olding, L.B., Murgita, R.A., Wigzell, H.: Mitogen-stimulated lymphoid cells from human newborns suppress the proliferation of maternal lymphocytes across a cell-impermeable membrane. J. Immunol. *119*, 1109–1114 (1977)

Oldstone, M.B.A., Tishon, A., Moretta, L.: Active thymus derived suppressor lymphocytes in human cord blood. Nature *269*, 333–335 (1977)

Parkman, R., Mosier, D., Umansky, I.: Cochran, W., Carpenter, C.B., Rosen, F.S.: Graft-verus-host disease after intrauterine and exchange transfusions for hemolytic disease of the newborn. New Eng. J. Med. *290*, 359–363 (1974)

Peavy, D.L., Pierce, C.W.: Cell-mediated immune responses in vitro. I. Suppression of the generation of cytotoxic lymphocytes by Concanavalin A and Concanavalin A-activated spleen cells. J. Exp. Med. *140*, 356–369 (1974)

Pellegrino, M., Pellegrino, A., Kahan, B.: Solubilization of fetal HL-A antigens. A preliminary report. Transplantation *10*, 425–430 (1970)

Perlmann, P., Perlmann, H., Wigzell, H.: Lymphocyte mediated cytotoxicity in vitro. Induction and inhibition by humoral antibody and nature of effector cells. Transplant. Rev. *13*, 91–114 (1972)

Purtilo, D.T., Hallgren, H.M., Yunis, E.J.: Depressed maternal lymphocyte response to phytohaemagglutinin in human pregnancy. Lancet *1972 I*, 769–771

Revillard, J.P., Beutel, H., Robert, M.: Effects of alloantibodies on lymphocyte proliferation in vitro. Cell Immunol. *8*, 339–355 (1973)

Rich, R.R., Rich, S.S.: Biological expressions of lymphocyte activation. IV. Concanavalin A-activated suppressor cells in mouse mixed lymphocyte reactions. J. Immunol. *114*, 1112–1115 (1975)

Robert, M., Beutel, H., Revillard, J.P.: Inhibition of the mixed lymphocyte reaction by sera from multipara. Tissue Antigens *3*, 39–56 (1973)

Schröder, J., De la Chapelle, A.: Foetal lymphocytes in the maternal blood. Blood *39*, 153–162 (1972)

Searle, R.F., Sellens, M.H., Elson, J., Jenkinson, E.J., Billington, W.D.: Detection of alloantigens during pre-implantation development and early trophoblast differentiation in the mouse by immunoperoxidase labeling. J. Exp. Med. *143*, 348–359 (1976) (1976)

Siegal, F.P., Siegal, M., Good, R.A.: Suppression of B-cell differentiation by leukocytes from hypogammaglobulinemic patients. J. Clin. Invest. *58*, 109–122 (1976)

Skowron-Cenrzak, A., Ptak, W.: Suppression of local graft-versus-host reactions by mouse fetal and newborn spleen cells. Eur. J. Immunol. *6*, 451–452 (1976)

Spear, P.G., Edelman, G.M.: Maturation of the humoral immune response in mice. J. Exp. Med. *139*, 249–263 (1974)

Stigbrand, T., Damber, M.G., Schoultz, B.v.: Biochemistry and properties of the immunosuppressive pregnancy zone protein (PZ). In: Protides of the Biological Fluids. 24th Colloquium (Bruges 1975). Peeters, H. (ed.), pp. 181–188. Oxford: Pergamon Press 1976

Stites, D.P., Carr, M.C., Fudenberg, H.H.: Development of cellular immunity in the human fetus: dichotomy of proliferative and cytotoxic responses of lymphoid cells to phytohemagglutinin. Proc. Natl. Acad. Sci. USA *69*, 1440–1444 (1972)

Stobo, J.D., Paul, R.-E., Van Scoy, Hermans, P.E.: Suppressor thymus-derived lymphocytes in fungal infection. J. Clin. Invest. *57*, 319–328 (1976)

Strelkauskas, A.J., Wilson, B.S., Dray, S., Dodson, M.: Inversion of levels of human T and B cells in early pregnancy. Nature *258*, 331–332 (1975)

Tada, T., Taniguchi, M., Takemori, T.: Properties of primed suppressor T cells and their products. Transplant. Rev. *26*, 106–129 (1975)

Tamerius, J., Hellström, I., Hellström, K.E.: Evidence that blocking factors in the sera of multiparous mice are associated with immunoglobulins. Int. J. Cancer *16*, 456–463 (1975)

Tiilikainen, A., Schröder, J., De la Chapelle, A.: Foetal leukocytes in the maternal circulation after delivery. II. Masking of HL-A antigens. Transplantation *17*, 355–360 (1974)

Turner, J.H., Wald, N., Quinlivan, W.L.: Cytogenetic evidence concerning possible transplacental transfer of leukocytes in pregnant women. Am. J. Obst. Gynec. *95*, 831–833 (1966)

Waldmann, T.A., Broder, S., Blaese, R.M., Durm, M., Blackman, M., Strober, W.: Role of suppressor T cells in pathogenesis of common variable hypogammaglobulinaemia. Lancet *1974 I*, 609–613

Walknowska, J., Conte, F.A., Grumbach, M.M.: Practical and theoretical implications of fetal/maternal lymphocyte transfer. Lancet *1969 I*, 1119–1122

Wallis, W.J., Goldberg, E.H., Krco, C.J., Williams, R.C.: Suppression of stimulation in mixed lymphocyte reaction by newborn splenic lymphocytes. Fed. Proceed. *35*, 734 (1976)

Weller, T.H.: The cytomegaloviruses: ubiquitous agents with protean clinical manifestations (I). New Engl. J. Med. *285*, 203–214 (1971a)

Weller, T.H.: The cytomegaloviruses: ubiquitous agents with protean clinical manifestations (II). New Engl. J. Med. *285*, 267–278 (1971b)

Transfer of Humoral Secretory and Cellular Immunity from Mother to Offspring*

J.P. KRAEHENBUHL, C. BRON, and B. SORDAT

I. Introduction 106
II. Transfer of Humoral Immunity 106

   1. Transfer Before Birth 107

      a) Transfer via the Yolk Sac in Lagomorphs 107
      b) Transfer via the Hemochorial Placenta in Primates 109

   2. Transfer After Birth 112

      a) Short-Term Intestinal Transmission of Antibodies in Ungulates 112
      b) Long-Term Transmission in Rodents 117

   3. Mechanism for the Specific Uptake and Transport of IgG 123

      a) Structure of Immunoglobulin G 123
      b) Fc Receptors and Specific Binding of IgG 123
      c) Endocytosis and Intracellular Transport 125

   4. Protection 128

III. Transfer of Secretory Immunity 129

   1. Secretory Immune System 129

      a) Structure of Secretory Immunoglobulins 130
      b) Processing of Secretory Immunoglobulins 130
      c) Local Antigenic Stimulation and Secretion of Secretory Immuno-
         globulins 130

   2. Milk Secretory Immunity 131

      a) Origin of IgA-Secreting Plasma Cells in the Mammary Gland 131
      b) Mechanism for the Transfer of Secretory Immunoglobulins into Milk . 132
      c) Fate of Secretory Immunoglobulins in the Newborn 134

IV. Transfer of Cellular Immunity 136

   1. Transfer Before Birth 136

      a) The Fetal-Maternal Barrier 136
      b) Transplacental Exchange of Cells 137

         α) Passage into the Mother 137
         β) Passage into the Fetus 138

      c) Potential Consequences of Cell Exposure 138

* From the Institute of Biochemistry, University of Lausanne, and the Swiss Institute for Experimental Cancer Research, 1066 Epalinges, Switzerland

2. Transfer After Birth   140

    a) The Cellular Components of Milk   140
    b) Characteristics of Milk Cells in vitro   145

        α) Monocytic Cells   145
        β) T and B Lymphocytes   145
        γ) In vitro Tests   145
        δ) Epithelial Cells   146

    c) Evidence for Access of Milk Cells to the Neonate   146
    d) Possible Significance of Cell Transmission via Milk   147

        α) Protective Responses   147
        β) Occurrence of Runting Disease   147

V. Conclusions   148

References   148

I. Introduction

Birth represents a drastic change in the environment of young mammals. During gestation the fetus is protected from contact with foreign antigens and microorganisms to which the mother is exposed. At birth when newborns begin to breathe and ingest food, they are challenged by a large variety of antigens and microorganisms. The young develop a primary immune response that does not afford significant protection against infection. Its inability to adequately respond immunologically is not entirely a consequence of immunologic immaturity, but also results from a lack of prior immunologic experience. Thus, survival is ensured by the newborn's early feeble response as well as by transfer of humoral, secretory, and cellular immunity of maternal origin.

This review provides a synthesis of current knowledge concerning basic molecular and cellular mechanisms involved in the transfer of antibodies and immunocompetent cells from mother to offspring. We also analyze the role of humoral, secretory, and cellular immunity in protecting newborns against pathogens.

II. Transfer of Humoral Immunity

Brambell and his co-workers were the first to recognize the importance of maternal transfer of humoral immunity and to establish the time of transmission to the young in different orders of mammals (*Brambell*, 1970). In primates and lagomorphs transfer of antibodies occurs exclusively before birth through fetal membranes including the yolk sac or hemochorial placenta. In ungulates (i.e., artiodactyls and perissodactyls) fetal tissues are impermeable to maternal antibodies, and transmission of humoral immunity occurs only after birth via the newborn's intestine by absorption of maternal antibodies present in milk. Finally, in rodents and carnivores transfer occurs both before and after birth. The time and principal routes of transmission of humoral immunity from mother to young are summarized in Table 1.

Table 1. Time and route of transmission of humoral immunity

Animal order	Species	Transmission		Duration of postnatal transfer
		Prenatal	Postnatal	
Primates	Man	Hemochorial	–	
	Monkey	placenta		
Lagomorphs	Rabbit	Yolk sac	– –	
Rodents	Guinea pig	Yolk sac		20 days
	Rat	Yolk sac	Proximal intestine	26 days
	Mouse	Yolk sac	Proximal intestine	
Carnivores	Cat	Placenta and/or	Gut	1–2 days
	Dog	yolk sac	Gut	1–2 days
Artiodactyls	Cow	–	Entire small intestine	24 h
Ruminants	Goat	–	Entire small intestine	24 h
	Sheep	–	Entire small intestine	24 h
Suiformes	Pig	–	Entire small intestine	24–36 h
Perrissodactyls	Horse	–	Entire small intestine	24 h

Source: Compiled from *Brambell* (1970) and *Schlamowitz* (1976).

1. Transfer Before Birth

The first attempt to correlate uptake of macromolecules by the fetus with the anatomic structure of fetal membranes was made by *Needham* in 1931. It was based on
a classification of eutherian mammalian placentas described by *Grosser* (1909, 1927).
The placenta was viewed as an ultrafilter that passively selects molecules according
to size and to number of tissue layers. Thus, the absence of prenatal transmission of
antibodies in artiodactyls and perissodactyls was explained by the persistence of the
uterine epithelium, which remains intact during gestation. More recent experimental
evidence indicates that transfer of antibodies is an active process depending on
special features of both maternal and fetal membranes (*Schlamowitz*, 1976). The
mechanism of prenatal transfer of antibodies has been well investigated in primates
(*Gitlin* et al., 1964a, b; *Virella* et al., 1972), lagomorphs, and rodents (*Sonoda* and
Schlamowitz, 1972a, b; *Wild*, 1976). In contrast, it is still not clear whether absence
of transmission before birth in ungulates is due to impermeability to antibodies by
maternal or fetal membranes.

a) Transfer via the Yolk-Sac in Lagomorphs

Transmission of antibodies via the splanchnopleure of the yolk-sac has been described
in rabbits, guinea pigs, and rats. Most work has been performed in the rabbit. A de-

tailed description of the development and structure of fetal membranes in the rabbit is available in works by *Mossman* (1926), *Amoroso* (1952), *Brambell* (1970), *Larsen* (1962, 1963), and *Larsen* and *Davies* (1962).

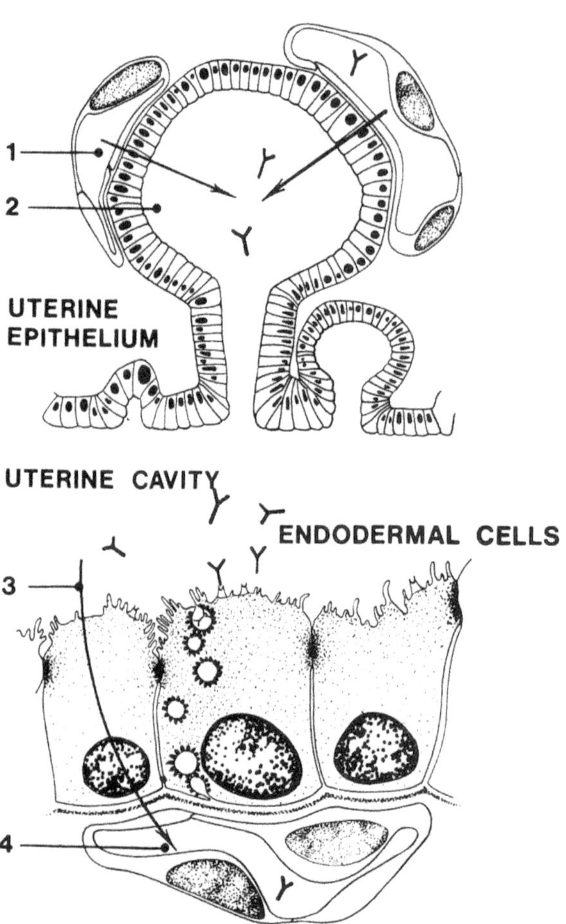

Fig. 1. Transfer of IgG molecules through rabbit maternofetal membranes. IgG molecules injected intravenously in a pregnant rabbit cross the following structures: *1:* The endothelial cells of uterine capillaries. It is not known if the process occurs passively by transudation or actively via specific recognition sites. *2:* The uterine epithelium. The cells, i.e., glandular epithelium or regenerated surface epithelium involved in secretion or transfer of IgG, have not been identified. *3:* From the uterine cavity IgG molecules interact with Fc receptors exposed on endodermal cells of the yolk sac splanchnopleure. IgG molecules are endocytosed and transported in coated vesicles and released in the mesenchymal space. *4:* The endothelial cells of the vitelline capillaries. This process has not been characterized.

The bilaminar omphalopleure, which forms the wall of the yolk-sac in rabbits, is composed of the trophoblast and endoderm and desintegrates between the 10th and the 13th day of gestation, opening up the yolk-sac cavity to the uterine lumen and exposing the endodermal cells of the splanchnopleure. The splanchnopleure is vascularized by vitelline vessels and lined by a continuous sheet of endodermal cells sealed at their apical end by tight junctions that restrict intercellular diffusion of macromolecules. The cells, polarized so that their numerous microvilli face the uterine lumen, contain a great number of vesicles, including coated vesicles and pits.

The yolk-sac becomes a functional placenta, as defined by *Mossman* (1937), in the second half of pregnancy when humoral immunity can be transmitted. In the rabbit the rate of transmission of antibodies increases from the 3rd week of gestation and reaches a maximum a few days before parturition (*Kulungara* and *Schechtmann,* 1962). In the rabbit (*Brambell,* 1948) and in the guinea pig (*Barnes,* 1959) transfer of antibodies occurs exclusively via the yolk sac since ligating the vitelline vessels completely abrogates passage of maternal antibodies into the fetal circulation. The mechanism of transfer has been extensively investigated at the level of the fetal membranes (*Sonoda* and *Schlamowitz,* 1972a, b; *Sonoda* et al., 1973), whereas the cells and cell organelles mediating transport through the maternal membranes have not been clearly identified. Once recruited into the uterine cavity, antibodies of the IgG class interact with specific recognition sites exposed on endodermal cells of the splanchnopleure. Binding is followed by endocytosis of IgG molecules and their translocation across the cells. These different stages are schematically represented in Figure 1. A similar mechanism has been reported in other organs mediating transfer of antibodies, such as the hemochorial placenta of primates, the gut of newborn rodents, and the mammary gland of ruminants. The general mechanism of specific uptake and transcellular transport of antibodies of the IgG class will be discussed in a later section.

b) Transfer via the Hemochorial Placenta in Primates

The development of placenta and fetal membranes of primates, extensively reviewed by *Hill* (1932), *Amoroso* (1952), and *Brambell* (1970), differs from that of other mammals considered in the preceding section. The yolk sac is rudimentary and at no stage constitutes an organ involved in uptake and transport of antibodies. There is no entry into the fetus except by traversing the chorionic trophoblast either within the placenta or the chorioamnion, a membrane constituted by the chorion and the amnion which adheres to the uterine wall. One mechanism suggests that antibodies are secreted across the chorioamnion into the amniotic fluid and transmitted to the fetus via the gut. However, concentrations of antibodies in the amniotic fluid vs the fetal serum after intravenous injection into the mother indicate that the principal route is via the hemochorial placenta (*Usategui-Gomes* et al., 1966). Thus, IgG molecules can be detected in the serum of the human embryo as early as the 38th day of gestation. The level remains under 100 mg% until the 17th week and then increases rapidly during the 3rd trimester of intrauterine life to reach term levels superior to maternal serum IgG level by 5%–10% (*Hyvarinen* et al., 1973).

110

The structure of the hemochorial placenta in primates has been examined with the light microscope by *Wislocki* and *Bennett* (1943) and the electron microscope by *Strauss* (1967). In the last trimester of pregnancy the chorionic villi project into the lacunae of maternal blood. The outermost layer of villi forms the continuous syncytiotrophoblast, which is polarized with irregular microvilli facing the maternal blood and lies on a basement lamina or on cytotrophoblast cells (Fig. 2). Fetal endothelial cells of the chorionic

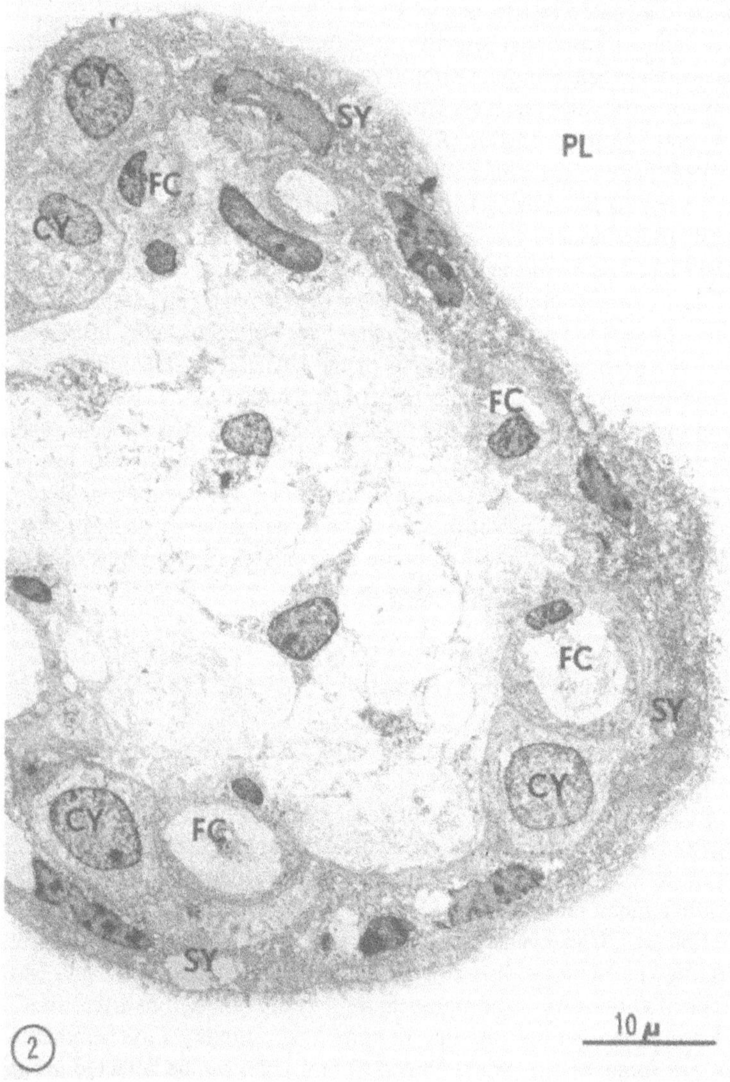

Fig. 2. Lower-power micrograph of a human trophoblastic villus (∿ 12th week of gestation). Microvilli of the syncytiotrophoblast *(SY)* face the placental lacunae *(PL)*. Underlying cytotrophoblastic cells *(CY)* are frequently in contact with fetal capillaries *(FC)* stained with alcian blue. Courtesy of *Ockleford* and *Whyte*. x 2400 (reduced to 75%)

capillaries are frequently in direct contact with the basement lamina of the syncytiotrophoblast, the structural features of which are characteristic of adsorptive pinocytosis and similar to those described for endodermal cells of the yolk-sac splanchnopleure. The syncytiotrophoblast possesses recognition sites for immunoglobulins G (*Gitlin* et al., 1964a, b; *Virella* et al., 1972; *Matre* et al., 1975) and numerous coated vesicles. Their distribution and relation to specific uptake have been analyzed by

TRANSMISSION VIA HEMOCHORIAL PLACENTA

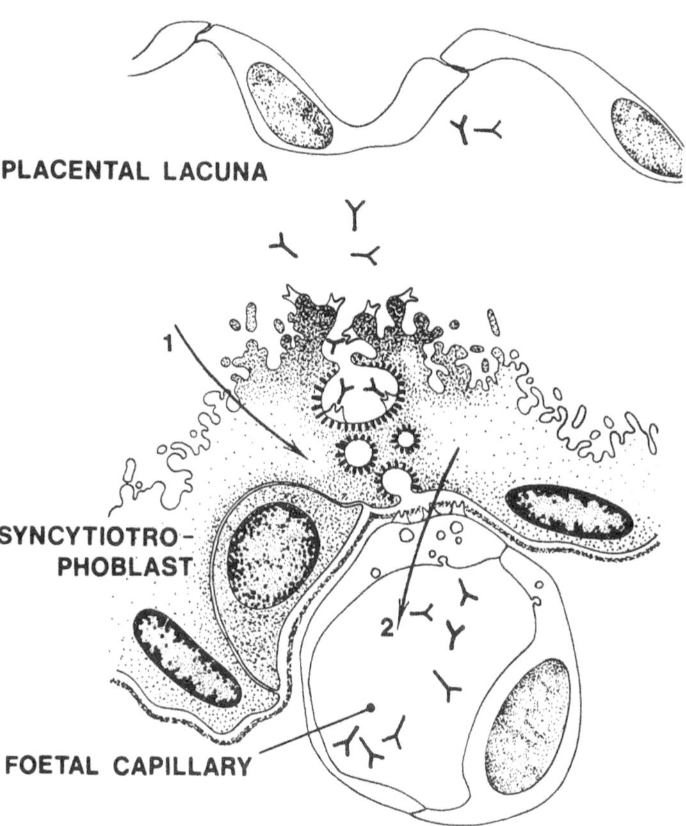

Fig. 3. Transfer of IgG molecules through hemochorial placenta. Maternal IgG present in the placental lacunae are transported into the fetal circulation across the following tissue layers: *1:* The syncytiotrophoblast. Upon interaction with Fc γ receptors exposed on the luminal plasma membrane, IgG molecules are endocytosed and transported across the syncytium via coated vesicles. The latter step has not been demonstrated with the electron microscope; however, the great number of coated vesicles and pits strongly suggests that these organelles mediate transport. *2:* Fetal capillaries. Fc γ receptors are present on endothelial cells and may play a role in transfer, thus explaining the higher concentration of IgG in fetal vs. maternal blood

112

Ockleford and *Whyte* (1977). The stages in the uptake and transfer of antibodies by the hemochorial placenta are summarized in Figure 3.

2. Transfer After Birth

Maternal antibodies are virutally unable to cross the maternal fetal barrier in utero in ungulates, and the newborn acquires humoral immunity from the milk during the first few hours of life. Since the newborn's gut is rather nonselective, adequate supply of antibodies depends upon concentration in milk, which is enriched by the mammary gland that selects antibodies of a given class from the maternal blood stream.

In rodents and carnivores, although significant amounts of antibodies are transmitted before birth via the yolk sac splanchnopleure or the placenta, greater concentrations are transported after birth via milk. In these species, transmission is not restricted to the first hours of life, but persists for several days; specificity is mediated by intestinal cells of the newborn.

The mode of transmission of immunity after birth will be analyzed in both groups of mammals in terms of specificity of uptake by the gut of the young, the site and route of transfer, and the mechanism of termination of transfer. The role of the mammary gland in providing specific antibodies will also be discussed.

The different steps of uptake and transmission of IgG molecules both in ungulates and rodents are diagramatically represented in Figure 4.

a) Short-Term Intestinal Transmission of Antibodies in Ungulates

Transmission of maternal IgG antibodies concentrated in colostrum across the gut of cattle, sheep, goat, pig, horse, and donkey is an extremely rapid process confined to a very short interval, i.e., the first 24–36 h after birth.

Specificity. A large number of reports indicate that intestinal absorption in piglets and cattle includes homologous and heterologous antibodies, with specificities directed against viruses or bacteria (*Nelson*, 1932; *Hoerlein*, 1957; *Speer* et al., 1959; *Royal* et al., 1968). Enzymes (*Balconi* and *Lecce,* 1966), hormones (*Asplund* et al., 1962; *Pierce* et al., 1964), or inert macromolecules (*Lecce* et al., 1961) are also transported, when fed orally, with the same efficiency as homologous milk antibodies. The biologic activity of antibodies, enzymes, or polypeptide hormones is preserved in the newborn circulation after intestinal absorption at least during the first hours of suckling.

Site and route of absorption. The entire length of the small intestine is involved in protein uptake in pigs and cattle (*Sibalin* and *Björkman,* 1966; *Kraehenbuhl* and *Campiche,* 1969; *Staley* et al., 1969). The cell compartments mediating transmission of antibodies have been described (*Kraehenbuhl* and *Campiche,* 1969). Proteins present in the lumen are endocytosed and accumulated in an elaborate tubulovesicular system located in the apex of absorptive cells just beneath the brush border. By fusion of vesicles, larger vacuoles are formed which move to the basolateral membranes and release their contents by exocytosis. The antigen-binding activity of antibodies is preserved in the intracellular

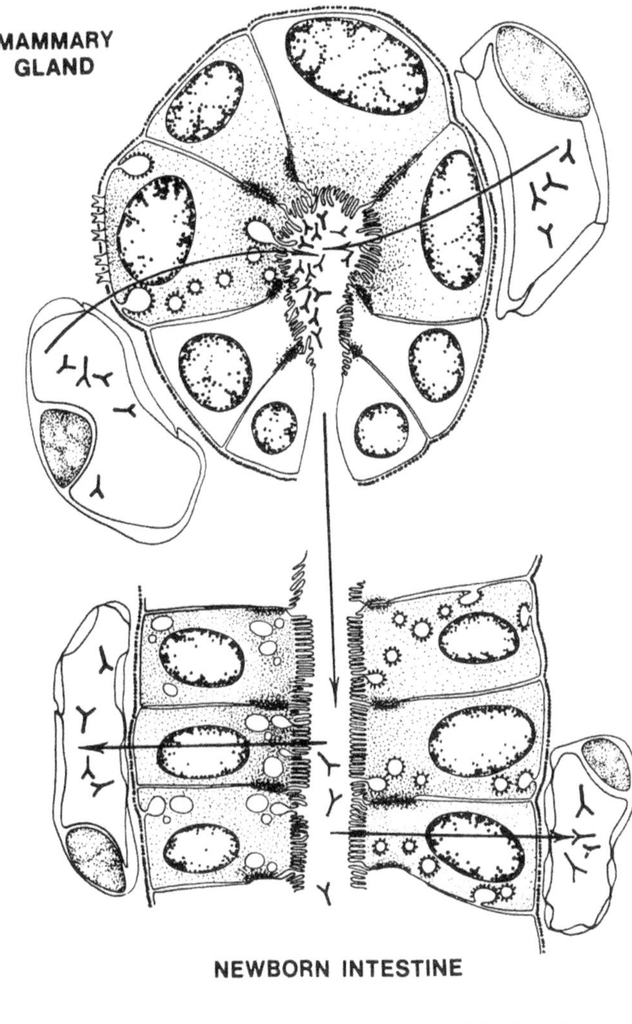

Fig. 4. Postnatal transmission of IgG molecules in ungulates and rodents. Maternal IgG are first secreted into milk (*upper part* of the drawing) and then absorbed in the circulation of the young by intestinal absorptive cells (*lower part*). *In ungulates (left part):* serum IgG are enriched in colostrum or milk. Fc receptors have been identified on alveolar mammary cells. The large number of coated vesicles suggest that transfer is mediated by these organelles. The entire length of the small intestine of the newborn is involved in uptake of IgG. Vesicles and large vacuoles transport nonspecifically milk proteins including IgG, which are then released into the interstitial space. IgG molecules are found both in blood and lymphatic vessels. *In rodents (right part):* serum IgG are not enriched in colostrum or milk. The mechanism of transfer has not been established. The entire small intestine takes up IgG molecules, but only the proximal absorptive cells express Fc receptors and transport intact IgG via coated vesicles. In the distal gut, IgG are degraded in lysosomes

tubules, vesicles, and vacuoles as illustrated in Figure 5. Thus, proteins including antibodies cross the absorptive cells nonselectively and intact via vesicles and vacuoles and are released in the lamina propria where they pass into the systemic or lymphatic circulation.

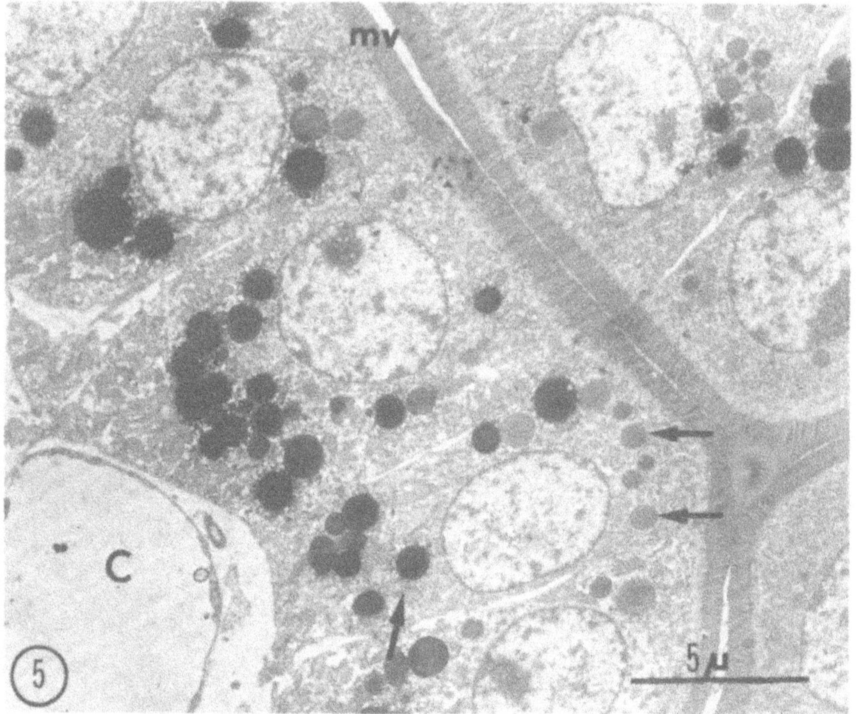

Fig. 5. Electron micrograph of jejunal cells of a newborn pig. Anti-peroxidase IgG antibodies were injected into the lumen. 60 min later the tissue was fixed, incubated with peroxidase, the enzyme activity of which was revealed using H_2O_2, and diaminobenzidine. The tissue was post-fixed with osmium, dehydrated, and embedded. Reaction product, indicating the presence of anti-peroxidase antibodies, appears electron opaque. Note the presence of IgG with preserved antibody activity in apical tubules and vesicles as well as in large apical and basolateral vacuoles (*arrows*). *mv*, microvilli; *C*, capillary. Stained with lead citrate. x 5000

Termination of uptake. Transmission of antibodies by the gut of the newborn declines rapidly and ceases after a few hours. The mechanism of termination has not been completely elucidated. A heat-stable, low molecular weight factor identified in the protein fraction of bovine milk seems to induce termination of uptake (*Lecce* et al., 1964). In jejunal and ileal absorptive cells, lysosomal activity, almost completely absent at birth (Fig. 6), is induced by endocytosis following protein ingestion (Fig. 7). After a few hours the vacuoles begin to fuse with lysosomes, and their content undergoes proteolytic digestion. Transmission of immunity is probably restricted to the first hours of life as a consequence of immaturity of the lysosomal system. Induction of lysosomal

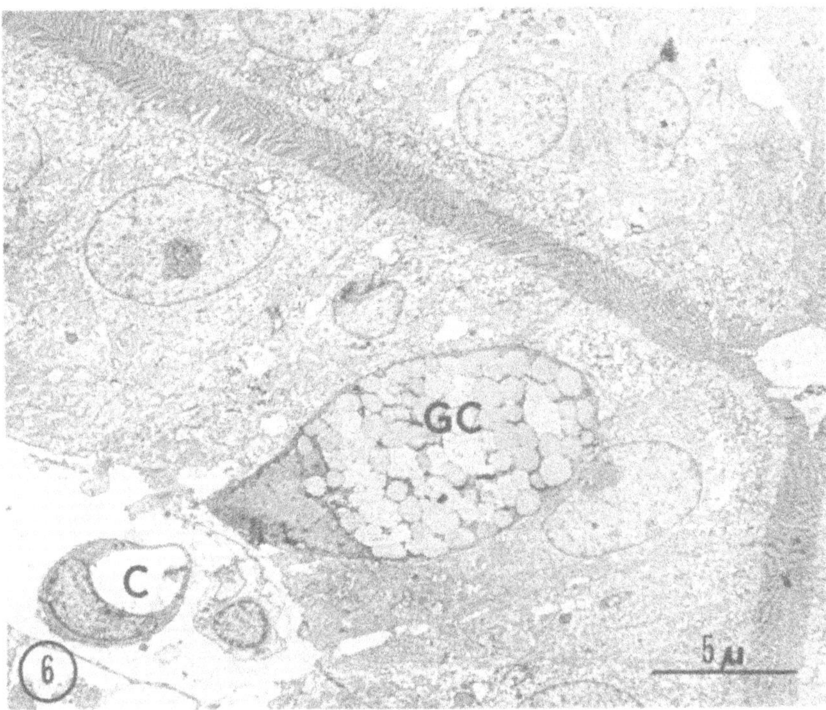

Fig. 6. Electron micrograph of jejunal cells of a newborn pig immediately after birth. The tissue was processed for acid phosphatase activity, a marker of lysosomal activity. Note the absence of reaction product in the cells. *GC*, goblet cells; *C*, capillary. Stained with uranyl acetate and lead citrate. x 4000

activity requires uptake of protein by absorptive cells (*Kraehenbuhl* and *Campiche*, 1969). Termination of transmission in this group of mammals is due to a maturation of the lysosomal system in absorptive cells of the small intestine which is induced by endocytosis but which might also be stimulated by exogeneous factors, such as the heat-stable factor (*Lecce* et al., 1964).

Role of the mammary gland. Since the gut of newborn ungulates appears to transmit proteins nonselectively, it follows that all proteins occurring naturally in milk will be found in the circulation of the young. Transmission of immunity in ungulates will therefore depend upon the presence in milk of antibodies selectively absorbed and secreted by the mammary gland. Much work has been devoted to this problem, and it has been reviewed by *Brambell* (1970).

Concentrations of different classes of immunoglobulins vary considerably in the early milk, termed colostrum, and in milk secreted after a few days (Table 2). The milk proteins include caseins and whey proteins, which remain in the supernatant after precipitation of caseins. The whey proteins are derived directly from blood (albumin, immunoglobulin G) or are synthesized and secreted by the mammary gland (α lactalbumin, lactoferrin). In ungulates the whey proteins of colostrum account for 150 mg per ml, of which 65% are immunoglobulins (*Morgan* and *Lecce,* 1964). The concentration

Table 2. Comparison of immunoglobulin concentration in serum, colostrum, and milk of mother and serum of young in various animal species

Order	Species	Immunoglobulin isotype	Immunoglobulin concentrations in mg/ml					
			Serum	Colostrum	Milk	Serum at birth	Serum after suckling	
Primates	Human	IgG$_1$	5.2–10.4					
		IgG$_2$	1.8– 3.7					
		IgG$_3$	0.6– 1.3 8–16	0.43	0.04	9	9	a
		IgG4	0.3– 0.6					
		IgA	1.4– 4	17.3	1.0	0	<0.5	
		IgM	0.5– 2	1.6	0.1	0.2	0.3	
Lagomorphs	Rabbit	IgG	5–10	1–2	0.1	5–10	5–10	a
		IgA	0.005	30	5	0	0.005	
		IgM	0.01	0.01	traces	traces	traces	
Artiodactyls	Pig	IgG	21.5	58.7	3.0	1.4	32	b
		IgA	1.8	10.7	7.7	–	–	
		IgM	1.1	3.2	0.3	–	–	
	Cow	IgG$_1$	11 (10.5)	47.6 (75)	0.59 (0.3)	0.15	1.3–2.5	b
		IgG$_2$	7.9	2.9	0.02	–	–	
		IgA	0.5	4.4	0.05	–	–	
		IgM	2.6	4.9	0.04	–	–	
Rodents	Mouse	IgG$_1$	1.4		0.25[c]			a
		IgG$_2$a	13		2.34			
		IgG$_2$b	–		–			
		IgA	0.5		0.34			
		IgM	4.3		0.59			

Rat	IgG$_2$a	6.91	0.67	0.99/1.19/ 1.53	1.0[d]	6.0
	IgG$_2$b	0.89	0.05	0.26	—	—
	IgA	0.18	1.15	1.26/1.42/ 0.59[d]	—	0
	IgM	0.95	—	0.002	—	<0.25

[a] Serum concentrations 2 weeks after birth. [b] Serum concentrations 12–72 h after birth. [c] Milk concentrations: average values between day 1 to 15 after parturition. [d] Milk concentrations at day 2, 4, and 19, respectively.

Source: Compiled from *Lecce* and *Matrone* (1960; *Franck* and *Rika* (1964), *Wang* et al. (1970), *Virella* et al. (1972), *McGhee* et al. (1975), *Humbert* et al. (1978).

of whey proteins decreases to 50 mg per ml after 1 day of suckling with 20% immunoglobulins. In ungulates the major immunoglobulin class in colostrum and milk is IgG. Recognition sites (Fc receptors) specific for the IgG subclass are expressed on the surface of mammary cells, mediating their transport into colostrum and milk to account for the high degree of IgG$_1$ over immunoglobulins of other classes and subclasses (*Dixon* et al., 1961; *Brandon* et al., 1971; *Brandon,* 1976; *Sasaki* et al., 1977). This mechanism of specific transfer of IgG is particularly efficient in ruminants 2–3 weeks before parturition, since enrichment of IgG$_1$ in colostrum is concomitant with an abrupt decrease of IgG$_1$ in maternal serum (*Brandon* et al., 1971).

b) Long-Term Transmission in Rodents

Unlike the situation in ungulates, intestinal absorption of antibodies from colostrum and milk in rodents and carnivores continues for a significant time during lactation (2–3 weeks).

Specificity. The intestine of newborn rodents is highly selective for homologous immunoglobulin G antibodies transmitted intact into the newborn's circulation. The high degree of selection led *Brambell* (1966) to postulate the existence of receptors at the surface of absorptive cells which selectively bind immunoglobulins. Several years were required to demonstrate that the structural basis of binding and transport in the gut is similar to that of fetal membranes (see Sect. C.II.2).

Route and site of absorption. Uptake of antibodies occurs along the entire length of the small intestine, as in ruminants. However, the fate of endocytosed proteins varies between the proximal and distal gut. *Jones* and *Waldman* (1972) were the first to describe binding sites for IgG in the proximal cells of the rat intestine. *Rodewald* (1970, 1973, 1978) localized the site of immunoglobulin uptake to the duodenal and jejunal absorptive cells and described the cell organelles mediating the transport (Figs. 8–10). Whereas antibodies in the proximal gut are transported intact in the circulation of the young, all internalized proteins undergo

118

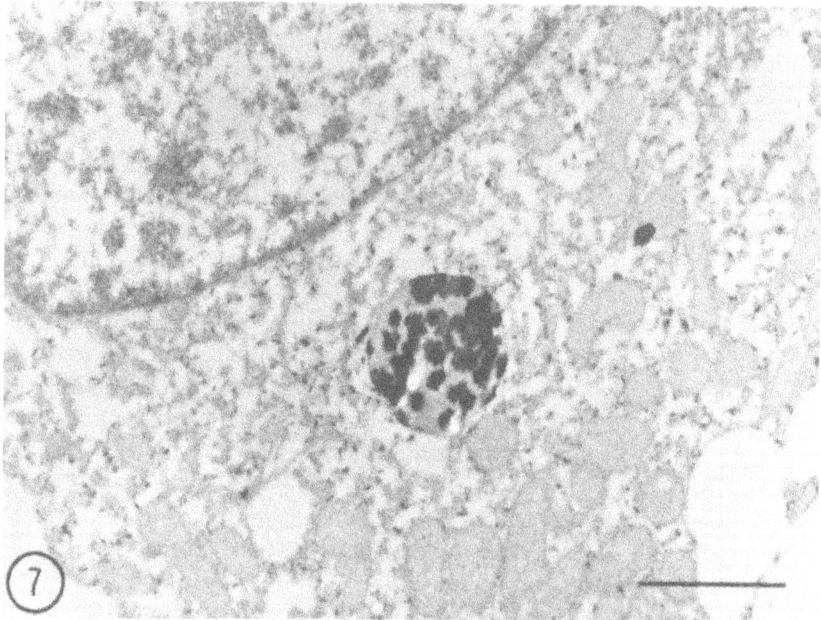

Fig. 7. Electron micrograph of a jejunal cell of a piglet fed 8 h with milk. A vacuole containing milk proteins contains acid phosphatase reaction product. Stained with uranyl acetate and lead citrate. x 20,000

enzymatic digestion in the lysosomal system of the distal intestine (Fig. 11) (*Morris* and *Morris*, 1977a, b), which after birth is immediately efficient in trapping and degrading exogeneous proteins in contrast to the system of ungulates which requires a few hours in order to become effective.

Termination of transmission. Disappearance of specific uptake and transport of antibodies is concomittant with morphologic changes in the proximal cells of the newborn. The absorptive cells containing a well-developed tubulovesicular and vacuolar apparatus disappear progressively and are replaced by new cells originating from the crypts, the site of cell proliferation. Moreover specific binding of monomeric IgG to newborn's jejunal cells decreases progressively, so that after 19 days no significant bindings can occur (*Borthistle* et al., 1977). These results suggest that specific receptors are expressed only on these cells present at birth which will be completely replaced in $\sim$ 3 weeks by cells bearing no receptors.

Role of the mammary gland. Neither colostrum nor milk is enriched in antibodies when compared with serum (Table 2), although selective uptake of proteins by mammary alveolar cells has been reported (*Jordan* and *Morgan,* 1967; *Gitlin* et al., 1976). Despite the absence of high concentration of antibodies in milk, the young acquires its immunity by sorting out IgG contained in milk and concentrating it in its circulation over a long period of time.

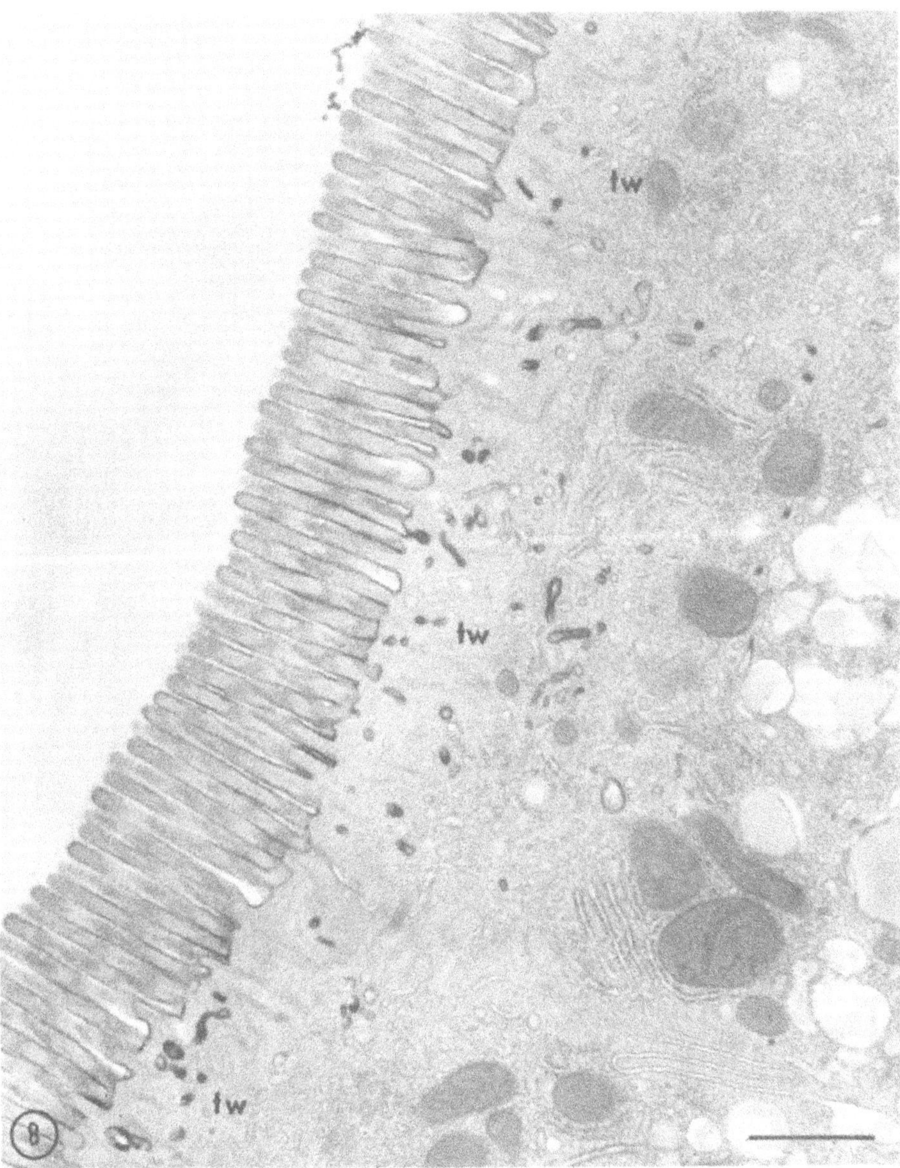

Fig. 8. A segment of 10-day-old rat jejunum was injected in situ with Fc fragments of rat IgG conjugated to horseradish peroxidase (HRP-Fc). The enzyme activity of the conjugate was revealed with H_2O_2 and diamine benzidine. Stained with uranyl acetate and lead citrate. After 15 min HRP-Fc is confined to the luminal plasma membrane and vesicles in the terminal web region *(tw)* of a jejunal absorptive cell. x 26,000; reduced to 80%. Courtesy of R. Rodewald

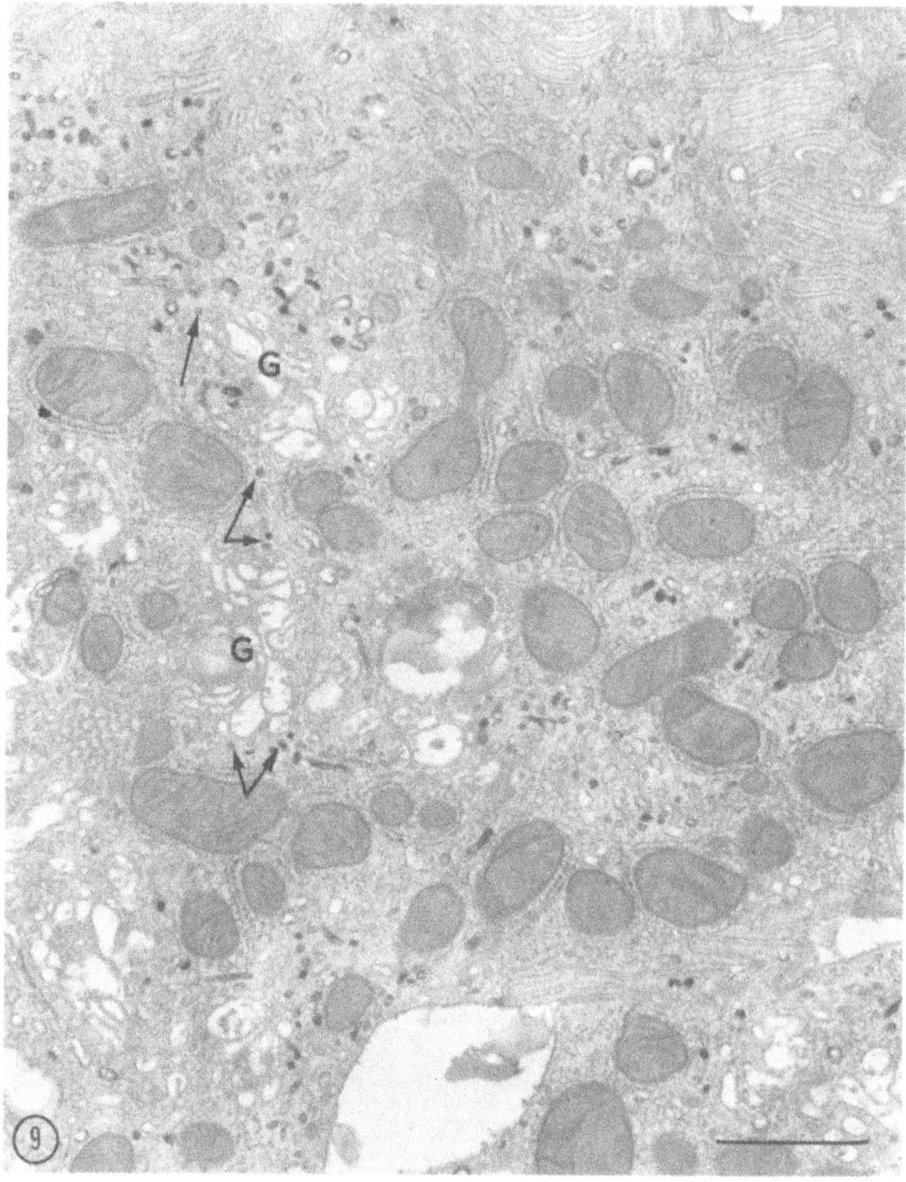

Fig. 9. Same protocol as described in Figure 8. 30 min after injection, HRP-Fc appears in vesicles including many coated vesicles. Vesicles *(arrows)* in Golgi region *(G)* contain Fc molecules, but Golgi cisternae are free of HRP-Fc. x 26,500; reduced to 80%.
Courtesy of R. Rodewald

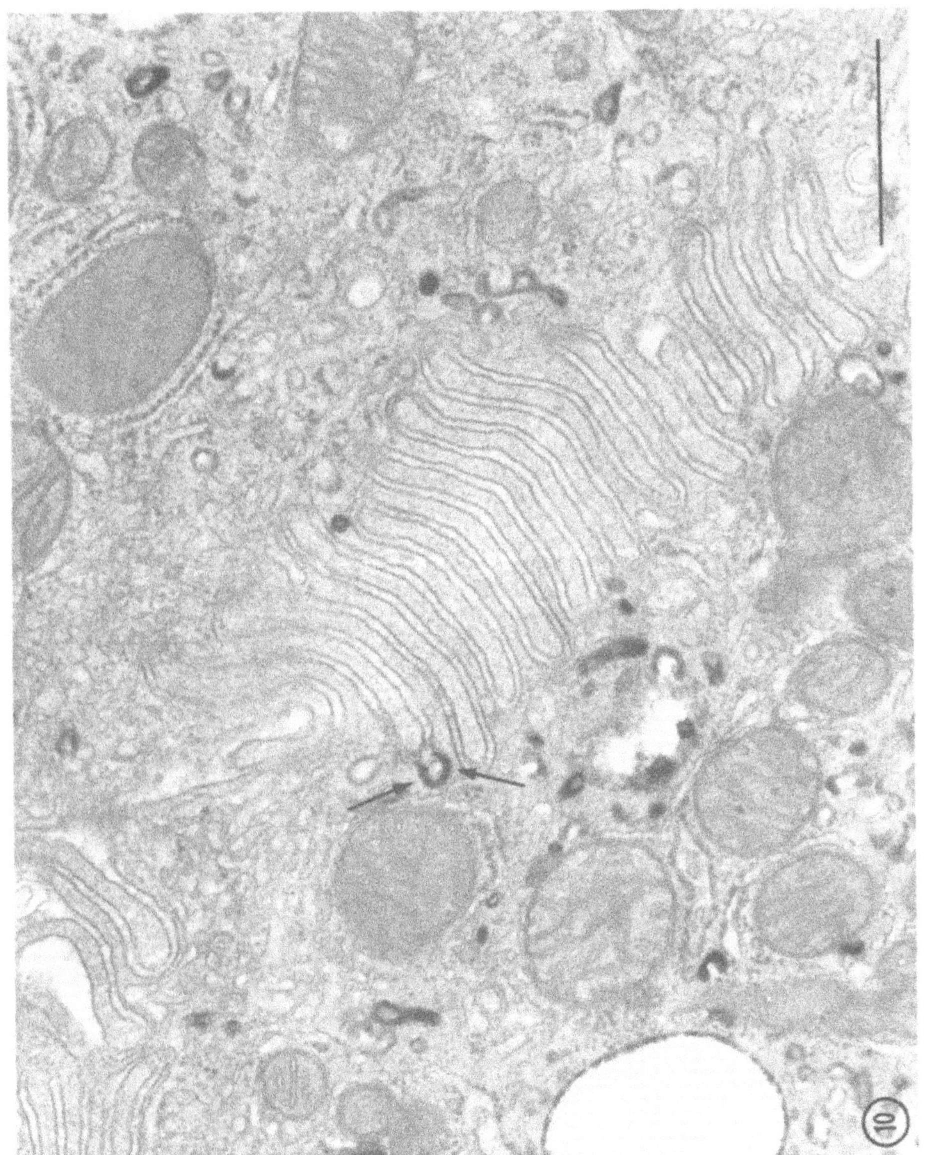

Fig. 10. Same protocol as in Figure 8. 30 min after injection, **HRP-Fc** is released from coated vesicles into the interstitial space of lateral cell surface. x 34,000; reduced to 80%. Courtesy of R. Rodewald

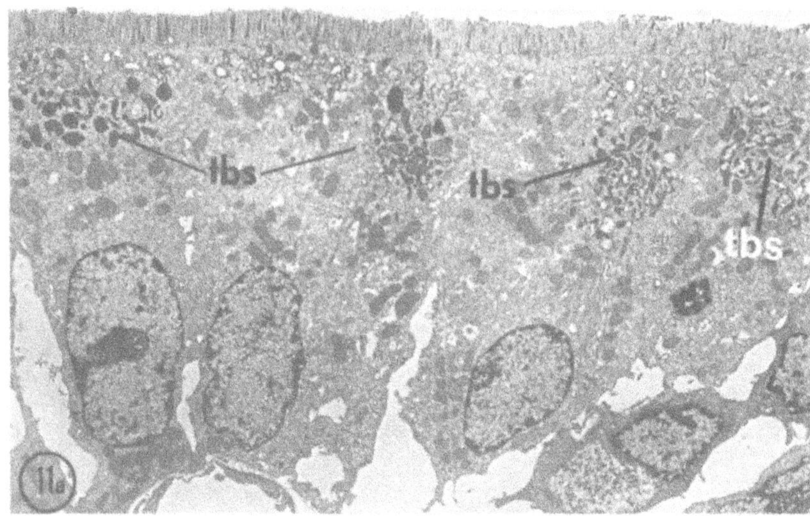

Fig. 11a. Electron micrograph through the distal intestine of a newborn rat. Anti-peroxidase IgG molecules were injected into the lumen; 4 h later the tissue was processed as in Figure 5. x 6000

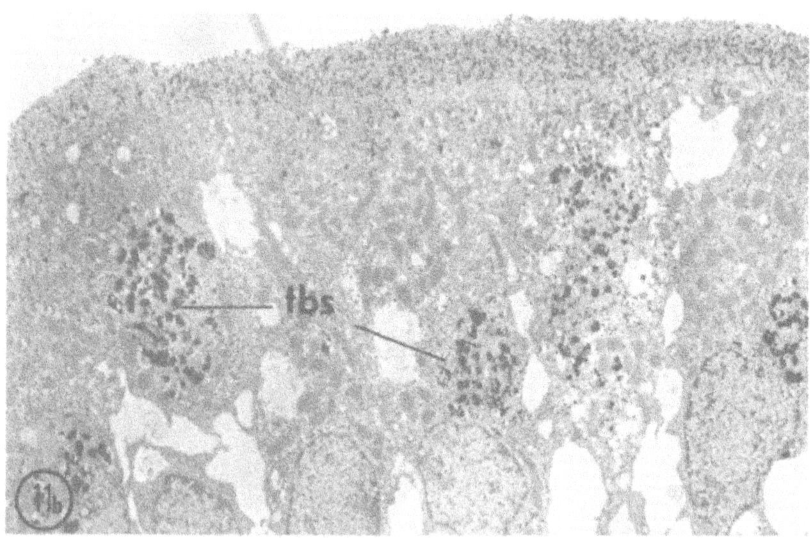

Fig. 11b. Same tissue processed for acid phosphatase. Anti-peroxidase IgG molecules are detected in an elaborate tubulovesicular system *(tbs)* that exhibits also acid phosphatase activity. This suggests that, upon endocytosis, IgG are accumulated in lysosomes where they undergo proteolytic digestion. x 6000

3. Mechanism for Specific Uptake and Transport of Immunoglobulins

Cells of different ontogeny, i.e., endodermal cells of the yolk-sac splanchnopleure and intestine as well as ectodermal cells of hemochorial placenta and mammary gland, share a common and saturable transport mechanism mediated by specific receptors restricted to IgG class and subclasses. A brief outline of the structure and function of the IgG class and subclasses will help to understand the process of antibody translocation. We shall then examine the molecular basis for selective uptake of IgG molecules and finally describe their route of transmission across absorptive cells.

a) Structure of Immunoglobulin G

In mammals IgG is the predominant class of immunoglobulins, having a molecular weight of $\sim$ 150,000 daltons. IgG is composed of two light polypeptide chains shared by all immunoglobulin classes (λ, κ) and two class-specific heavy chains (γ) linked together by interchain disulfide bonds. Subjecting IgG to proteolytic cleavage by papain yields three fragments. Two of these are able to combine with antigens (Fab); the third crystallizable fragment (Fc), although not involved in antigen binding, directs a number of other biologic activities of IgG. These include (1) binding of the first component of complement which requires combination of IgG with antigen for its activation (*Müller-Eberhard*, 1969), (2) binding to the surface of monocytes, thus stimulating ingestion of opsonized microorganisms by phagocytosis (*Spiegelberg* and *Weigle*, 1966), and (3) selective passage of IgG across the fetal membrane or the gut barrier (*Gitlin* et al., 1964a, b; *Jones* and *Waldman*, 1972; *Wild*, 1976)

IgG subclasses have been identified in several species including human (IgG_1, IgG_2, IgG_3, IgG_4), cow (IgG_1 and IgG_2), and rodents (IgG_1, IgG_{2a}, IgG_{2b}, IgG_{2c}) (Table 2). Each of these molecular species possesses several of the properties located on the Fc portion, but all the properties are not shared by all subclasses. IgG molecules are divided into variable and constant regions, depending on the degree of homology in the amino acid sequence of each polypeptide chain. In addition the constant region of IgG heavy chains is in turn divided into three homology regions compactly folded in globular domains (C_H1, C_H2, C_H3) (*Cunningham* et al., 1971), the two latter domains bearing the Fc active sites. Moreover studies on the reactivity of Fc subfragments in blocking the activity of whole IgG or Fc indicate that the C_H2 domain is implicated in complement fixation and activation (*Kehoe* and *Fougereau*, 1969), whereas the cytophilic properties are located on the C_H3 domain (*Yasmeen* et al., 1973).

b) Fc Receptors and Specific Binding of IgG

By using Fc and Fab fragments derived from papain-digested IgG, the Fc piece has been shown to be transmitted across absorptive cells to the fetal circulation, almost as readily as intact IgG molecules, whereas transmission of the Fab fragment occurs at a much lower rate (*Brambell* et al., 1960). Variable transmission rates indicate that IgG molecules interact via the Fc portion with recognition sites also termed Fc receptors exposed on the surface of absorptive cells. The specificity of Fc receptors for different immunoglobulin classes has been analyzed by competition and kinetic studies, which have shown that only IgG molecules bind with high affinity. The cellular distribution of Fc receptors in organs implicated in the transmission of humoral immunity has been established by morphologic means using fluoresceinated ligands. The distribution reveals that at least five cell types bind IgG molecules, i.e., syncytiotrophoblastic and fetal endothelial cells of chorial placentas in primates, proximal intestinal absorptive cells in rodents, endodermal cells of the yolk-sac splanchnopleure in lagomorphs, and mammary cells in ruminants. Finally some parameters such as pH variations that control binding of immunoglobulins to receptors have been characterized. These aspects shall now be examined in more detail.

Selectivity. Selectivity of transfer depends upon the specificity of binding of proteins to cell surface receptors. Immunoglobulins such as IgA or IgM, which do not bind to surface receptors on absorptive cells, are thus only minimally transferred across cells. Binding of IgG is not species restricted, but where binding of homologous IgG occurs, binding of heterologous IgG also occurs, though usually with less efficiency (*Morris,* 1976). In any given species, the affinity of different subclasses of IgG for Fc receptors varies.

In human placenta a single class of Fc receptors has been identified which binds IgG_1 and IgG_3 strongly, but IgG_2 and IgG_4 weakly. Binding is not restricted to one domain of the constant region (C_H3) as it is for Fc receptors of lymphoid cells and macrophages. The affinity constant, measured by competition studies and Scatchard analysis, is of the order of $5 \times 10^6/M$. The linearity of the Scatchard plot indicates a single binding site (*McNabb* et al., 1975).

In the rabbit yolk-sac Fc receptors bind IgG molecules from different species according to the chemical similarity of their Fc portion (*Schlamowitz,* 1976). The carbohydrate moiety of the IgG molecule seems to play a role, too, in its interaction with the Fc receptor, since the affinity of IgG separated by ion exchange chromatography is inversely related to the sialic acid content (*Schlamowitz* et al., 1975a, b).

Intestinal cell receptors with a single specificity directed against Fc determinants of monomeric IgG have been identified in rodents (*Jones* and *Waldman,* 1972; *Waldman* and *Jones,* 1973; *Guyer* et al., 1976; *Borthistle* et al., 1977). IgG subclass molecules differ in their affinity for these receptors, and the order of binding constants correlates with their relative concentration in the newborn circulation (*Guyer* et al., 1976).

The presence of binding sites with association constants of $\sim 5–10 \times 10^8/M$ for IgG_1 and IgG_2 have been detected in the bovine mammary gland near parturition. A week before parturition a new group of sites numbering about 5000 per cell with a strong binding for IgG_1 (Ka $\sim 4.5 \times 10^9/M$) appears on the mammary cells (*Sasaki* et al., 1977).

Cellular distribution. Preferential binding of labeled IgG molecules is associated with endodermal cells of rabbit splanchnopleure (*Sonoda* and *Schlamowitz,* 1972a, b; *Sonoda* et al., 1973; *Wild,* 1975; *Schlamowitz,* 1976), syncytiotrophoblast of human placenta (*Matre* et al., 1975; *Moskalewski* et al., 1975; *Wald,* 1970, 1973, 1976). It has not been established whether the distribution of Fc receptors on all these cells is polarized, e.g., if the receptors are segregated on the apical plasma membrane at the exclusion of the basolateral membrane. The vectorial translocation of IgG across cells may suggest that polarization causes IgG to interact with the microvilli, which face the compartment containing the maternal molecules, e.g., the intestinal lumen, the blood lacunae of hemochorial placentas, and the uterine cavity. However, in some organs (hemochorial placenta) receptors are not restricted to the absorptive cells, but are also found on fetal endothelial cells (*Matre,* 1977).

Control of the binding of IgG molecules. Binding of IgG to jejunal absorptive cells is pH dependent in rats and mice. Thus, acidic pH (6–6.5) in the lumen of the proximal gut favors binding of IgG, whereas physiologic pH in the interstitial space induces dissociation (*Jones* and *Waldman,* 1972; *Rodewald,* 1976, 1978). An important role in transfer of IgG molecules is probably played by pH gradients across epithelia by allowing their binding on one side of the cells and their release on the other side. Such a pH gradient is also present in the mammary gland between the interstitial space (pH 7.4) and the milk space (pH 6.0). However, since IgG are transported from the mammary blood vessels into milk, one must postulate that binding is favored by physiologic pH in contrast to the gut and that low pH induces dissociation (Fig. 12). A pH dependency of IgG binding in the yolk-sac splanchnopleure and in the hemochorial placentas has not been established. More work is still necessary to determine if variation of pH is the unique mechanism controlling binding of IgG to receptors on one side of the cells and release on the other side.

c) Endocytosis and Intracellular Transport

Binding of IgG molecules to Fc receptors present on the cell surface constitutes the first step in specific transport of antibodies. Binding first triggers endocytosis, which is followed by transcellular transport. It is essential that antibody activity of IgG molecules is preserved in the course of their transcellular route. In most cells endocytosed proteins undergo proteolysis upon fusion of phagosomes with lysosomes. The following question is pertinent: How do IgG molecules escape lysosomal degradation during transfer? Two models for explanation have been proposed; these are schematically represented in Figure 13.

Phagolysosome-mediated transport. This model, proposed by *Brambell* (1966), postulates that specific receptors of IgG are uniformly distributed on the absorptive cell surface, and endocytosis consecutive to binding occludes both IgG and unrelated macromolecules. The phagosomes formed fuse in the course of their transcellular route with primary lysosomes. In the phagolysosomes, proteolytic enzymes (cathepsins) digest all but receptor-bound molecules, which are then released from the cells by exocytosis at the opposite surface of the cell. Selection and proteolysis are intimately related; indeed both IgG molecules and unrelated proteins can be often detected in the same phagosomes, but only IgG, in the interstitium. Transferable IgG and nontransferable proteins were detected in the rabbit splanchnopleure in the same phagosomes of endodermal cells, whereas only transferable IgG were found in the vascular mesenchyme and the fetal vessels (*Wild,* 1976). Assuming *Brambell*'s hypothesis to be correct, one would expect first to find tight binding of transferable IgG to phagosome membranes and, second, fusion of phagolysosomes with the basolateral membrane of absorptive cells; such fusion has not been observed by electron microscopy (*Wild* et al.,

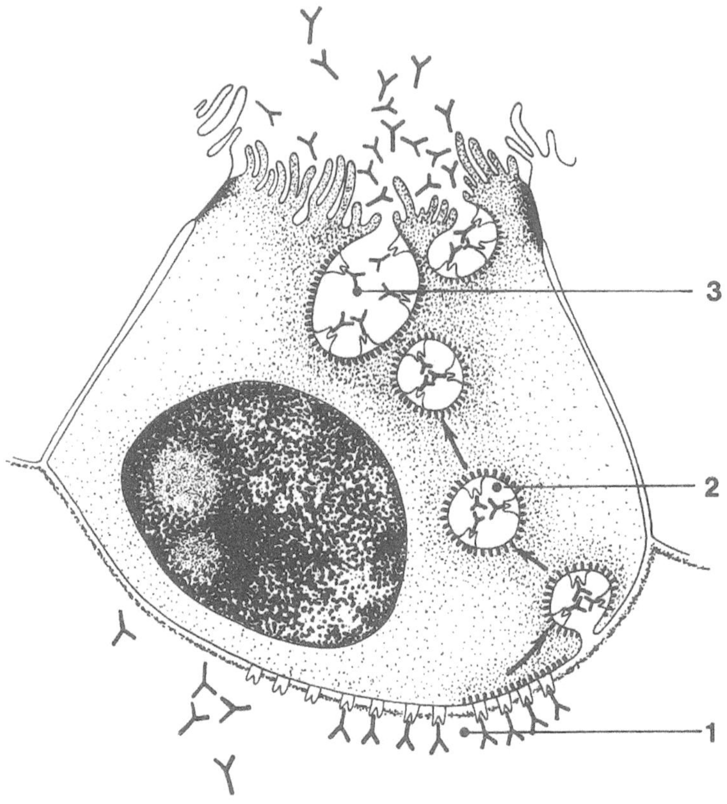

Fig. 12. Transfer of IgG molecules across the mammary gland. In ungulates, maternal IgG interact with Fc receptors: *(1)*, endocytosis occurs; *(2)*, transport may occur via coated vesicles, which are numerous in the mammary epithelial cells; *(3)*, the IgG molecules are released in the gland lumen by exocytosis. The mechanisms controlling binding and release have not been characterized

1972). In addition release of lysosomal enzymes following fusion has not been detected in the underlying mesenchyme (*Wild* et al., 1972; *Wild,* 1976). These observations raise doubts as to whether phagolysosomes ever discharge a protected fraction of contained IgG molecules. An alternative pathway may involve budding off of vesicles from phagolysosomes, which contain tightly bound IgG molecules and fuse with the basolateral membrane and then release their contents.

Coated-vesicle mediated transport. Wild proposed another model (1976) in which two transport mechanisms coexist in the same cell: (1) a *nonspecific* pathway mediated by phagosomes that fuse with lysosomes to form phagolysosomes, the content of which is completely degraded; and (2) a *specific* pathway in which IgG molecules are endocytosed into organelles, termed coated vesicles, which do not fuse with lysosomes, but with the basolateral cell membrane directly. *Roth* and *Porter* (1964) first demonstrated specialized coated vesicles possessing an electron-dense "bristle-like" coating on their cytoplasmic surfaces. Coated vesicles have been identified in all tissues involved in specific transfer of immunoglobulins.

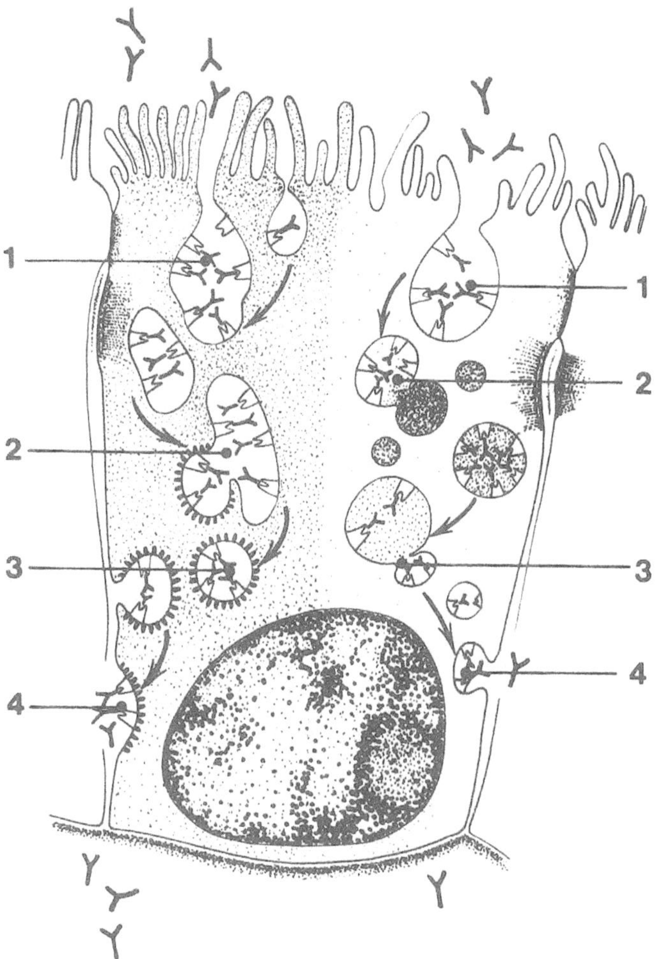

Fig. 13. Mechanism for the transfer of IgG molecules across epithelial cells (intestine, yolk-sac splanchnopleure, and syncytiotrophoblast). Two pathways are diagramatically represented. On the *left, the coated vesicle pathway:* IgG bind to Fc receptors exposed on the microvillous plasma membrane *(1)*. IgG are endocytosed in vesicles *(2)* that become coated *(3)*. The coating may prevent fusion with lysosomes. Coated vesicles ultimately release their contents in the interstitial space by fusion with the basolateral membrane *(4)*. On the *right, the phagolysosome pathway:* IgG interact with Fc receptors *(1)* and are internalized in phagosomes, which fuse with lysosomes *(2)*. In phagolysosomes, proteolytic enzyme digest all but receptor-bound IgG molecules *(3)*. Release in the interstitial space may result from fusion of phagolysosomes with the basolateral membrane or from vesicles that budd off from phagolysosomes and contain tightly bound IgG *(4)*. In the intestine, pH controls binding and release of IgG molecules

Binding of IgG molecules to a localized membrane receptor (Fc receptor) has been correlated with their sequestration and transport in coated vesicles. This was established

128

in the absorptive cells of the neonatal rat intestine (*Rodewald*, 1970, 1973), in the rabbit yolk-sac endoderm (*Slade*, 1975; *Moxon* and *Wild*, 1976), and in the fetal chick yolk-sac (*Linden* and *Roth*, 1978). How is fusion with lysosomes prevented? *Wild* (1976) suggested that the bristle coat of the vesicles may function so as to prevent membrane contact and fusion between the two organelles. However, coated vesicles do fuse with the basolateral membrane, and loss of the bristle coat must precede membrane fusion. Thus, in the low density lipoprotein (LDL) receptor system, fusion of coated vesicles, formed after endocytosis of LDL by fibroblasts with lysosomes, occurs with loss of the bristle coat (*Anderson* et al., 1976, 1977). So far the mechanism directing assembly and disassembly of coated vesicles has not been characterized. However, recent progress in isolating coated vesicles (*Pearse*, 1975; *Woods* et al., 1978) and their biochemical characterization (*Pearse*, 1976; *Woods* et al., 1978) should provide an approach to investigating the role of this coating in preventing or allowing membrane fusion. At the present time, it is difficult to favor either of these two models. It may very well be that IgG are transported via the two pathways and that in any given cell type one is predominant.

In conclusion, transfer of IgG molecules through an epithelial cell layer involves a number of processes; there is interaction with recognition sites (Fc receptors) that are exposed on the membrane facing the compartment containing IgG, and this is followed by endocytosis and intracellular transport via coated vesicles or phagolysosomes. Antibody activity of IgG molecules is preserved during transport either by lysosomal escape in the coated vesicle pathway or by protection from proteolysis by tight association of IgG to Fc receptors in the phagolysosome pathway. Binding and release of IgG molecules have been related to changes in the environment on each side of the absorptive cell layer.

4. Protection

The ability to elicit an immunologic response is fully acquired in utero by the 3rd trimester of fetal development, thus providing the fetus with a potentially active defense mechanism. The synthesis of IgM in human can already be detected after 10.5 weeks of gestation (*Gitlin* and *Blasucci*, 1969), whereas fetal lymphocytes are immunologically responsive at the 18th week of gestation as judged by phytohaemagglutin-induced blast transformation (*Carr* et al., 1973).

Under normal conditions the fetal immune system remains unchallenged due to the relative impermeability of fetal membranes to pathogens. Under abnormal conditions pathogens such as common viral agents have access to the fetus and may elicit direct or indirect damage (*Catalano* et al., 1971; *Ruben* et al., 1973). In addition, prenatal sensitization of the fetus can also occur during normal pregnancies without placental damage. Human fetuses were shown to be sensitized to antigenic determinants of various infectious agents including tuberculosis, mumps, *Escherichia coli*, *Salmonella typhosa* without fetus infection (*Cramer* et al., 1974). In utero exposure of the fetus to antigens inoculated into the mother was further proven in animal models (*Kruger* and *Stoppolman*, 1971; *Stastny*, 1965). Although the mammalian acquires the capacity for immunologic responsiveness early in its development, the defense system is fully active only after birth when the neonate comes in contact with foreign substances.

The transfer of preformed immunity provides the newborn with a large repertoire of protective antibodies to a variety of antigens. This confers efficient although temporary immunity, reflecting the maternal immunologic experience against most infecting agents disseminated via the blood. For instance, efficient transfer is observed in the case of antibodies to diphtheria, tetanus, and erythrogenic toxins, staphylococcus, streptolysins, and antibodies to viral diseases (*Bellanti* and *Jurlado*, 1976). Moreover passively acquired immunoglobulins may function as opsonins, which enhance phagocytosis by macrophages and polymorphonuclear leukocytes, thus stimulating the primitive defense mechanism.

III. Transfer of Secretory Immunity

The defense of mucous surfaces, e.g., in the digestive, respiratory or urogenital tracts, and secretory epithelia such as salivary, lacrimal, and mammary glands is in mammals determined by complex interactions of both immune and nonimmune mechanisms. Immune interactions are mediated by the secretory immunologic system characterized by local production of an 11S immunoglobulin A antibody, termed secretory IgA, which is found in secretion fluids. Transfer of secretory immunity from the mother to the young is of great importance since the newborn is unable to build up its own secretory immune response due to lack of previous experience and because the mucous surfaces, particularly those of the intestinal and respiratory tracts, are the first sites to experience major antigenic challenge.

1. The Secretory Immune System

The concept of local immunity, introduced at the beginning of the century, is based on observations that suggest discrepancies between degree of immunity and serum antibody level. Local immunity was first reviewed by *Besredka* (1927) in a monograph entitled "Local Immunization," but then the possibility of a local secretory immune system was not considered. Evidence for an independent secretory immune system came from the work of *Burrows* (1948), who showed the importance of antibodies present in stools. These antibodies, referred to as coproantibodies, were considered important in the recovery from and subsequent protection against experimental cholera in guinea pigs. An important step forward was made by the discovery by *Heremans* et al. (1958) of the IgA class of antibodies and by *Tomasi* et al. (1965) that IgA is the predominant immunoglobulin in secretions, where it is structurally different and where it possesses an extra antigenic component not present in circulating serum IgA. Much biologic and biochemical data in the literature have now been reported which suggest that (1) secretory IgA molecule has a unique structure in all species, (2) specific cell types are involved in the processing of this molecule, and (3) production of specific antibodies results from local antigenic stimulation. These aspects will be briefly reviewed in the next sections.

130

a) Structure of Secretory Immunoglobulins

Secretory immunoglobulins have been identified in the secretion fluid of several mammals, but their chemical structure has been worked out mainly in humans (*Newcomb* et al., 1968; *Tomasi* and *Grey,* 1972) and rabbits (*Cebra* and *Robbins,* 1966; *Cebra* and *Small,* 1967).

The secretory IgA antibody (sIgA) is an 11S molecule composed of a dimer of serumlike IgA and a glycoprotein, called secretory component (SC), secretory piece, transport piece, or T piece. The polypeptide structure, the size, and the bonding of SC to the IgA dimer vary from one species to another (*Tomasi* and *Grey,* 1972; *Heremans* and *Vaerman,* 1971). The serumlike IgA is characterized by two class-specific heavy chains (α) and two light chains common to all class of immunoglobulins. Dimerization is mediated by the J chain (joining chain), a small glycoprotein, via disulfide bridges between the J chain cysteine residues and the penultimate cysteine of the heavy chain of IgA (*Mestecki* et al., 1974). Clearly sIgA is the main carrier of mucoantibody activity. Other immunoglobulins may also contribute such as IgM, which replaces IgA in IgA-deficient individuals (*Crabbé,* 1967). IgM is also found in the secretions of neonates (*Allen* and *Porter,* 1973; *Porter* et al., 1974).

b) Processing of Secretory Immunoglobulins

Most of the immunofluorescence studies, radioactive tracer, and organ culture experiments, reviewed by *Tomasi* and *Grey* (1972), *Hurlimann* (1971), and *Lamm* (1976), have demonstrated that sIgA is processed locally by different cell types. The IgA moiety is synthesized in local plasma cells present in the *lamina propria* of mucous membranes and in the interstitium of exocrine glands. Prior to secretion into the interstitial fluid, the IgA are dimerized by addition of the J chain (*Parkhouse* and *Della Corte,* 1976). From the extracellular space dimeric IgA gain access to the gland lumen by crossing the epithelial cells, since intercellular diffusion is restricted by the presence of tight junctions sealing the cells at their apical ends. SC is synthesized by the epithelial cells of the mucous membranes and the exocrine gland and secreted into their lumen (*Brandtzaeg,* 1974, 1977; *Lamm,* 1976; *Kraehenbuhl* et al., 1975). Very little is known about the mechanisms in secretory tissues which are responsible for the uptake and transport of secretory immunoglobulins. In the mid 60s SC was already postulated to act as a recognition site or receptor which triggers the uptake of dimeric IgA by epithelial cells and transport into secretions (*South* et al., 1966) as Fc receptors mediate transfer of IgG in the different organs described in the preceding sections. Recently experimental evidence indicates that SC binds the mammary epithelial cells (*Kraehenbuhl* et al., 1977); these aspects will be discussed later.

c) Local Antigenic Stimulation and Secretion of Secretory Immunoglobulins

A secretory immune response is elicited in response to local antigenic stimulation that is restricted to the same site and or to a distant mucosal surface in contrast to the humoral immune response, which is systemic. The cellular events leading to a secretory immune response have been extensively investigated, but a brief review is helpful in understanding secretory immunity transferred from mothers to newborns. Numerous specialized lymphoid aggregations and organs are associated with the digestive (e.g., tonsils, Peyer's patches, appendix) and respiratory tracts (*Bienenstock* et al., 1973a, b, 1974). These lymphoid organs are characterized by the existence of a specialized overlying epithelium (*Joel* et al., 1970; *Owen* and *Jones,* 1974). They contain the precursors of IgA secreting plasma cells which will ultimately populate the *lamina propria* of mucous membranes and the interstitium of exocrine glands. As shown previously (*Hess* et al., 1973; *Cottier* et al., 1975), antigen crosses the thin epithelium covering the gut- or bronchial-associated lymphoid tissues (GALT or BALT), enters the lymphoid structures, and triggers mitotic activity and the formation of germinal centers. Primed lymphoid cells emigrate into efferent lymphatics, become part of the pool of circulating lymphocytes, seed then the lamina propria of interstitium of the secretory organs where they differentiate into IgA-secreting plasma cells (*Guy-Grand* et al., 1974; *Cebra* et al., 1976; *Roux* et al., 1977). The basic mechanism for homing in secretory organs, especially the gut, appears to be antigen independent, since seeding of immunoblasts to antigen-free grafts or fetal gut has been described (*Guy-Grand* et al., 1974).

2. Milk Secretory Immunity

a) Origin of IgA-Secreting Plasma Cells in the Mammary Gland

Attempts to induce a local secretory immune response within the mammary gland by direct immunization have failed. Usually the antibody produced is of the IgG and not IgA class and is not restricted to colostrum or milk (*Hurlimann* and *Lichaa,* 1976). Furthermore the mammary gland has no lymphoid structures similar to those associated with the gut and respiratory systems. Studies on antibody specificity of secretory immunoglobulins present in milk indicate that milk immunity is derived from a site different from the breast (*Allardyce* et al., 1974; *Montgomery* et al., 1974; *Ahlstedt* et al., 1975; *Arnold* et al., 1976).

Oral immunization of pregnant swine with gastroenteritis virus induced the appearance of specific IgA antibodies in colostrum, whereas intramammary immunization elicited a systemic response with IgG antibodies detected in colostrum and serum (*Bohl* et al., 1974). Similar observations have been reported in other species as well as man, thus indicating that colostral IgA antibodies have specificities directed against intestinal or respiratory antigens or microorganisms (*Allardyce* et al., 1974; *Arnold* et al., 1976; *Hanson* et al., 1978). Recently *Lamm* and his group (*Roux* et al., 1977) have obtained experimental evidence supporting the view that lymphoid cells producing milk or colostral antibodies originate from distant sites. Thus mesenteric lymph node blasts when injected in syngeneic mice home to the mammary gland during late pregnancy and lactation, and here they differentiate into plasma cells secreting IgA antibodies. The migration pattern of lymphoid cell precursors to the mammary gland is schematically represented in Figure 14.

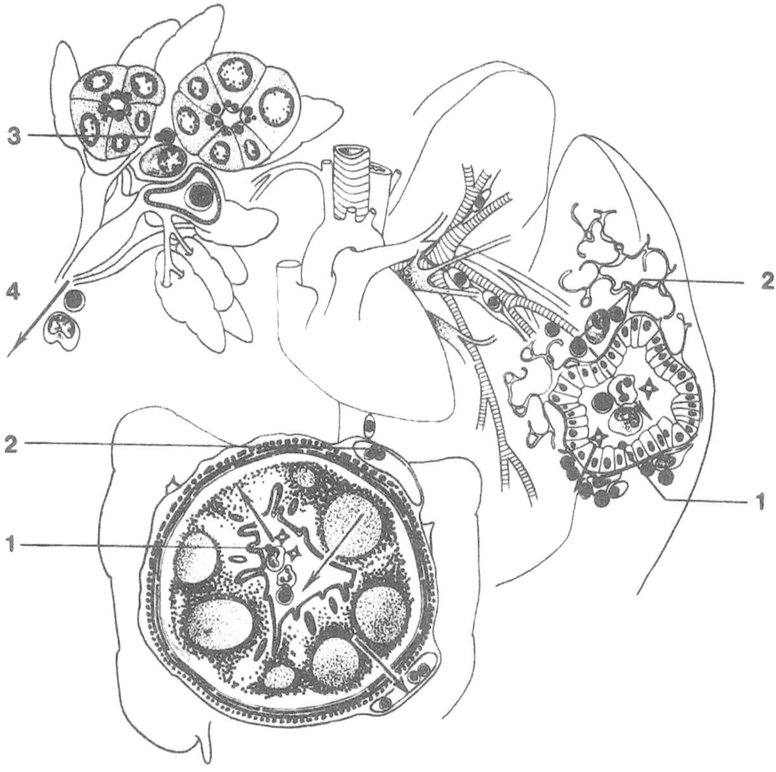

Fig. 14. Migration pattern of lymphoid cell precursors to the mammary gland. *1,* The gut- and bronchial-associated lymphoid tissues are the sites of antigenic stimulations; *2,* primed lymphoid cells emigrate into efferent lymphatics and become part of the pool of circulating lymphocytes; *3,* lymphoid cells eventually seed the interstitial space where they differentiate into IgA secreting plasma cells; *4,* some cells (B or T lymphoid cells) cross the mammary epithelium and are found in colostrum or milk

b) Mechanism for the Transfer of Secretory Immunoglobulin into Milk

The cell organelles in local plasma cells and epithelial cells, involved in the processing of sIgA by the mammary gland, have been identified through the electron microscope with immunocytochemical means (*Kraehenbuhl* et al., 1975). The IgA moiety was detected in cisternae of the rough endoplasmic reticulum and Golgi elements of plasma cells, in apical vacuoles of epithelial cells, and in the gland lumen. SC was found exclusively in the mammary epithelial cells and in the gland lumen.

The presence of SC in the rough endoplasmic reticulum, in Golgi elements, and in apical vacuoles indicates that SC is synthesized and secreted by mammary epithelial cells, following the same pathway as other milk protein such as caseins or α lactalbumin. SC has also been found associated with the basolateral membrane of mammary cells (*Kraehenbuhl* et al., 1977) (Fig. 15). Since SC cannot diffuse backward from its site of secretion, i.e., the gland lumen, due to the presence of tight junctions that seal

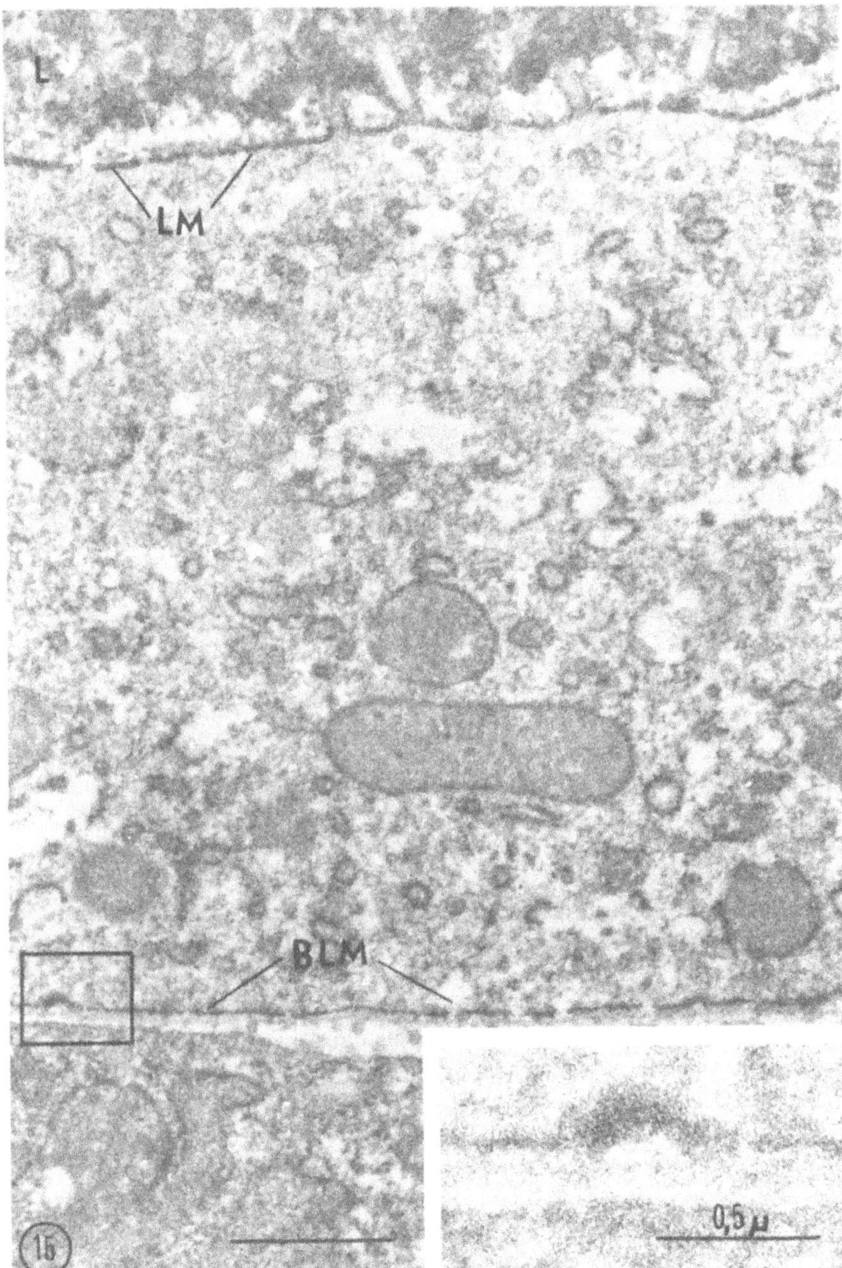

Fig. 15. Electron micrograph of mammary gland of a midpregnant rabbit. The tissue was fixed with formaldehyde, thick sectioned, and incubated with goat F(ab')$_2$ anti-rabbit SC, followed by sheep F(ab')$_2$ anti-goat F(ab')$_2$ coupled to a heme octapeptide, the peroxidatic activity of which was revealed by H_2O_2 and diaminobenzidine. SC was found in the gland lumen *(L)* and associated with the luminal plasma membrane *(LM)*. SC is also bound to the basolateral membrane *(BLM)*. x 25,000. *Inset:* high magnification showing the presence of SC associated with the epithelial plasma membrane and a coated pit. The surface of an adjacent plasma cell remains unstained. x 50,000

the epithelial cells, one must postulate that SC is actively transported from the lumen to the basolateral cell surface, where it may act as a recognition site for dimeric $(IgA)_2$. Epithelial cells have been dissociated from mammary gland and enriched by isopyknic centrifugation in dense albumin solutions (*Kraehenbuhl*, 1977). Free SC isolated from milk binds specifically to mammary cells with an affinity constant of the order of $10^8/M$ and approximately 2000 sites per cell as shown by competitive studies and Scatchard analysis (*Kraehenbuhl* et al., 1977). Moreover the binding is pH dependent with an optimum at pH 6.0, which corresponds to the pH of milk. SC also interacts specifically with dimeric $(IgA)_2$ but not with IgG or monomeric IgA, and an affinity constant of $10^8/M$ was calculated. These findings suggest the following pathway for transfer of secretory immunoglobulins into milk as summarized in Figure 16. Upon secretion into the milk space, SC binds to the luminal plasma membrane since the pH is optimum (6–6.5). Binding triggers endocytosis and bound SC is transported through the cell within vesicles which move to the basolateral membrane where fusion occurs. Membrane-bound SC is then exposed to the interstitial space and can interact specifically with dimeric $(IgA)_2$ secreted by local plasma cells. The complex $SC - (IgA)_2$ is in turn internalized and transported via the reverse pathway. At the luminal surface, the complex $SC - (IgA)_2$ is released by competition with free SC. Experiments are underway to identify the vesicles mediating transport through mammary cells and the binding constants and pH dependency of dimeric $(IgA)_2$ for membrane-associated SC.

c) Fate of Secretory Immunoglobulins in the Newborn

Breast feeding and oral administration of colostrum has been found to confer upon newborns of various mammals a significant degree of immunity against a number of naturally acquired or vaccine-induced enteric and upper respiratory infections (*Mata* and *Urrutia*, 1971; *Winberg* and *Wessner*, 1971; *Guinchat* et al., 1972; *Gerrard*, 1974; *Goldblum* et al., 1975). The protection appears to be mediated largely through secretory immunoglobulins in colostrum (*Hanson* and *Winberg*, 1972), although a number of host-resistance factors have been identified (*Goldman* and *Smith*, 1973), including the presence of viable leukocytes.

Little information is available regarding the fate of orally administered colostral secretory immunoglobulins in the young. Conflicting results have been reported as to whether secretory immunoglobulins are absorbed into the circulation by the newborn's intestine (*Ogra* et al., 1977). It is generally agreed, however, that the great majority of secretory immunoglobulins remain in the gastrointestinal tract where they provide the most relevant means of control of enteropathogens, which are generally noninvasive and operate by the production of toxins. Secretory immunoglobulins in gastrointestinal secretions play an important role in the colonization by intestinal flora of the newborn gut which occurs during the first hours of life. Colostral IgA agglutinate a wide range of enteric organisms which enhances their elimination by intestinal peristalsis (*Porter* et al., 1974), prevent attachment of pathogenic microorganisms (*McClelland* et al., 1972; *Williams* and *Gibbons*, 1972), lyse *E. coli* in the presence of complement and lysozyme (*Adinolfi* et al., 1966; *Bollen* et al., 1972), and enhance phagocytosis (*Girard* and *Kalbermatten*, 1970; *Wernet* et al., 1971). Furthermore secretory IgA may reduce the intestinal

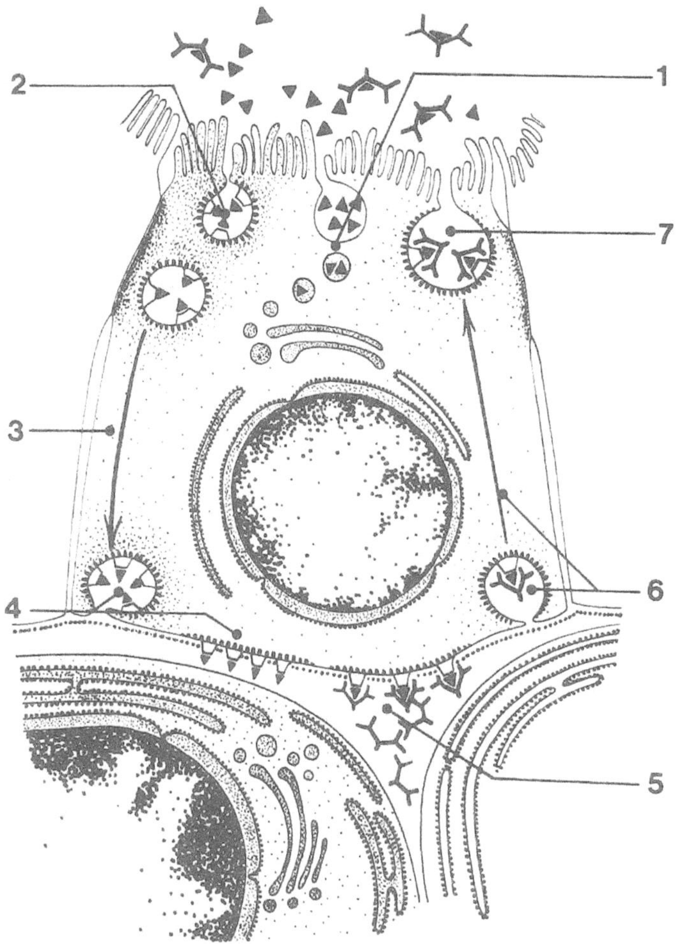

Fig. 16. Proposed mechanism for the transfer of secretory IgA: *1*, Secretory component is synthesized, processed, and secreted by the mammary epithelial cells; *2*, in the lumen SC binds to a membrane receptor (binding is favored by acidic pH); *3*, binding triggers endocytosis and transcellular transport via coated vesicles, but it has not been clearly demonstrated that coated vesicles mediate transport; *4*, upon fusion with the basolateral membrane, membrane-bound SC is exposed and *5*, can interact with dimeric IgA, which is secreted by local plasma cells; *6*, binding triggers again endocytosis and transcellular transport; fusion occurs between vesicles and the luminal plasma membrane; *7*, the complex SC − (IgA)$_2$ is released from its receptor by competition with free secretory component

absorption of food antigens responsible for allergic reactions (*Walker*, 1975). An appropriate supply of colostral secretory immunoglobulins is particularly important in the first days of life, when the secretory immune system of the newborn is still inefficient (*Mata* and *Urrutia*, 1971; *Winberg* and *Wessner*, 1971; *Hanson* and *Winberg*, 1972).

IV. Transfer of Cellular Immunity

Substantial evidence exists for the exchange of soluble, particulate, or cellular material between the mother and fetus or offspring. The extent and actual or potential consequences of antibody, antigen, and cellular traffic, either across the placenta in both directions or as a result of suckling, is of increased interest for investigators, particularly immunologists and clinicians. The hemolytic anemia resulting from Rh incompatible pregnancies is one clear example of immunologic interaction between mother and fetus. In addition transfer of viable cells via maternal milk to the neonate is more recently documented and such an instance of natural transplantation suggests important immunologic consequences for the offspring.

1. Transfer Before Birth

Due to the unique fetal maternal relationships, there is need to understand the (1) role of the trophoblastic-decidual barrier, (2) ontogeny of fetal immunocompetence, (3) maternal capacity to express immunologic reactions during pregnancy, and (4) extent and consequences of antigenic and cell exchange across the placental barrier. Since some of these subjects have been reviewed extensively (*Kirby,* 1968; *Beer* and *Billigham,* 1976), attention in this section will be directed to the (1) physiologic barrier between mother and fetus, (2) nature and degree of cell exchange before and after birth, and (3) possible adverse or beneficial effects of such cell exposure.

a) The Fetal-Maternal Barrier

With the exception of syngeneic conditions in inbred animal strains, pregnancy may be considered as the unique success of transplanting a natural F_1 hybrid. Previous attempts to demonstrate the effects of presensitizing mothers with paternal transplantation antigens or their adoptive immunization were unsuccessful despite the presence of maternal cytotoxic antibodies in the circulation. Apparently the maternal capacity to fully express immunologic reactions is modified during pregnancy. However, only limited alteration occurs in some components of maternal immunocompetence against fetal or embryonic tissue antigens of paternal origin (*Gudson,* 1976). Transplantation antigens in mice appear very early in ontogeny, and their density on cell surfaces increases until parturition. HLA antigens in man are probably present on all tissues by $\sim$ 5 months.

Fetal and maternal circulations are apparently always completely separate despite a wide range of structural variation between species (*Grosser,* 1927). As regards structure, the placental-maternal-fetal relationships vary from (1) a trophoblast apposed to the endometrium (pig, horse) to (2) an invasive penetration deep into the vascular and connective submucosal tissue (e.g., hemochorial placenta of humans and rodents). In the latter instance trophoblastic tissue is in immediate contact with maternal blood containing immunocompetent lymphoid cells. Thus, if the fetus expresses transplantation antigens and progressively develops its own immunocompetence and if the mother is recognized as being fully immunocompetent too, the trophoblastic tissue must provide an immunologic buffer zone between the host and the natural graft.

The role of the mucoprotein coating (*Kirby*, 1968) that frequently surrounds trophoblast cells is still another hypothetical barrier for protection. This fibrinoid material containing sialic acid may be considered either to promote cellular interactions between the trophoblast and endometrium or to mask transplantation antigens expressed by trophoblastic cells. Recognition of trophoblast tissue by the mother has been suggested by histology (*Beer* et al., 1971) and by observations showing variations in placental size and vascularity. Both conditions are associated with degrees of histocompatibility between mother and fetus, at least in rodents and possibly in humans. The concentration of human chorionic gonadotrophin (HCG) produced locally by trophoblast cells may also play a role in preventing maternal immune recognition, but the functional relationship between HCG and the presence of a fibrinoid coating requires further elucidation.

After extensive experiments, mechanisms of immunologic enhancement in preventing trophoblast rejection have been proposed. A specific enhancing role of maternal serum components was suggested by *Kaliss* and *Dagg* (1964). Their view assumes that antibody against transplantation antigens which is produced by the host can coat the trophoblast surface to interfere with or weaken maternal cellular immune responses and the production of effector cells (*Heron*, 1973). Prolonged acceptance of cardiac allograft from paternal or F_1 hybrid donors has been demonstrated in rats and rabbits when grafting is performed during late pregnancy or the immediate postpartum period. This acceptance could be partially abolished by preimmunizing with alloantigens before or during the course of gestation. Although evidence exists and views are based upon unrelated findings, the relative importance of mechanisms explaining persistence of the fetus allograft remains unsettled.

b) Transplacental Exchange of Cells

Although vascular anastomoses are not directly established between the maternal-fetal circulations, the placenta, especially the hemochorial type, is apparently not impermeable to cells passing across the trophoblastic barrier. In addition to cellular elements, subcellular antigens may also enter the maternal circulation.

α) Passage into the Mother

The shedding of syncytiotrophoblast from the placental villi, possibly reaching 1 g trophoblast tissue per day, has been documented in man and the chinchilla (*Douglas* et al., 1959). The syncytiotrophoblast presumably undergoes enzymatic degradation within the maternal blood, but some of it may reach the pulmonary capillaries without evidence of any local histologic host reactions. The functional significance of this trophoblastic deportation is still unresolved. Fetal red cells enter the maternal circulation in increasing numbers from the 8th week of gestation up to the time of delivery. They can be detected in maternal bloodsmears since fetal hemoglobin resists alcali or acid denaturation (technique of *Kleihauer* and *Betke*).

The passage of fetal leukocytes has been indirectly identified by the presence of leukocyte-isoagglutinins or more directly by cytogenetic analysis. *Walknowska* et al. (1969), using cytogenetic analysis, detected the presence of XY karyotypes among maternal leukocytes in the circulation of mothers who gave birth to male fetuses. Further examination using the fluorescent Y chromosome revealed the presence of these cells, first detectable at 15 weeks of gestation, in the maternal circulation throughout pregnancy and after delivery in some cases. The passage of cells across the placenta may lead to a transient spontaneous chimerism in the mother due to the persistence of fetal lymphocytes (*Gill*, 1977).

β) Passage into the Fetus

Little evidence exists concerning the incidence and extent of passage of maternal erythrocytes into the fetal circulation. As regards other cell types, malignant melanoma may metastatize across the placenta and occasionally is associated with the disseminated disease in infants.

Evidence has been presented by *Tuffrey* and co-workers (1969) suggesting a maternal-to-fetal cell passage in mice. These results, obtained with the aid of the T6 chromosome marker, could not be confirmed by other researchers and clearly from other investigations large-scale traffic of cells does not occur between the mother and fetus. Perhaps immune reactions in the developing fetus can interfere with circulating cells of maternal origin, thus impeding their detection. To test this experimental models in rats have been developed by *Beer* and *Billingham* (1973) in which active (skin grafting) or adoptive (transfer of sensitized syngeneic cells) immunization of females against paternal transplantation antigens is indeed possible. This immunization procedure performed shortly before parturition induces a high incidence of runting disease within subsequent litters. According to their interpretation, migrating lymphocytes from the maternal circulation are the cause of pathologic manifestations. *Beer* and *Billingham* also obtained similar results in mice, hamsters, guinea pigs, and rabbits. Timing the immunization proved to be an important parameter for developing runt disease.

In a more recent study (*Kramer* and *Gershwin*, 1976), the homing characteristics of 51Cr-labeled thymocytes prepared from heterozygote individuals in pregnant athymic nude mice have been studied. The small percentage of radioactivity recovered from placentas and fetuses was attributed to placental transfer of allogeneic maternal lymphocytes.

c) Potential Consequences of Cell Exposure

It is not clear if antigenic fetal material gaining access to the maternal circulation will induce an immune response. However, certain known consequences in the mother suggest prior exposure to fetal cells. For example, enlarged lymph nodes regional to the uterus have been reported during pregnancy (*Beer* et al., 1971). As regards humoral components, serum leukocyte-isoagglutinins have been detected in multiparous women (up to 25% of the women with more than three pregnancies). They show responses to HL-A fetal leukocyte antigens by antibodies mainly of the IgG type which can readily cross the placenta. Although they do not appear to frequently induce leukopenia, they may have deleterious effects during subsequent pregnancies, as suggested by the higher-than-expected incidences of congenital anomalies in offspring of mothers producing such cytotoxic antibodies (*Terasaki* et al., 1970). The mother's reactivity may be otherwise altered by additonal factors, such as elevated concentration of corticosteroids and/or estrogen and progesterone. The problems of maternal tolerance, alteration in T cell and allograft reactivities, and the demonstration of immunologic enhancement have been reviewed in detail (*Beer* and *Billingham,* 1976; *Bernard,* 1977).

As demonstrated in Rh incompatibility, the consequences to the fetus of transplacental exchange of cells may be quite deleterious (*Zipursky* et al., 1963). Hemolytic disease of the newborn, not caused by ABO blood group incompatibility, is due to the strong D antigen of the Rh blood group system. If red cells from a Rh+ fetus gain access to the circulation of a Rh− mother, they may induce the formation of IgG antibody that crosses the placenta. We should recall here the success in preventing maternal sensitization by passive administration of anti-D antibody. Evidence supporting a natural passage of leukocytes through the placenta are far from certain. However, if it were to occur early in gestation, the consequences clearly would lead to tolerance or graft-versus-host (GVH) reactions causing a variety of pathologic disorders.

To test for transplacental passage of "sensitized" maternal cells, *Stastny* (1965) mated Sprague-Dawley female rats with males of the same stock; when pregnant, they received a Lewis-strain skin allograft. When grafted with Lewis skin, the offspring showed an accelerated rejection. These findings have been subsequently confirmed using inbred pregnant Fischer female rats exposed to Lewis alloantigens. *Billingham* and his co-workers (*Beer* and *Billingham,* 1976) have performed detailed experiments during the past 10 years designed to analyze, on the one hand, the maternal induction of tolerance and, on the other, elicitation of GVH in the fetus by either passive or active immunization against histocompatibility antigens during pregnancy. They treated virgin Fischer rats with high doses of cyclophosphamide and then reconstituted and made them chimeric with adult Lewis bone marrow cells. Following mating with Fischer males, about half of the Fischer offspring died of a wasting syndrome within the 1st week of life, whereas the survivors were unresponsive to Lewis skin grafts. The wasting syndrome was characterized by pathologic manifestations usually associated with GVH disease (*Elkins,* 1971; *Grebe* and *Streilein,* 1976), such as ruffled fur, hunched position, occasional dermatitis. Histopathology revealed abnormal differentiation and hypocellularity of lymphoid tissues. The maternally induced runt disease was attributed to placental transmission of Lewis lymphoid cells into the fetal circulation. Recent results by *Milgrom* et al. (1977), who studied the fetal and neonatal mortality in rat hybrids from mother stimulated with paternal skin, further substantiate passage of sensitized cells from mother to fetus.

Such factors as genetic disparity between host and donor as well as the magnitude and timing of cell exposure during gestation are believed to influence the outcome of cell transfer to the fetus. Following the suggestion made earlier by *Clarke* and *Kirby* (1966) that antigen incompatibility might be beneficial to the offspring, *Palm* demonstrated in rats (1970) that fetuses possessing a major histoincompatibility with respect to maternal lymphoid tissues had a selective advantage prior to birth. Thus, after conducting breeding in rats, *Palm* (1974) also showed that compatibility of fetus to maternal antigens may be deleterious with respect to reproductive performance in rat colonies. Moreover, paternally derived antigens other than Ag-B (the major histocompatibility complex in rats) may play a role in the genesis of runt disease and fetal mortality, since progeny were either not obtained or failed to survive until weaning if matings involved Ag-B compatible parental strains which differed for other antigens.

The passage of maternal cells, documented at least in part in rodents, appears to produce a wide variety of responses ranging from tolerance to GVH reactions. Runting disease has been observed in deficient infants after attempts to restore their immunologic functions. Attenuated GVH reactions in mice have been reported to increase the incidence of malignant lymphoma in this species (*Cornelius,* 1972), possibly by unmasking oncogenic viruses (*Schwartz,* 1972). According to one view, transplacental cell contribution of maternal origin may influence the incidence of lymphoma in children (*Beer* and *Billingham,* 1976). As *Palm* (1970) pointed out: "The possibility that migration of significant numbers of maternal cells may be a normal feature of mammalian gestation, with beneficial or adverse consequences depending upon histocompatibility antigen interrelationships, provides a new conceptual approach for interpreting the immunological abnormalities associated with infancy."

2. Transfer After Birth

Prior to birth the placenta performs a nutritive role, which after birth is fulfilled by the mammary gland, an exocrine gland. Besides nutrition, the mammary gland participates in various functions that may be of immunologic importance to the offspring. It may (1) select from the maternal circulation and secrete certain immunoglobulins, (2) produce locally IgA antibodies, and (3) contain and release various types of viable leukocytes, including lymphocytes. Both antibodies and cells will eventually be transmitted to the infant via the colostrum and milk. As the significance of antibodies and immunoglobulins during lactation has been emphasized in preceding sections, we will review observations dealing with the presence and characterization of lymphoid cells in milk (milk cells) and their in vitro responses to mitogens and/or antigens. We will then include recent findings obtained in young rodents indicating that milk cells may actually gain access to tissues of sucklings and affect subsequent development.

a) The Cellular Components of Milk

The association of nonepithelial cells with mucous surfaces has long been recognized histologically. The relative abundance of intraepithelial leukocytes and their presence in exocrine secretions, particularly in colostrum and milk, have drawn attention to the physiologic and pathologic significance of these cells. It has been repeatedly documented that leukocytes infiltrate the mammary secretory epithelium during gestation and, to a lesser degree, after parturition. This observation is illustrated in the mammary gland of lactating mice (Fig. 17).

Following the original description by *Donné* in 1844 of colostral corpuscles (macrophages that have engulfed fat droplets), continued early findings were concerned pri-

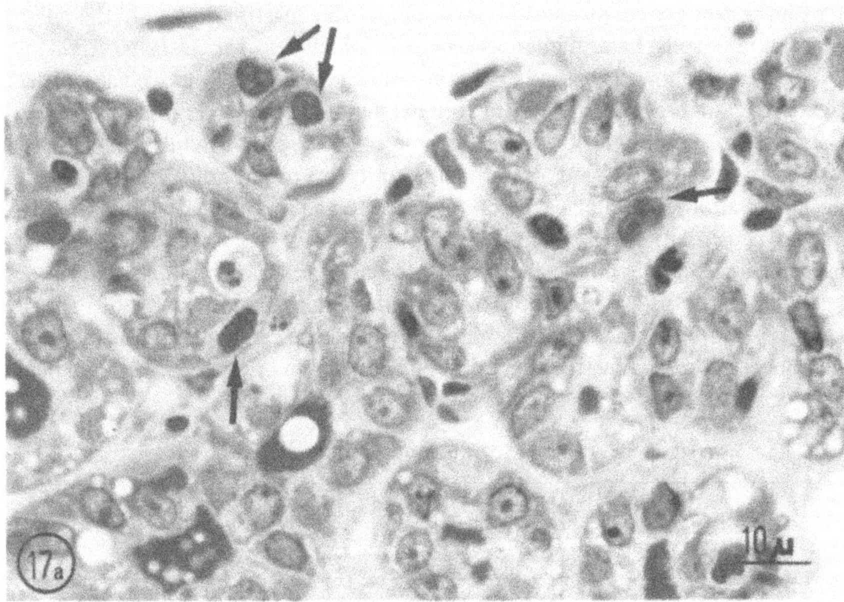

Fig. 17a and b. Light micrographs of mammary gland, 2 days post partum. **a** Presence of interepithelial lymphocytes and monocytoid cells *(arrows)* in nu/nu Balb/c mouse (nude mouse). Note the absence of plasmacytic cells in the stroma

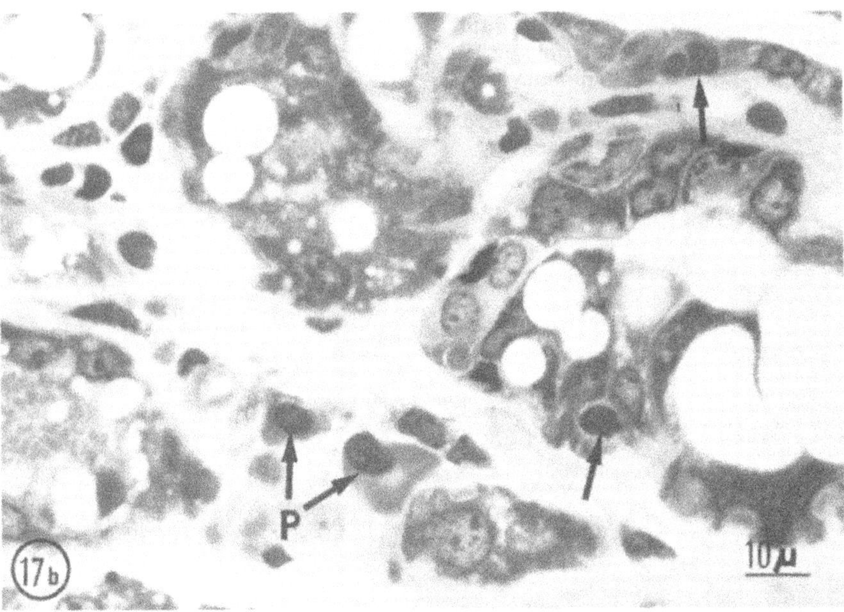

Fig 17b. Presence of interepithelial lymphoid cells in nu/+ heterozygote Balb/c mouse *(arrows)*. Presence of plasmacytic cells in the stroma *(P)*. Giemsa staining. x 1200

marily with the sanitary conditions of cow's milk, bovine mastitis, and only the relative abundance of milk cells. Later numerous morphologic studies (*Varrier-Jones*, 1924; *Duran-Jorda*, 1944) showed that milk contains intact epithelial cells as well as anucleate cell fragments, granulocytes (mostly neutrophils), lymphocytes, and monocytic cells, which phagocytize fat droplets (colostral corpuscles). The relative number of these cells, in cow milk for instance, may vary within wide limits due to physiologic (the breed, the stage of lactation), pathologic (infectious disease), and mechanical factors (milking).

The total cell counts show variability (see Table 3) at various stages of lactation, between species, and the way milk cells are enumerated. Morphologic studies show intact ultrastructural features such as endoplasmic reticulum, mitochondria and Golgi apparatus (Fig. 18). Moreover there are also numerous anucleate cell bodies with abundant endoplasmic reticulum; these are assumed to be epithelial in origin (Fig. 19). Milk leuko-

Table 3. Cell composition of milk among different mammals

Source		Total/differential cell count (range/ml) x 10^6		Authors
Human	Colostrum	Macrophages Lymphocytes Neutrophils	0.5 −3.0 0.08−0.25 0.8 −9.0	*Smith* and *Goldman*, 1968
	Colostrum	Total leukocytes Mononuclear cells Granulocytes	2.2 −4.1 1.5 −4.0 0.05−0.3	*Mohr* et al., 1970
	Colostrum	Total cell count Macrophages Lymphocytes	1.6 −2.4 1.2 −1.8 0.18−0.24	*Diaz-Jouanen* and *Williams*, 1974
	Milk	Total nucleated cells Lymphocytes	1.3 0.026−0.3	*Parmely* et al., 1976
Cow	Milk	Total cell count	0.3 −0.5	*Smith* and *Schultz*, 1977
	Milk	Total cell count Lymphocytes	0.06−0.1 160−300/ml	*Concha* et al., 1978
Rat	Milk	Total cell count	0.23−1.06	*Parmely*, 1976 (unpubl. observ.)
Mouse	Milk	Total cell count	0.26−6.0	*Head*, 1976 (unpubl. observ.)
(Swiss albino)	Milk	Total cell count	0.2 −2.0	*Humbert*, 1978 (unpubl. observ.)
Rabbit	Milk	Total cell count Macrophages Lymphocytes	0.2 −3.0 0.03−0.45 0.01−0.3	*Kraehenbuhl*, 1978 (unpubl. observ.)

cytes represent, in part, a population of peripheral blood cells which passes through the stroma and epithelial lining of the mammary gland. Conditions that affect the kinetics of their passage are not known; but recent findings suggest that some cells may represent selected populations originating from specific areas within lymphoreticular tissues (see below).

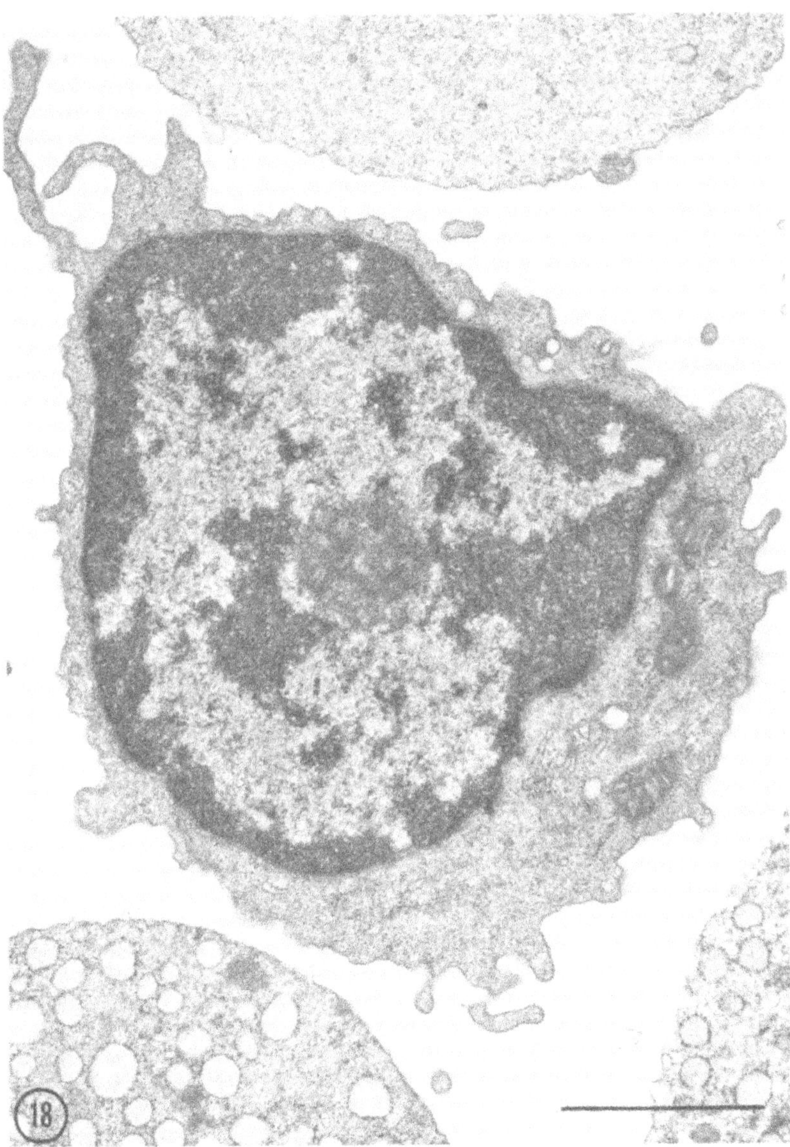

Fig. 18. High magnification electron micrograph of a typical human milk lymphocyte. Stained with uranyl acetate and lead citrate. x 30,000

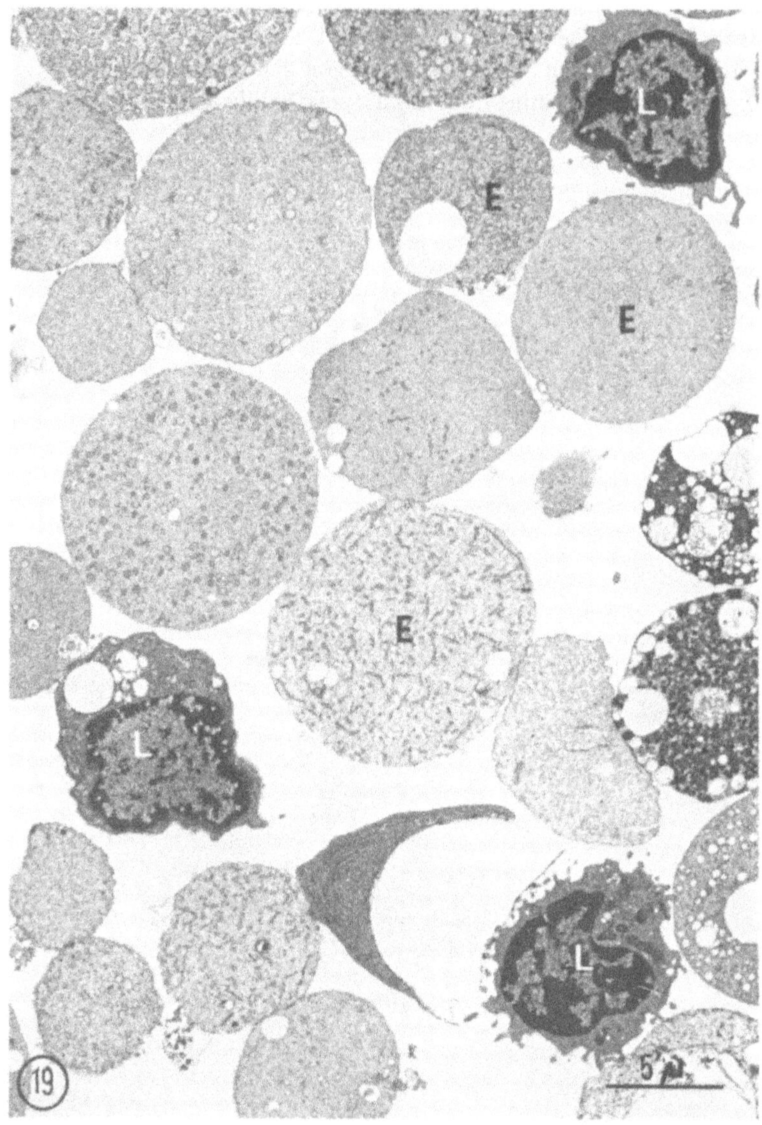

Fig. 19. Electron micrograph of human milk cells. Fresh human milk was diluted with 2 volumes of medium M_{199}, centrifuged ($100\,g$) and washed twice. The majority of the cells are epithelial *(E)*. In the field, three lymphocytes *(L)* are present, which represent $\sim 5\% - 8\%$ of the total nucleated cells. x 5000

b) Characteristics of Milk Cells in vitro

α) Monocytic Cells

Human monocytic cells in colostrum display amoeboid movements, attach to glass, and possess phagocytic activities and lysosomal structures (*Mohr* et al., 1970). The milk macrophage has even recently been considered a potential cell for immunoglobulin transport (*Pittard* et al., 1977).

β) T and B Lymphocytes

Both T and B lymphoid cells have been demonstrated in the colostrum and milk of various species, including humans. *Diaz-Jouanen* and *Williams* (1974) showed in human colostrum that ∿ 40%–50% of lymphocytes were T cells, as identified by E rosetting or anti-T cell antiserum, and 35%, B cells, as shown by the presence of surface immuno-globulins. A third category (constituting ∿ 15%) could not be defined by these methods. As regards B lymphocytes and the immunoglobulin class, half of colostrum cells were positive for surface IgA, a distribution higher than that of peripheral blood B lympho-cytes. As regards milk, results by *Smith* and *Schultz* (1977) indicate that both T and B cells are present in bovine and canine milk since they can be stimulated by T and B mitogens. Using more direct quantitation, *Concha* et al. (1978) reported proportions of T and B lymphocytes in bovine milk, 45% and 20%, respectively, similar to distribu-tion in peripheral blood. They also detected a third lymphocyte population, not defin-able with T and B reagents.

γ) In vitro Tests

Milk lymphoid cells can be purified and tested in the presence of mitogens or antigens in vitro. Human colostral lymphocytes can undergo blast transformation when exposed to phytohemagglutinin (PHA) (*Smith* and *Goldman,* 1968) and pokeweed mitogen (PWM) (*Diaz-Jouanen* and *Williams*, 1974), but the proliferative responses were weaker than those obtained with peripheral blood lymphocytes. This hyporesponsiveness has been subsequently confirmed by *Parmely* et al. (1976) using milk lymphocytes that function both as stimulator and responder cells in mixed lymphocyte cultures (MLC). Similar to mitogen responsiveness, MLC responses were lower than those of blood lymphocytes from the same donors. In additional experiments, milk lymphocytes were unresponsive to antigenic challenge with *Candida albicans,* whereas the K1 cap-sular antigen of *E. coli* induced proliferation of milk lymphocytes, but failed to stim-ulate blood lymphocytes. The authors assumed that differential reactivities may re-flect local accumulations of selected lymphocytes in the mammary gland (*Parmely* et al., 1977). To support this view, the possibility that cell-mediated immunity could be acquired by breast-feeding has already been evaluated by *Mohr* in 1973 and other results by *Schlesinger* and *Covelli* (1977) suggested, indeed, that breast-fed infants may passively acquire T cell responsiveness to specific antigens by ingestion of milk.

Bovine and canine milk contain lymphocytes responsive to PHA, concanavalin A (ConA), PWM, and lipopolysaccharide (LPS) (*Smith* and *Schultz*, 1977). Individual responses of milk lymphoid cells were also not identical to proliferation index obtained using blood lymphocytes. Moreover specifically sensitized animals were shown to possess antigen-sensitive cells in milk. Specific anti-*E. coli* plaque-forming cells were demonstrable following oral immunization of the mother, although no systemic antibody response was detectable (*Goldblum* et al., 1975). Thus antibody-producing cells present in colostrum may originate within gut-associated lymphoid tissue (GALT) and then migrate to the breast.

δ) Epithelial Cells

In addition to cells associated with immunity, epithelial cells have been grown in vitro from human early-lactation milk to provide a source of normal mammary epithelium for comparative experiments. These cells were used to compare the behavior of hyperplastic and malignant cells obtained from breast tumors (*Taylor-Papadimitriou* et al., 1977). Morphologic and growth criteria identified epithelial-like colonies growing in vitro, but as a functional test the actual demonstration of milk-protein synthesis by these cells has not yet been provided.

c) Evidence of Access of Milk Cells to the Neonate

During suckling the gastrointestinal tract of infants is exposed to maternal milk proteins and allogeneic cells. Since the transfer of maternal immunoglobulins has been discussed in the preceding sections, in this and in the following section we will provide some aspects of current investigations relative to the infant's exposure to maternal cells. This exposure could represent a new aspect of maternal-neonatal relationships. Transmission of cells should be mostly dependent on their survival within the infant's alimentary tract. After histologic analysis of gastric content in rodents at day 2 after birth, macrophages, neutrophils, lymphoid and plasmacytic cell types were localized (*Head* et al., 1977). This relative abundance of cells suggests that conditions in the rodent stomach (peptic activity, pH), at least at an early age, are not incompatible with the cell survival. The ability of cells to move through epithelial layers in newborn rabbits is supported by the observations of *Kmetz* et al. (1970), demonstrating that their activities are not restricted since trypan-blue labeled bovine leukocytes inoculated orally into colostrum-deprived rabbits have been shown to invade and penetrate the mucosa of the upper digestive tract.

It has been suggested that milk from heterozygous nu/+ mothers is the source of small numbers of circulating theta-alloantigen bearing cells detected in nude mice. A recent report by *Hale* et al. (1976) refers to the existence of T cell helper activity, which may be transmitted during lactation: nude mice born from and suckled by homozygous nude mothers exhibited a plaque-forming cell response to SRBC which was tenfold less than that of nudes raised by heterozygous mothers.

d) Possible Significance of Cell Transmission via Milk

α) Protective Responses

Milk macrophages may participate in the protection of neonates by functioning in the gastrointestinal tract. A transient daily hypoxia in the newborn rat may induce a form of necrotizing enterocolitis which has been proposed as a model of the disease in infants. *Pitt* et al. (1974) demonstrated in the rat that protection against the disease may be accomplished through breast-feeding. This beneficial effect was dependent on the presence of viable macrophages derived from milk.

β) Occurrence of Runting Disease

Despite the presence of milk cells, experimental evidence for the possible roles is mostly indirect. *Head* and *Beer* (1978) suggest that milk cells may express selected maternal immune reactivities and, in specific strain combinations, manifest competence in the suckling. Their original observation (reviewed by *Beer* and *Billingham,* 1976) showed in rats that milk from allogeneic foster mothers (Lewis strain) may modify the reactivity of the neonate (Fischer strain) to Lewis skin allografts and, in some cases ($\sim$ 30% of the offspring) cause the development of GVH disease. These results imply that cells are transferred into and proliferate in tissues of the offspring. *Uphoff* (1977), using certain strain combinations, also observed runting disease in mice among suckling hybrids which was attributable to transfer of maternal leukocytes. Neonates were normal at birth and required a week or more to develop symptoms, but they recovered after removal from nursing females. In contrast, *Trentin* et al. (1977), using the mouse T6 chromosome marker, were unable to detect mitotic maternal cells in the bone marrow, spleen, thymus, and mesenteric lymph nodes of F1 hybrid mice after 14 days or 21 days of suckling. Similarly, *Silvers* and *Poole* (1975) failed to find evidence that foster nursing can alter the survival or immune competence of offsprings in several strains of mice and rats. Further studies are certainly required to explain these contradictory results and to substantiate more directly the incorporation of milk cells into the tissues of sucklings.

To test for the potential effect of T cell transfer, *Head* (1977) reported that milk from allogeneic C57 foster mothers may affect the development of BALB/c newborn nude mice. Fostered nudes exhibited erythrodermia, 50% died by day 15, and none lived longer than 35 days. In contrast, using a similar allogeneic strain combination of nude mouse (colony at the Ludwig Institute for Cancer Research in Lausanne), we were unable to confirm this mortality rate and timing among the fostered nude offspring (*Merenda* and *Sordat,* 1977, unpublished observation). From a total of 16 nude BALB/c neonates, transferred to C57 nu/+ females from the day of birth, all were alive at day 90 after birth. Genetic aspects in the nude gene transfer experiments as well as maintenance conditions might influence the outcome of results among nude mice colonies.

V. Conclusions

Transfer of maternal immunity is of great importance for the subsequent survival of the young mammal when suddenly exposed to an aggressive environment after birth. Transfer, which includes secretory, humoral, and cellular immunity, may occur before and/or after birth, depending on the species.

Transfer of secretory immunity from the mother to the young constitutes a first line of defense because the newborn's mucous surfaces are the first sites to experience major antigenic challenge. Protection is ensured by a special class of immunoglobulins, i.e., secretory immunoglobulins, which are secreted into milk. These immunoglobulins possess specificities against microorganisms, pathogens, or antigens present in the lumen of the mother's intestinal, respiratory, and urogenital tracts. The mechanism of secretion into milk is poorly understood; however, recent immunocytochemical and kinetic studies suggest that epithelial translocation occurs by adsorptive pinocytosis mediated by a glycoprotein synthesized in epithelium.

A second line of defense is provided by maternal humoral antibodies, which confer immunity and reflect the maternal immunologic experience against most infecting agents. Transfer occurs in primates and lagomorphs exclusively before birth via fetal membranes, but is restricted to a few hours after birth in ungulates and is mediated by milk; transmission occurs before and after birth in rodents and carnivores. All cells involved in translocation of humoral antibodies (yolk-sac splanchnopleure, hemochorial placenta, jejunal and duodenal absorptive cells, mammary gland cells) share a common and saturable mechanism mediated by specific recognition sites, i.e., Fc receptors, restricted to IgG class and subclasses.

Finally, maternal immunocompetent cells may also be transmitted to the young before birth; no direct evidence favors a transfer of maternal immunocompetent cells, although a degree of cell traffic has been established. B and T lymphocytes as well as macrophages have been found in milk after birth. No direct evidence shows that lymphocytes enter the newborn's circulation; thus their role in mediating protection is poorly understood and open to investigations.

Acknowledgment: We wish to thank E.L. Cooper, on sabbatical leave (University of California, Los Angeles) at the Ludwig Institute for Cancer Research, Unit of Cancer Immunology, for kindly revising the manuscript and Marie-Claude Knecht for typing it.

This work was supported by Swiss National Science Foundation, grants 3.122-0-77 and 3—136-077.

References

Adinolfi, M., Glynn, A.A., Lindsay, M., Milne, C.M.: Serological properties of γ-A antibodies to *Escherichia coli* present in human colostrum. Immunology *10*, 517—521 (1966)

Ahlstedt, S., Carlsson, B., Hanson, L.A., Goldblum, R.M.: Antibody production by human colostral cells. I. Immunoglobulin class, specificity and quantity. Scan. J. Immunol. *4*, 535 (1975)

Allardyce, R.A., Shearman, D.J.C., McClelland, D.B.L., Marwick, K., Simpson, A.J., Laidlaw, R.B.: Appearance of specific colostrum antibodies after clinical infection with *Salmonella typhimurium*. Brit. med. J. *1974 III*, 307

Allen, W.D., Porter, P.: The relative distribution of IgM and IgA cells in intestinal mucosa and lymphoid tissues of the young unweaned pig and their significance in ontogenesis of secretory immunity. Immunology *24*, 493–501 (1973)

Amoroso, E.C.: Placentation. In: Marshall's physiology of reproduction, 3rd ed. A.S. Parkes (ed.), Vol. 2. London: Longmans & Green 1952

Anderson, R.G.W., Goldstein, J.L., Brown, M.S.: Localization of flow density lipoprotein receptors on plasma membrane of normal human fibroblasts and their absence in cells from a familial hypersholesterolemia homozygote. Proc. Natl. Acad. Sci. USA *23*, 2434–2438 (1976)

Anderson, R.G.W., Brown, M., Goldstein, J.L.: Role of the coated endocytic vesicle in the uptake of receptor bound low density lipoprotein in human fibroblasts. Cell *10*, 351–364 (1977)

Arnold, R.R., Mestecky, J., McGhee, J.R.: Naturally occurring secretory immunoglobulin A antibodies to *Streptococcus mutans* in human colostrum and saliva. Infect. Immun. *14*, 355 (1976)

Asplund, J.M., Grummer, R.H., Philips, P.H.: Absorption of colostral γ-globulins and insulin by the newborn pig. J. Anim. Sci. *21*, 412–413 (1962)

Balconi, I.R., Lecce, J.G.: Intestinal absorption of homologous lactic dehydrogenase isoenzymes by the neonatal pig. J. Nutr. *88*, 233–238 (1966)

Barnes, J.M.: Antitoxin transfer from mother to foetus in the guinea pig. J. Pathol. Bacterial. *77*, 371–380 (1959)

Beer, A.E., Billingham, R.E.: Maternally acquired runt disease. Science *179*, 240–243 (1973)

Beer, A.E., Billingham, R.E.: The immunobiology of mammalian reproduction. Englewood Cliffs, N.J.: Prentice Hall 1976

Beer, A.E., Billingham, R.E., Hoerr, R.A.: Elicitation and expression of transplantation immunity in the uterus. Transplant. Proc. *3*, 609–611 (1971)

Bellanti, J.A., Jurlado, R.C.: Immunology and resistance to infection. In: Infectious diseases of the fetus and newborn infants. Remington, R.E., Klein, A.S. (eds.), pp. 33–20. Philadelphia: Saunders 1976

Bernard, O.: Possible protecting role of maternal immunoglobulins on embryonic development in mammals. Immunogenetics *5*, 1–15 (1977)

Besredka, A.: Local immunization. Baltimore: Williams & Wilkins 1927

Bienenstock, J., Johnson, N., Perrey, D.Y.E.: Bronchial lymphoid tissue. I. Morphological characteristics. Lab. Invest. *28*, 686–692 (1973a)

Bienenstock, J., Johnson, N., Perey, D.Y.E.: Bronchial lymphoid tissue. II. Functional characteristics. Lab. Invest. *28*, 693–695 (1973b)

Bienenstock, J., Rudzik, O., Clancy, R.L., Perey, D.Y.E.: Bronchial lymphoid tissue. Adv. Exp. Med. Biol. *45*, 47–58 (1974)

Bohl, E.H., Saif, L.J., Gupta, R.K.P., Frederick, G.T.: Secretory antibodies in milk of swine against transmissible gastroenteritis virus. Adv. Exp. Med. Biol. *45*, 337 (1974)

Bollen, J.J., Rogers, H.J., Loigh, H.: Iron Binding protein in milk and resistance to *Escherichia coli* infection in infants. Brit. med. J. *1972 I*, 69–75

Borthistle, B.K., Kubo, R.T., Brown, W.R., Grey, H.M.: Studies on receptors for IgG on epithelial cells of the rat intestine. J. Immunol. *119*, 471–476 (1977)

Brambell, F.W.R.: The transmission of immunity from mother to young and the catabolism of immunoglobulins. Lancet *1966 II*, 1087–1093

Brambell, F.W.R.: The transmission of passive immunity from the mother to young. Frontiers of Biology. Vol. 18, pp. 1–385. Amsterdam, London: North Holland 1970

Brambell, F.W.R., Hemmings, W.A., Rowlands, W.T.: The passage of antibodies from the maternal circulation into the embryo in rabbits. Proc. R. Soc. Lond. (Biol.) *135*, 390–403 (1948)

Brambell, F.W.R., Hemmings, W.A., Oakley, C.L., Porter, R.R.: The relative transmission of the fractions of papain hydrolyzed homologous γ-globulin from the uterine cavity to the foetal circulation in the rabbit. Proc. R. Soc. Lond. (Biol.) *151*, 478–482 (1960)

Brandon, M.R.: Selective transfer and catabolism of IgG in the ruminant. In: Maternofoetal transmission of immunoglobulins. Hemmings, W.A. (ed.). London, New York: Cambridge University Press 1976

Brandon, M.R., Watson, D.L., Lascelles, A.K.: The mechanism of transfer of immunoglobulins into mammary secretion of cows. Aust. J. Exp. Biol. Med. Sci. *49*, 613–624 (1971)

Brandtzaeg, P.: Mucosal and glandular distribution of immunoglobulin components: differential localization of free and bound SC in secretory epithelial cells. J. Immunol. *112*, 1553–1563 (1974)

Brandtzaeg, P.: Immunohistochemical studies on various aspects of glandular immunoglobulin transport in man. In: Histochemistry of secretory processes. Garrett, J.R., Harrison, J.-D., Stoward, P.J. (eds.), pp. 73–92. London: Chapman & Hall 1977

Burrows, W., Harens, I.: Studies of immunity of asiatic cholera. V. The absorption of immune globulin from the bowel and its excretion in the urine and feces of experimental animals and human volonteers. J. Infect. Dis. *82*, 231 (1948)

Carr, M.C., Stiles, D.P., Fundenberg, H.H.: Dissociation of responses to phytohaemagglutinin and adult allogeneic lymphocytes in human foetal lymphoid tissues. Nature New Biol. *241*, 279–281 (1973)

Catalano, L.W., Sever, J.L.: The role of viruses as causes of congenital defects. Annu. Rev. Microbiol. *25*, 255–282 (1971)

Cebra, J.J., Robins, J.B.: Gamma A-immunoglobulin from rabbit colostrum. J. Immunol. *97*, 12–24 (1966)

Cebra, J.J., Small, P.A.: Polypeptide chain structure of rabbit immunoglobulins. 3. Secretory gamma A-immunoglobulin from colostrum. Biochemistry *6*, 503–512 (1967)

Cebra, J.J., Craig, S.W., Jones, P.P.: Natural History of the lymphocytes responsible for the secretory immunological response. In: The role of immunological factors in infections, allergic and autoimmune processes. Beers, R.F., Bassett, E.G. (eds.), pp. 403–417. New York: Raven 1976

Clarke, B., Kirby, D.R.S.: Maintenance of histocompatibility polymorphism. Nature *211*, 999-1000 (1966)

Concha, C., Holmberg, O., Morein, B.: Proportion of B- and T-lymphocytes in normal bovine milk. J. Dairy Res. *45* (1978) (in press)

Cornelius, E.A.: Induction of both host and donor-type tumors as a result of the graft-versus-host reaction. Transplantation *13*, 589–591 (1972)

Cottier, H., Schaffner, Th., Chanana, A.D., Joel, D.D., Sordat, B., Bryant, B.J., Hess, M.W.: Species differences in the effectiveness of intestinal barriers against penetration of inert particulates and bacteria. In: Gram-negative bacterial infections and mode of endoxin actions. Pathophysiological, Immunolgical and clinical aspects. Urbaschek, B., Urbaschek, R., Neter, E. (eds.) New York: Springer 1975

Crabbé, P.A.: Signification du tissue lymphoide des muqueuses digestives. Brussels: Arscia, Paris: Maloine 1967

Cramer, D.V., Kunz, H.W., Gill, Th.H.: Immunologic sensitization prior to birth. Am. J. Obstet. Gynecol. *120*, 431–439 (1974)

Cunningham, B.A., Gottlieb, P.D., Pflumm, M.N., Edelman, G.M.: Immunoglobulin structure: diversity, gene duplication and domains. In: Progress in immunology. Amos, B. (ed.), pp. 3–24. New York: Academic Press 1971

Diaz-Jouanen, E., Williams, R.C.: T and B lymphocytes in human colostrum. Clin. Immunol. Immunopathol. *3*, 248–255 (1974)

Dixon, F.J., Weigle, W.O., Vasquez, Y.Y.: Metabolism and mammary secretion of serum proteins in the cow. Lab. Invest. *10*, 216–237 (1961)

Donné, A.: Cours de Microscopie. Vol.1 and Atlas No. 1. Paris: Baillière 1844

Douglas, G.W., Thomas, L., Carr, M., Cullen, N.M., Morris, R.: Trophoblast in the circulating blood during pregnancy. Am. J. Obstet. Gynecol. *78*, 960–969 (1959)

Duran-Jorda, F.: Cell contents of milk. Nature *154*, 704–705 (1944)

Elkins, W.L.: Cellular immunology and the pathogenesis of graft-versus-host reactions. Prog. Allergy *15*, 78–187 (1971)

Franck, F., Rika, I.: Purification and structural characterization of 7S γ-globulin in newborn pigs. Immunochemistry *1*, 49–63 (1964)

Garrard, J.W.: Breast-feeding: second thoughts. Pediatrics *54*, 757–764 (1974)

Gill III, T.J.: Chimerism in humans. Transplant. Proc. *IX/2*, 1423–1431 (1977)

Girard, J.P., Kalbermatten, A.: Antibody activity in human duodenal fluid. Eur. J. Clin. Invest. *1*, 188 (1970)

Gitlin, B., Biasucci, A.: Development of IgG, IgA, IgM, beta 1_C, beta 1_A, C_1 esterase inhibitor, ceruloplasmin, transferrin, hemopexin, haptoglobin, fibrinogen, plasminogen, alpha-1-antitrypsin, mucoid beta-lipoprotein, alpha-2-macroglobulin and prealbumin in the human conceptus. J. Clin. Invest. *48*, 1433–1446 (1969)

Gitlin, D., Kumate, J., Urrusti, J., Morates, C.: The selectivity of the human placenta in the transfer of plasma proteins from mother to foetus. J. Clin. Invest. *43*, 1938–1951 (1964a)

Gitlin, D., Kumate, J., Urrusti, J., Morates, C.: Selective and directional transfer of 7S γ2-globulin across the human placenta. Nature *203*, 86 (1964b)

Gitlin, Y.D., Gitlin, Y.I., Gitlin, D.: Selective transfer of plasma proteins across mammary gland in lactating mouse. Am. J. Physiol. *230*, 1594–1602 (1976)

Goldblum, R.M., Ahlstedt, S., Carlson, B.: Antibody production in human colostrum cells. Pediatr. Res. *9*, 336 (1975)

Goldman, A.S., Smith, C.W.: Host resistance factors in human milk. J. Pediatr. *82*, 1082–1090 (1973)

Grebe, S.C., Streilein, J.W.: Graft-versus-host reactions: a review. Adv. Immunol. *22*, 119–222 (1976)

Grosser, O.: Vergleichende Anatomie und Entwicklungsgeschichte der Eihaut und Plazenta. Vienna: Braumüller 1909

Grosser, O.: Frühentwicklung, Eihautbildung und Plazentation der Menschen und der Säugetiere. Munich: Bergmann 1927

Guinchat, J.J., Gothefors, L., Hanson, L., Winbergs, A.: Antibodies in human milk against *E. coli* of the serogroups most commonly found in neonatal infections. Acta Paediatr. (Upsala) *61*, 587–590 (1972)

Gusdon, J.P.: Maternal immune responses in pregnancy. In: Immunology of human reproduction. Scott, J.S., Jones, W.R. (eds.), pp. 103–125. London: Academic Press 1976

Guy-Grand, D., Griscelli, C., Vassali, P.: The gut associated lymphoid system: nature and properties of the large dividing cells. Eur. J. Immunol. *4*, 435–447 (1974)

Guyer, R.L., Koshland, M.E., Knopf, I.: Immunoglobulin binding by mouse intestinal epithelial cell receptors. J. Immunol. *117*, 587 (1976)

Hale, M.L., Hanna, E.E., Hansen, C.T.: Nude mice from homozygous nude parents show smaller PFC responses to sheep erythrocytes than nude mice from heterozygous mothers. Nature *260*, 44–45 (1976)

Hanson, L.A., Winberg, J.: Breast milk and defense against infection in the newborn. Arch. Dis. Child. *47*, 845 (1972)

Hanson, L.A., Ahlstedt, S., Carlsson, B., Kaigser, B., Svanborg Eden, C.: Recent developments in local immunity against bacteria. Acta Pathol. Microbiol. Scand. (1978) (in press)

Head, J.R., Beer, A.E.: The immunologic role of viable leukocytic cells in mammary exosecretions. In: Lactation. Larson, B.L., Smith, V.R. (eds.), Vol. IV, pp. 337–364. New York: Academic Press 1978

Head, J.R., Beer, A.E., Billingham, R.E.: Significance of the cellular component of the maternal immunologic endowment in milk. Transplant. Proc. 9, 1465–1471 (1977)

Heremans, J.F., Vaerman, J.P.: Biological significance of IgA antibodies in serum and secretions. Prog. Immunol. 1, 875–859 (1971)

Heremans, J.F., Heremans, M.-Th., Schultze, H.E.: Isolation and description of a few properties of the γ2A-globulin of human serum. Protides. Biol. Fluids 6, 166 (1958)

Heron, J.: Is transplantation tolerance in the rat serum-mediated? Transplantation 15, 534–539 (1973)

Hess, M.W., Cottier, H., Sordat, B., Joel, D.D., Chanana, A.D.: The intestinal barrier to bacterial invasion. In: "Non specific" factors influencing host resistance. Braun, W., Ungar, J. (eds.), pp. 447–451. Basel: Karger 1973

Hill, J.P.: The developmental history of the primates. Philos. Trans. R.Soc. B 221, 45–178 (1932)

Hoerlein, A.B.: The influence of colostrum on antibody response in baby pigs. J. Immunol. 78, 112–117 (1957)

Humbert, J., Kraehenbuhl, J.P., Bron, C.: Unpublished results, 1978

Hurlimann, J.: Immunoglobulin synthesis and transport by human salivary glands. Immunological mechanisms of the mucous membrane. Curr. Top. Pathol. 55, 69–108 (1971)

Hurlimann, J., Lichaa, M.: Local immunization in the mammary glands of the rabbit. J. Immunol. 116, 1295–1301 (1976)

Hyvarinen, M., Zeltzer, P., Oh, W., Stiehm, R.: Influence of gestational age on serum levels of α-1 fetoprotein, IgG and albumin in newborn infants. J. Pediatr. 82, 430 (1973)

Joel, D.D., Sordat, B., Hess, M.W., Cottier, H.: Uptake and retention of particles from the intestine by Peyer's patches in mice. Experientia 26, 694 (1970)

Jones, E.A., Waldman, T.A.: The mechanism of intestinal uptake and transcellular transport of IgG in the neonatal rat. J. Clin. Invest. 51, 2916 (1972)

Jordan, S.M., Morgan, E.H.: Albumin, transferrin and gamma globulin metabolism during lactation in the rat. Q. J. Exp. Physiol. 52, 422–429 (1967)

Kaliss, N., Dagg, M.K.: Immune response engendered in mice by multiparity. Transplantation 2, 416–425 (1964)

Kehoe, J.M., Fougereau, M.: Immunoglobulin peptide with complement fixing activity. Nature 224, 1212–1213 (1969)

Kirby, D.R.S.: Immunological aspects of pregnancy. Adv. Reprod. Physiol. 3, 34–79 (1968)

Kmetz, M., Dunne, H.W., Schultz, R.D.: Leukocytes as carriers in the transmission of bovine leukemia invasion of the digestive tract of the newborn by ingested cultured leukocytes. Am. J. Vet. Res. 31, 637–641 (1970)

Kraehenbuhl, J.P.: Dispersed mammary gland epithelial cells. I. Isolation and separation procedures. J. Cell Biol. 72, 390–405 (1977)

Kraehenbuhl, J.P., Campiche, M.A.: Early stages of intestinal absorption of specific antibodies in the newborn. An ultrastructural cytochemical and immunological study in the pig, rat and rabbit. J. Cell Biol. 42, 345–365 (1969)

Kraehenbuhl, J.P., Racine, L., Galardy, R.E.: Localization of secretory IgA, secretory component and α chain in the mammary gland of lactating rabbits by immunoelectron microscopy. Ann. N.Y. Acad. Sci. 254, 190–202 (1975)

Kraehenbuhl, J.P., Suard, Y., Kuhn, L.: Specific uptake of secretory immunoglobulins by mammary epithelial cells. (Abstract Am. Soc. Cell Biol.) J. Cell Biol. 75, ST 108 (1977)

Kramer, M.H., Gershwin, M.E.: Immune competency of nude mice bred from homozygous and heterozygous mothers. Transplantation 22, 539–544 (1976)

Kruger, G., Stoppelman, H.J.: Postnatal development of lymph nodes in mice after prenatal antigenic stimulation. Z. Immunitätsforsch. *142*, 115–121 (1971)

Kulungara, A.C., Schechtmann, A.M.: Passage of heterologous serum proteins from mother into fetal compartments in the rabbit. Am. J. Physiol. *203*, 1071–1080 (1962)

Lamm, M.E.: Cellular aspects of immunoglobulin A. Adv. Immunol. *22*, 233 (1976)

Larsen, J.F.: Electron microscopy of the chorioallantoic placenta of the rabbit. Am. J. Anat. *1112*, 269–284 (1962)

Larsen, L.F.: Electron microscopy of the chorioallantoic placenta of the rabbit. 2. The decidua and the maternal vessels. J. Ultrastruct. Res. *8*, 327–338 (1963)

Larsen, J.F., Davies, J.: The paraplacental chorion and accessory fetal membranes of the rabbit. Histology and electron microscopy. Anat. Rec. *143*, 27–46 (1962)

Lecce, J.G., Matrone, G.: Porcine neonatal nutrition: the effect of diet on blood serum proteins and performance of the baby pig. J. Nutr. *70*, 13–20 (1960)

Lecce, J.G., Matrone, G., Morgan, D.O.: Porcine neonatal nutrition: absorption of un-altered non porcine proteins and polyvinyl pyrrolidone from the gut of piglets and the subsequent effect on the maturation of the serum protein profile. J. Nutr. *73*, 151–166 (1961)

Lecce, J.G., Morgan, D.O., Matrone, G.: Effect of feeding colostral and milk components on the cessation of intestinal absorption of large molecules (closure) in neonatal pigs. J. Nutr. *84*, 43–48 (1964)

Linden, L.D., Roth, T.F.: IgG receptors on fetal chick yolk sac. *33*, 317–328 (1978)

Mata, L.J., Urrutia, J.H.: Intestinal colonization of breastfed children in a rural area of low socio-economic level. Ann. N.Y. Acad. Sci. *176*, 93–109 (1971)

Matre, R.: Similarities of Fcγ receptors on trophoblasts and placental endothelial cells. Scand. J. Immunol. *6*, 953–958 (1977)

Matre, R., Tunder, O., Enderssen, C.: Fc receptors in human placenta. Scand. J. Imm Immunol. *4*, 741 (1975)

McClelland, D.B.L., Samson, R.R., Parkin, D.M., Shearman, D.J.C.: Bacterial agglutination studies with secretory IgA prepared from human gastrointestinal secretions and colostrum. Gut *13*, 450 (1972)

McGhee, J.R., Michalek, S.M., Ghauta, V.K.: Rat immunoglobulins in serum and secretions: purification of rat IgM, IgA and IgG and their quantitation in serum, colostrum, milk and saliva. Immunochemistry *12*, 817–823 (1975)

McNabb, T., Kuh, T.Y., Dorrington, K.J., Painter, R.H.: Structure and function of immunoglobulin domains. V. Binding of immunoglobulin G and fragments to placental membrane preparations. J. Immunol. *117*, 882–888 (1975)

Merenda, C., Sordat, B.: Unpublished results, 1977

Mestecky, J., Schrohenloher, R., Kulhavy, R., Wright, J.P., Tomana, M.: Site of J chain attachment to human polymeric IgA. Proc. Natl. Acad. Sci. USA *71*, 544–549 (1974)

Milgrom, F., Comini-Andrada, E., Chaudhry, A.P.: Fetal and neonatal fatality in rat hybrids from mothers stimulated with paternal skin. Transplant. Proc. *9*, 1409–1415 (1977)

Mohr, J.A.: The possible induction and/or acquisition of cellular hypersensibility associated with ingestion of colostrum. J. Pediatr. *82*, 1062–1064 (1973)

Mohr, J.A., Leu, R., Mabry, W.: Colostral leukocytes. J. Surg. Oncol. *2*, 163–167 (1970)

Montgomery, P.C., Cohn, J., Lolly, E.T.: The induction and characterization of secretory antibodies. Adv. Exp. Med. Biol. *45*, 453 (1974)

Morgan, D.O., Lecce, J.G.: Electrophoretic and immunoelectrophoretic analysis of the proteins in the sow's mammary secretions throughout lactation. Res. Vet. Sci. *5*, 332–339 (1964)

Morris, I.G.: Intestinal transmission of IgG subclasses in suckling rats. In: Maternofoetal transmission of immunoglobulins. Hemmings, W.A. (ed.), pp. 341–357. London, New York: Cambridge University Press 1976

154

Morris, B., Morris, R.: Fractionation studies of the absorption of labelled immunoglobulin G by the gut of young rats. J. Physiol. *265*, 429–442 (1977a)

Morris, B., Morris, R.: The digestion and transmission of labelled immunoglobulin G
by enterocytes of the proximal and distal regions of the small intestine of young
rats. J. Physiol. *273*, 427–442 (1977b)

Moskalewski, S., Ptak, W., Czannik, Z.: Demonstration of cells with IgG receptors in
human placenta. Biol. Neonate *26*, 268 (1975)

Mossman, H.W.: The rabbit placenta and the problem of placental transmission. Am.J.
Anat. *37*, 433–437 (1926)

Mossman, H.W.: Comparative morphogenesis of the fetal membranes and accessory
uterine structure. Contrib. Embryol. *479*, 129–246 (1937)

Moxon, L.A., Wild, A.E.: Localization of proteins in coated micropinocytotic vesicles
during transport across rabbit yolk sac endoderm. Cell Tissue Res. *171*, 175–193
(1976)

Müller-Eberhard, J.J.: Complement. Annu. Rev. Biochem. *38*, 389–414 (1969)

Needham, J.: Chemical Embryology. Vol. 3. Biochemistry of the placental barrier.
Cambridge: Cambridge University Press 1931

Nelson, J.B.: The maternal transmission of vaccinal immunity in swine. J. Exp. Med.
56, 835–840 (1932)

Newcomb, R.W., Normansell, D., Stanworth, D.R.: A structural study of human exocrine IgA globulin. J. Immunol. *101*, 905–914 (1968)

Ockleford, C.D., Whyte, A.: Differentiated regions of human placental cell surface
associated with exchange of materials between maternal and fetal blood: coated
vesicles. J. Cell Sci. *25*, 293–312 (1977)

Ogra, S.S., Weintraub, D., Ogra, P.L.: Immunologic aspects of human colostrum and
milk. III. Fate and absorption of cellular and soluble components in the gastrointestinal tract of the newborn. J. Immunol. *119*, 245–248 (1977)

Owen, R.L., Jones, A.L.: Epithelial cell specialization within human Peyer's patches:
An ultrastructural study of intestinal lymphoid follicles. Gastroenterology *66*,
189–199 (1974)

Palm, J.: Maternal-fetal interactions and histocompatibility antigen polymorphisms.
Transplant. Proc. *2*, 162–173 (1970)

Palm, J.: Maternal-fetal histocompatibility in rats: an escape from adversity. Cancer
Res. *34*, 2061–2065 (1974)

Parkhouse, P.M.E., Della Corte, E.: Control of IgM biosynthesis. In: The role of
immunological factors in infections, allergic and autoimmune processes. Beers, R.F.,
Bassetts, E.G. (eds.). New York: Rave 1976

Parmely, M.J., Beer, A.E., Billingham, R.E.: *In vitro* studies on the T-lymphocyte
population of human milk. J. Exp. Med. *144*, 358–370 (1976)

Parmely, M.J., Reath, D.B., Beer, A.E., Billingham, R.E.: Cellular immune responses of
human milk T lymphocytes to certain environmental antigens. Transplant. Proc. *9*,
1477–1483 (1977)

Pearse, B.M.F.: Coated vesicles from pig brain: purification and biochemical characterization. J. Mol. Biol. *97*, 93–98 (1975)

Pearse, B.M.F.: Clathrin, a unique protein associated with intracellular transfer of
membrane by coated vesicles. Proc. Natl. Acad. Sci. USA *13*, 1255 (1976)

Pierce, A.E., Risdall, P.C., Shaw, B.: Absorption of orally administered insulin by the
newly born calf. J. Physiol. (Lond.) *171*, 203–215 (1964)

Pitt, J., Barlow, B., Heird, W.C., Santulli, T.V.: Macrophages and the protective action
of breast milk in necrotizing enterocolitis. Pediatr. Res. *8*, 110 (1974)

Pittard, W.B., Polmar, S.M., Fanaroff, A.A.: The breastmilk macrophage: a potential
vehicle for immunoglobulin transport. J. Reticuloendothel. Soc. *22*, 597–603 (1977)

Porter, P., Kenworthy, R., Noakes, D.E., Allen, W.D.: Intestinal antibody secretion in
the young pig in response to oral immunization with *Escherichia coli*. Immunology
27, 841–853 (1974)

Rodewald, R.: Selective antibody transport in the proximal small intestine of the neonatal rat. J. Cell Biol. *45*, 635–640 (1970)

Rodewald, R.: Intestinal transport of antibodies in the newborn rat. J. Cell Biol. *58*, 189–211 (1973)

Rodewald, R.: pH dependent binding of immunoglobulins to intestinal cells of the neonatal rat. J. Cell Biol. *71*, 666–670 (1976)

Rodewald, R.: Distribution of immunoglobulin G receptors in the small intestine of the young rat. (1978) (in press)

Roth, T.F., Porter, K.R.: Yolk protein uptake in the oocyte of the mosquito *Aedes aegypti* L. J. Cell Biol. *20*, 313–332 (1964)

Roux, M.E., McWilliams, M., Phillips-Quagliata, J.M., Weise-Carrington, P., Lamm, M.E.: Origin of IgA secreting plasma cells in the mammary gland. J. Exp. Med. *146*, 1311–1322 (1977)

Royal, W.A., Robinson, R.A., Duganzich, D.M.: Colostral immunity against *Salmonella* infection in calves. N.Z. Vet. J. *16*, 141–145 (1968)

Ruben, F.L., Jackson, G.G., Gotoff, S.P.: Humoral and cellular response in humans after immunization with influenza vaccine. Infect. Immun. 7, 594–596 (1973)

Sasaki, M., Larson, B.L., Nelson, D.R.: Kinetic analysis of the binding of immuno-globulins IgG_1 and IgG_2 to bovine mammary cells. Biochem. Biophys. Acta *497*, 160–170 (1977)

Sibalin, M., Bjorkman, N.: On the fine structure and absorptive function of the porcine jejunal villi during the early suckling period. Expl. Cell Res. *44*, 165–174 (1966)

Silvers, W.K., Poole, T.W.: The influence of foster nursing on the survival and immunol-ogic competence of mice and rats. J. Immunol. *115*, 1117–1121 (1975)

Slade, B.: The role of coated micropinocytotic vesicles in the transport of homologous immunoglobulins across the rabbit yolk sac endoderm. IRCS Med. Sci. *3*, 235 (1975)

Schlamowitz, M.: Membrane receptor in the specific transfer of immunoglobulins from mother to young. Immunol. Comm. *5*, 481–500 (1976)

Schlamowitz, M., Kaplan, M., Show, A., Tsay, D.D.: Preparation and characterization of rabbit IgG fractions. J. Immunol. *114*, 1590–1598 (1975a)

Schlamowitz, M., Hillman, K., Lichtiger, B., Ahearn, J.J.: Preparation of IgG binding membrane vesicles from the microvillar brush border of the fetal rabbit yolk sac. J. Immunol. *115*, 296–302 (1975b)

Schlesinger, J.J., Covelli, M.D.: Evidence for transmission of lymphocyte responses to tuberculin by breast-feeding. Lancet *1977 II*, 529–532

Schwartz, R.S.: Immunoregulation, oncogenic viruses and malignant lymphoma. Lancet *1972 I*, 1266–1269

Smith, C.W., Goldman, A.S.: The cells of human colostrum. I. *In vitro* studies of morphology and functions. Pediatr. Res. *2*, 103–109 (1968)

Smith, J.W., Schultz, R.D.: Mitogen- and antigen-responsive milk lymphocytes. Cell Immunol. *29*, 165–173 (1977)

Sonoda, S., Schlamowitz, M.: Kinetics and specificity of transfer of immunoglobulin G and serum albumin across rabbit yolk sac *in utero*. J. Immunol. *108*, 807–817 (1972a)

Sonoda, S., Schlamowitz, M.: Specificity of the *in vitro* binding of IgG and rabbit serum albumin (RSA) to rabbit yolk sac membrane. J. Immunol. *108*, 1345–1352 (1972b)

Sonoda, S., Shigematsu, T., Schlamowitz, M.: Binding and vesiculation of rabbit IgG by rabbit yolk sac membrane. J. Immunol. *110*, 1682–1692 (1973)

South, M.A., Cooper, M.P., Wolheim, F.A., Hong, R., Good, R.A.: The IgA system. I. Studies of the transport and immunochemistry of IgA in the saliva. J. Exp. Med. *123*, 615 (1966)

Speer, V.C., Brown, H., Quinn, L., Caltron, D.V.: The cessation of antibody absorption in the young pig. J. Immunol. *85*, 652–654 (1959)

Spiegelberg, H.L., Weigle, W.O.: The *in vivo* formation and fate of antigen-antibody complexes formed by fragments and polypeptide chains of rabbit γG-antibodies. J. Exp. Med. *123*, 999–1012 (1966)

Staley, T.E., Jones, E.W., Cordey, L.D.: Fine structure of duodenal absorptive cells in the newborn pig before and after feeding of colostrum. Am. J. Vet. Res. *30*, 567–581 (1969)

Stastny, P.: Accelerated graft rejection in the offspring of immunized mothers. J. Imm J. Immunol. *95*, 929–936 (1965)

Strauss, F.: Die normale Anatomie der menschlichen Plazenta. Handbuch der Speziellen Pathologischen Anatomie und Histologie, Vol. 7, pp. 1–96. Berlin, Heidelberg, New York: Springer 1967

Taylor-Papadimitriou, J., Shearer, M., Tilly, R.: Some properties of cells cultured from early-lactation human milk. J. Natl. Cancer Inst. *58*, 1562–1571 (1977)

Terasaki, P.I., Mickey, M.R., Yamazaki, J.N., Vredevoe, D.: Maternal-fetal incompatibility. I. Incidence of ML-A antibodies and possible association with congenital anomalies. Transplantation *9*, 538–543 (1970)

Tomasi, T.B., Grey, H.M.: Structure and function of immunoglobulin A. Progr. Allergy *16*, 81–213 (1972)

Tomasi, T.B., Tan, E.M., Soloman, A., Pendergast, R.A.: Characteristics of an immune system common to certain external secretions. J. Exp. Med. *121*, 101 (1965)

Trentin, J.J., Gallagher, M.T., Priest, E.L.: Failure of functional transfer of maternal lymphocytes to F_1 hybrid mice. Transplant. Proc. *9*, 1473–1475 (1977)

Tuffrey, M., Bishun, N.P., Barnes, R.D.: Porosity of the mouse placenta to maternal cells. Nature *221*, 1029–1030 (1969)

Uphoff, D.E.: Runt disease in suckling hybrid mice: substrain differences and litter seriation. Transplant. Proc. *9*, 1455–1458 (1977)

Usategui-Gomez, M., Morgan, F., Toolan, H.W.: A comparative study of amniotic fluid, maternal sera and cord sera by disc electrophoresis. Proc. Soc. Exp. Biol. Med. *123*, 547–551 (1966)

Varrier-Jones, P.C.: The cellular content of milk: variations met with under physiological and pathological conditions. Lancet *1924 II*, 537–542

Virella, G., Nunes, M., Tomaynini, G.: Placental transfer of human IgG subclasses. Clin. Exp. Immunol. *10*, 475–478 (1972)

Waldman, T.A., Jones, E.A.: The rate of cell surface receptors in the transport and catabolism of immunoglobulins. In: Protein turnover. Wolstenholme, G.E.W., O'Connor, M. (eds.). Ciba Foundation Symp. *9*, 5–18. Amsterdam: North Holland 1973

Walker, W.A.: Antigen absorption from the small intstine and gastrointestinal disease. Pediatr. Clin. North Am. *22*, 731–746 (1975)

Walknowska, J., Coute, F.A., Grumbach, M.: Practical and theoretical implications of fetal-maternal lymphocyte transfer. Lancet *1969 I*, 1119–1122

Wang, A.C., Faulk, W.P., Stuckey, M.A., Fudenberg, H.H.: Chemical differences of adult, fetal and hypogammaglobulinemic IgG immunoglobulins. Immunochemistry *7*, 703–708 (1970)

Wernet, P., Bren, H., Knop, J., Rowley, D.: Antibacterial action of specific IgA and transport of IgM, IgA and IgG from serum into the small intestine. J. Infect. Dis. *124*, 223 (1971)

Wild, A.E.: Role of the cell surface in selection during transport of proteins from mother to foetus and newly born. Philos. Trans. R. Soc. Lond. (Biol.) *271*, 395–410 (1975)

Wild, A.E.: Mechanism of protein transport across the rabbit yolk sac endoderm. In: Maternofoetal transmission of immunoglobulins. Hemmings, W.A. (ed.), pp. 155–167. London, New York: Cambridge University Press 1976

Wild, A.E., Stauber, V.V., Slade, B.S.: Simultaneous localisation of human γ-globulin I^{125} and ferritin during transport across the rabbit yolk sac splanchnopleure. Z. Zellforsch. *123*, 168–177 (1972)
Williams, R.C., Gibbons, R.J.: Inhibition of bacterial adherence by secretory immunoglobulin A: a mechanism of antigen disposal. Science *177*, 697–699 (1972)
Winberg, J., Wessner, G., Does breast milk protect against septicaemia in the newborn? Lancet *1971 I*, 1091–1094
Wislocki, G.B., Bennett, H.S.: The histology and cytology of the human and monkey placenta, with special reference to the trophoblast. Am. J. Anat. *73*, 345–350 (1943)
Woods, J.W., Woodward, M.P., Roth, T.F.: Common features of coated vesicles from dissimilar tissues: composition and structure. J. Cell Sci. *30*, 87–98 (1978)
Yasmeen, D., Ellerson, J.R., Donington, K.J., Painter, R.H.: Evidence for the domain hypothesis: Location of the site of cytophilic activity toward guinea pig macrophages in the C_H3 homology region of immunoglobulin G_1. J. Immunol. *110*, 1706–1709 (1973)
Zipursky, A., Pollack, J., Neelands, P., Chown, B., Israels, L.: The transplacental passage of foetal red blood cells and the pathogenesis of Rh isoimmunization during pregnancy. Lancet *1963 II*, 489–493

Single Umbilical Artrey with Congenital Malformations

H. SOMA

   I. The Frequency of SUA 160
  II. Sex and Birthweight 160
 III. Perinatal Mortality 162
 IV. Congenital Malformations 162
  V. Chromosomal Anomalies 163
 VI. Placental Features Associated with SUA 164
VII. Pathogenesis of SUA 166
VIII. Relationship to Acardiac Twin 168
 IX. Follow-up Studies 170

References 171

It is now recognized that the absence of one umbilical artery is an important index for detecting many congenital malformations at birth. Single umbilical artery (SUA), one of the most common malformations in man, can be found by the careful inspection of the cut surface of the umbilical cord and is frequently associated with other congenital malformations (Fig. 1). Since *Benirschke* and *Brown* (1955) emphasized that SUA was associated with an increased incidence of congenital anomalies, many publications concerning the incidence, the pathogenesis, and the clinical significance of SUA (*Benirschke* and *Bourne,* 1960; *Gömöri* and *Koller,* 1964; *Froehlich* and *Fujikura,* 1966; *Papadatos* and *Paschos,* 1965; *Peckham* and *Yerushalmy,* 1965; *Solnitzky,* 1967; *Cederqvist,* 1970; *Soma* and *Yoshida,* 1970; *Molz,* 1971; *Bryan* and *Kohler,* 1974 and *Phillipe,* 1974). The reported incidence of SUA, as well as the frequency and type of associated congenital malformations, varies widely. As *Benirschke* pointed out, there remain some question-

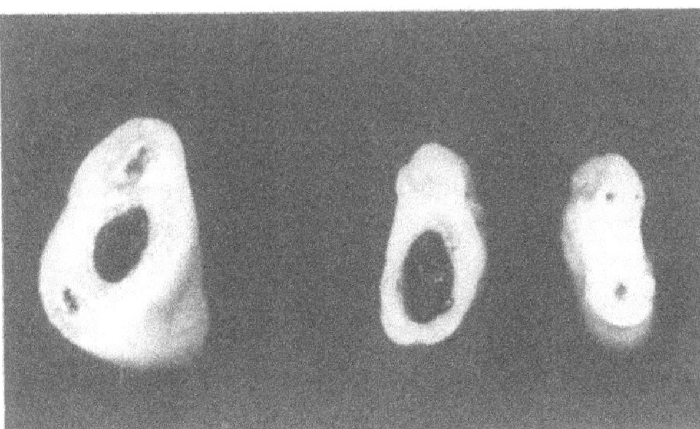

Fig. 1. Cross sections of umbilical cords with two arteries *(right)* and one artery *(middle, left)*

able points concerning the difference of the frequency of SUA in the numerous case reports, the difference of pathogenesis of SUA (whether resulting from primary aplasia or atrophy), the relationship between SUA and chromosome errors, the prognosis of infants with SUA; and follow-up studies of surviving infants (*Benirschke* and *Driscoll*, 1967; *Benirschke*, 1973). Therefore, the clinical and pathologic significance of SUA are reevaluated in this review.

I. The Frequency of SUA

Recent data since 1968, concerning the incidence of SUA, are summarized in Table 1. From these data it is apparent that there is variation in the incidence of SUA and that it occurs with a frequency of slightly less than 1%. It has been found that SUA is more frequent in whites than in blacks and orientals (*Peckham* and *Yerushalmy*, 1965; *Johnsonbaugh*, 1973), and in the present series it also appears that the incidence of SUA in Japanese is lower than in whites (*Itoh* et al., 1976; *Soma* and *Yoshida*, 1977). In addition, our recent data have been tended to be lower than previously ascertained incidence figures (*Soma* et al., 1963). It is suggested that such discrepancies in frequency of SUA reported by many authors might have arisen because of different methods of examination of the cords by various investigators. According to *Kristoffersen* (1969), the incidence of SUA is found to be significantly higher on macroscopic or microscopic examinations after fixation than that found by routine inspection of fresh cords at birth. It is concluded that the best way to discover all cases of SUA is to examine all cords macroscopically or microscopically after fixation in formalin or glacial acetic acid.

It has been generally stated that SUA is more frequently associated with twins: According to an analysis of 250 consecutive twin placentas, 18 infants exhibited SUA — a frequency of 3.6% (*Benirschke*, 1965). From our data of 108 twin placentas, SUA appeared with as high an incidence as 5.6% compared to 0.52% in the singleton placenta (*Matayoshi*, 1977).

II. Sex and Birthweight

Birth weight and duration of gestation seem to be determined at least in part by fetal factors. Diminished birth weight is a more important feature of SUA than is the duration of gestation (*Solnitzky*, 1967). It has also been noted that the incidence of SUA progressively decreases with increments of birth weight (*Froehlich* and *Fujikura*, 1966), and the highest incidence of SUA occurs in infants weighing 3.6 lb or less (*Peckham* and *Yerushalmy*, 1965). On the other hand, in our series of 34 SUA cases, the incidence of SUA in infants exceeding birth weights of 2500 g was 64.7% and correlated with gestational age (35 weeks and over) (*Soma* and *Yoshida*, 1977). However, the incidence of SUA in stillborn infants weighin 2100 g or less was consistently high. As reported by

Table 1. Summary of recent series of SUA

Authors	Total number of cases	Incidence	Perinatal mortality	Anomalies	Remarks
Harris and *Van Leeuwen* (1968)	17	17/4800 infants (0.35%)		3/17 (17.6%)	2: 16—18 Chromosome anomaly
Kristoffersen (1969)	41	41/7622 infants (0.37%)	11/41 (26.8%)	11/41 (26.8%)	15 infants, healthy, 2—5 years of age
Cederqvist (1970)	53	53/19442 deliveries (0.27%)		17/53 (32%)	
Molz (1971)	68	68/955 autopsies of stillborns and infants (7.12%)		66/68 (97%)	Multiple anomalies 52, single anomalies 14
Vlietinck et al. (1972)	29	29/2572 cords (1.1%)	6/29 (20.7%)	2/29 (7%)	23 still living
Johnsonbaugh (1973)	9	9/1152 (0.8%)	1/9 (11%)	1/9 (11%)	Angiography Pyelography
Froehlich and *Fujikura* (1973)	344	344/39773 single births (0.9%)	48/344 (14.0%)	19/36 dead infants (52.8%) 11/266 survivors (4.1%)	266: follow-up for 4 years
Bryan and *Kohler* (1974)	143	143/20000 placentas (0.72%)	25/143 (17.5%)	25/143 (17.5%)	4: twins 96: follow-up
Altshuler et al. (1975)	48 (19)	19/4138 placentas (0.45%)	12/48 (25%)	19/48 (39.5%)	
Itoh et al. (1976)	37	37/18108 infants (0.2%)	7/37 (18.9%)	16/37 (44%)	
Satoh (1977)	27	27/5784 autopsies of infants (0.45%)		24/27 (88.9%)	
Soma and *Yoshida* (1977)	34	34/7057 placentas (0.48%)	14/34 (41.1%)	14/34 (44.1%)	4: twins

many authors it seems that there is no definite connection between the occurrence of SUA and the infants sex (*Froehlich* and *Fujikura,* 1966; *Johnsonbaugh,* 1973).

III. Perinatal Mortality

In this review the overall perinatal mortality associated with SUA was found to be between 11% and 44% (Table 1). The perinatal mortality among infants born with SUA was approximately four times higher than among those with two arteries. The reasons for the higher perinatal mortality rates of SUA infants have been multiple and have included cases of stillbirth as well as congenital malformations, as quoted in Table 1.

IV. Congenital Malformations

The single artery syndrome is related to a 10- to 20-fold increase in the incidence of congenital malformations. *Benirschke* and *Brown* (1955) collected 55 cases with SUA from autopsy records and found other congenital anomalies in 27 of these, since which time many additional reports have been published concerning the relationship between SUA and congenital anomalies. *Papadatos* (1965) found that major congenital anomalies were present in 31.2% of infants with SUA, compared to a 1.15% incidence of congenital defects when two arteries are present. In the series collected here, the incidence of congenital anomalies with SUA varies from 17.5% to 88.9% (Table 1). As for a relationship between SUA and congenital anomalies, *Benirschke* has previously proposed the following theories: (a) SUA might be one of a number of malformations in the same child, all due to the same cause; (b) SUA might cause an increased resistance to the umbilical blood flow with possible fetal hypoxia and consequent multiple malformations.

The types of associated congenital malformations were classified according to organ systems and are listed in Table 2. Cardiovascular, musculoskeletal, gastrointestinal and

Table 2. Congenital anomalies by organ system associated with SUA (collected from 7 authors)

Abnormality	No. of infants
Cardiovascular	87
Genitourinary	72
Musculoskeletal	83
Gastrointestinal	74
Neurological	32
Respiratory	28
Miscellaneous	47

genitourinary malformations are encountered most frequently, but all organ systems are involved at times except, possibly, the endocrine system. However, most authors agree that concomitant congenital anomalies lack organ specificity. *Molz* (1971) studied the associated anomalies in 955 autopsied fetuses and newborns: In 68 instances one artery was lacking (7.12%) and this was associated with other anomalies in 97%; severe and fatal anomalies were found in 60%. In 885 autopsies with normal umbilical vessels, associated anomalies were found in 51%. Abnormally low birth weight and intrauterine growth retardation were more frequent in the cases with SUA. *Satoh* (1977) has also observed a high incidence of other anomalies (88.9%) in 27 autopsied fetuses with SUA.

V. Chromosomal Anomalies

The occurrence of SUA has been connected with such autosomal chromosomal aberrations as the 13–15 and 16–18 trisomy syndromes (*Lewis*, 1962; *Lenoski* and *Medory*, 1962; *Uchida* et al., 1962; *Seki* and *Strauss*, 1964; *Marin-Padilla* et al., 1964 *Van Leeuwen* and *Glenn*, 1967; *Khudr* and *Benirschke*, 1971; *Altshuler* et al., 1975). It has been suggested that SUA has a very high incidence in autosomal trisomies and other chromosomal errors (*Philippe*, 1974), yet relatively few consecutive studies have been made of the chromosomal constitution of infants with this anomaly when no obvious trisomy was present. Such studies should be encouraged and the chromosomal pattern of every case with this anomaly should be studied (Table 3). In other studies it is argued that a teratogenic etiology exists for this syndrome: This was suggested from the study of a malformed infant with SUA, born to a woman in whom ovulation had been induced (*Hack* et al., 1970). A case of pure gonadal dysgenesis associated with SUA at 14 weeks of gestation was reported by *Khudr* and *Benirschke* (1971). According to the data of *Vlietincks* et al. (1972) chromosomal studies were successfully carried out in 19 cases with SUA. In contrast to the frequency of an association reported above, all cases displayed 46 normal chromosomes without structural anomalies, excessive breaks, or recombinations. Furthermore, in 18 children the dermatoglyphics were analysed, revealing that the fingerprints of infants with SUA differ significantly from those found in the normal population. In particular, in SUA males the frequency of radial loops was three times that seen in normal infants, and in SUA girls the total finger ridge count was higher (156.5) than in normal controls (125). Although we have examined the cords of seven infants associated with such chromosomal aberrations as Down and E-trisomy syndromes, a lack of one artery was found in no case (*Matayoshi* et al., 1977).

SUA has bee found in the thalidomide embryopathy of man and in thalidomide-treated baboons (*Kajii* et al., 1963; *Thomas*, 1959; *Hendrickx* and *Katzberg*, 1967). More recently it has been found that one of two male infants presenting with abnormal genitalia as a sign of the hydantoin embryopathy syndrome also had a SUA (*Pinto* et al., 1977). With respect to the causation of the hydantoin embryopathy which appears to be due to phenytoin, it is possible that pregnant women who metabolize phenytoin at a slower rate in early pregnancy via their placenta would have children with malformations.

Table 3. Chromosomal anomalies associated with SUA

Authors	No. of cases	Chromosomal anomaly	Age at death	Sex
Richart and *Benirschke* (1958)	1	Gonadal dysgenesis	18 mo	female
Lewis (1962)	3	Trisomy 18 Atypical trisomy 18 Atypical mongolism	19 d 1 d	
German et al. (1962)	1	Trisomy 16–18	37 d	male
Lenoski and *Medovy* (1962)	3	Autosomal trisomy		
Uchida et al. (1962)	2	Trisomy 18 Trisomy 18	19 d	female
Miller et al. (1963)	1	Trisomy 13–15		male
Finley et al. (1963)	1	Trisomy 17–18	21 wk	male
Feingold et al. (1964)	1	Trisomy D-1		
Fujikura (1964)	1	Simian creases		
Seki and *Strauss* (1964)	9	2 Trisomy E 3 Trisomy D		
Marin-Padilla et al. (1964)	1	Trisomy 13–15	10 d	female
Van Leeuwen and *Glenn* (1967)	2	Trisomy 16–18		
Khudr and *Benirschke* (1971)	1	Gonadal dysgenesis	14 wk	male
Altshuler et al. (1975)	3	Trisomy 18 Trisomy 18 Trisomy 18	37 wk 38 wk 40 wk	 female female

VI. Placental Features Associated with SUA

Little (1961) reported that SUA is associated with some placental anomalies such as velamentous insertion of the umbilical cord and placental duplex. Moreover, there was a higher percentage of placentas weighing below 300 g in the SUA group (13.9%) than in a control group (3.7%) (*Froehlich* and *Fujikura,* 1966). Conversely, only 6.2% of SUA placentas weighed 550 g or more, compared to 13.3% of placentas with two umbilical arteries. Abnormalities of the placenta, especially velamentous insertion of the cord and infarcts, are found in association with SUA more frequently than one would expect (*Kristoffersen,* 1966). *Krone* (1963) has emphasized that malformations are highly correlated with eccentric or velamentous insertion of the cord and are more common than centrally inserted cords. Velamentous insertion of the cord is also more common in malformed infants with SUA than in thos with two arteries. Several investigators have suggested that the pathogenetic mechanism for the development of eccentric insertion is to be sought in an interference with the early expansion of the placenta (*Krone,* 1963; *Benirschke* et al., 1964).*Cipparone* (1966), studying 19 placentas associated with SUA, observed in 53% of the placentas gross abnormalities such as circumvallation, circummargination, velamentous insertion of the cord, and infarcts. Table 4 represents our macroscopic findings of the placentas with SUA and compares these to a control group also observed by us (*Soma* and *Yoshida,* 1977).

Table 4. Comparative findings of the placentas between SUA group and control group (*Soma* and *Yoshida,* 1977)

Gross findings	SUA group (34 cases)		Control group 4764 cases)
	(No.)	(%)	(%)
Infarction	7	20.6	32.8
Meconium stained	8	23.5	12.8
Intervillous thrombosis	2	5.9	10.0
Succenturiate lobe	4	11.8	10.9
Extrachorial placenta	6	17.6	10.0
Decidua necrosis	3	8.8	9.8
Squamous metaplasia	1	2.9	2.9
Chorionic cyst	3	8.8	2.6
Marked calcification	1	2.9	1.6
Marginal hemorrhage	1	2.9	2.7
Abnormal length of cord	6	17.6	4.1
Abnormal insertion of cord	3	8.8	1.8

In the SUA group significant differences were seen in abnormalities of the cord: abnormal length (17.6%) and eccentric insertion of cord (8.8%) compared to those of a control group (4.1% and 1.8%). *Bhargava* et al. (1971) demonstrated the anatomical characteristics of placental blood vessels with SUA by using an injection-corrosion technique. He found that the placentas with SUA had a significant reduction in the number of primary divisions of arteries and veins, exaggerated degrees of tortuosities of umbilical vein and artery, and often a reversal of arteriovenous relationships. His suggestion that these conditions lead to excessive slowing of placental circulation with resultant hypoxia should be considered as a potential background for abnormal states such as hydramnios and developmental defects. Finally, of the complications or maternal diseases during pregnancy associated with SUA infants, only diabetes mellitus, hydramnios, and multiple pregnancies have been incriminated (*Kristoffersen,* 1969; *Cipparone,* 1966; *Bhargava,* 1971).

VII. Pathogenesis of SUA

There remain questions of whether the absence of one umbilical artery is primarily absent (*Little*, 1961) or whether it atrophies at times, to disappear during fetal development. *Benirschke* et al. (1964) discussed the probability that this anomaly represents primary aplasia as well as atrophy and suggested that the SUA syndrome represents a divergent spectrum, in most cases caused by atrophy and in some by primary aplasia. In addition, postulated that aplasia is mostly associated with other congenital anomalies, whereas associated anomalies are less frequent when trophotropism has led to atrophy of the artery. In the course of studying the development of the umbilical arteries in embryos, *Monie* (1970) suggested that this anomaly resulted from failure of the single umbilical artery, normally present in the body stalks of 3.0–4.0 mm embryos, to shorten as gestation advances. Such a situation leads to atrophy of the second artery within the embryo. Consequently it has been suggested that the anomaly may arise from atrophy of one vessel: Experimental support for this thesis has come from *Monie* and *Khemman* (1973). In female rats given retinoic acid during gestation, the vitello-umbilical anastomosis persisted and the definitive umbilical arteries failed to develop completely. *Tanimura* (1977) confirmed that the prevalence of SUA in 1554 embryos examined at 4–8 weeks is approximately 0.1% and thus much lower than that reported in the Japanese newborn. Therefore, it is more likely that a majority of cases of SUA develop by secondary atrophy of a formerly present vessel.

In a study of three malformed stillborn infants, *Chaurasia* (1974) suggested that SUA can give rise to developmental anomalies in three ways: First, by replacing the greater part of the abdominal aorta and disturbing the blood supply of the caudal half of the body during early embryogenesis, it can give rise to visceral anomalies; second, by impairing the growth of the umbilical mesoderm it can disturb the formation of the infraumbilical portion of anterior abdominal wall and its correlates; third, by disturbing the hemodynamics of the embryo it can give rise to cardiovascular anomalies and possibly also to defects in the cephalic half of the body. This concept disagrees sharply with *Monie*'s theory and is based on dissection specimen.

The effects of single umbilical artery ligation have been studied in 20 lamb fetuses (*Emmanouilides* et al., 1968). Although fetuses in which ligation was undertaken near term did not survive the trauma, long-term survival (3–56 days) was observed in nine animals of earlier gestational age. After an initial period of hypoxia, acidosis, and hypercapnia, chronic fetal distress due to placental insufficiency occurred.

Thomas (1963) pointed out that there are variations of structural patterns of the abnormal umbilical artery, leading to an aplasia or an atrophic remnant. In many autopsied infants with this anomaly there is an atrophic remnant of a vessel in the abdominal portion, and occasionally the entire iliac bed of the affected side is hypoplastic (*Seki* and *Strauss*, 1964). On the other hand *Altshuler* et al. (1975) confirmed from 48 infants with SUA that there is no statistical difference between the relationship of atrophy or aplasia of an artery and type or incidence of fetal abnormalities. In other words, irrespective of the pathogenesis, fetal outcome is identical.

By means of transumbilical angiography, vascular anomalies, such as significant narrowing or atrophic remnant of common and internal iliac arteries, have been observed, often on the side where the umbilical artery is absent (Fig. 2). With SUA a

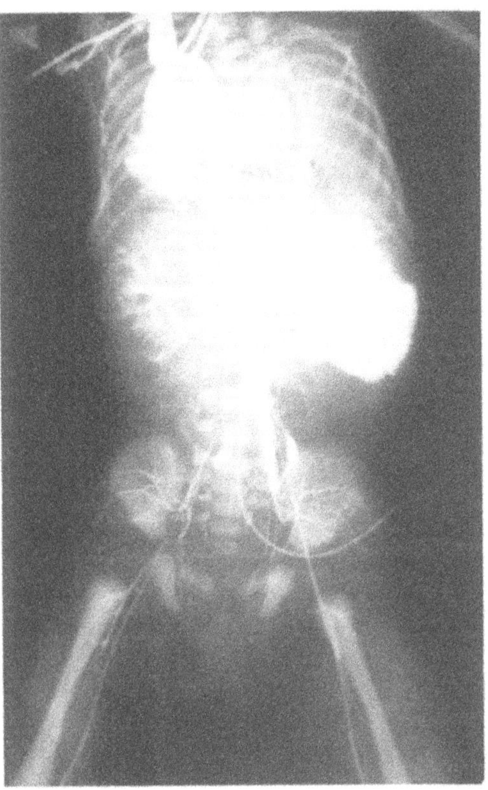

Fig. 2. Angiograph of a stillborn infant with SUA at 37 weeks of gestation. Note significant narrowing of the common and internal iliac arteries on the right side where umbilical artery is absent; also note diaphragmatic hernia on the left side

unique hemodynamic situation arises during fetal development resulting in a different caliber and structure of the iliac arteries on the two sides of the body. On the side of the SUA, the enlarged iliac arteries, which do not participate in the placental circuit, show the typical structure of muscular arteries (*Meyer* and *Lind,* 1974). These differences of arterial structure determine the morphologic patterns of early calcification, which are regularly present in the iliac arteries on both sides of the body but are usually more conspicuous in the large iliac arteries on the side of the SUA. In addition, atherosclerotic lesions were present in the common iliac artery on the side of the obliterated SUA in two children aged 18 months and 4 years. The author suggested that they are related to an adaptation to decreased blood flow.

According to studies using intravenous pyelography, unsuspected urinary abnormalities were revealed in 30% of cases with SUA (*Feingold* et al., 1964). They recommended routine intravenous pyelography in all newborn infants with SUA. However, abnormalities of the urogenital system, as investigated by pyelography, were not found in five infants with SUA in other series (*Johnsonbaugh,* 1973).

Berry et al. (1976) have measured arterial compliance of children with SUA at birth using a noninvasive ultrasonic Doppler technique. Anomalous compliance was found between the two iliac vessels, and it is suggested that this is the result of hemodynamic stress-induced changes during development. The demonstration that the form of large arteries may be changed by altered hemodynamic stress and that their physiological function is thus affected may have important implications in the pathogenesis of degenerative disease.

Kelber (1976) has recently disputed that the finding of a SUA 10 cm above the placenta is proof of its singularity in the entire course and that a SUA is a main pathogenetic fact or evidence for fundamental disorders in placenta and fetal development. In other words, he suggests that if there are only two vessels near the insertion of the umbilical cord into the placenta, it is possible that in the fetal end of the umbilical cord three vessels are present. In spite of this report, all authors agree that SUA is associated with a higher perinatal mortality and increased incidence of a variety of congenital anomalies as previously described. For example, when umbilical cord arterial anastomoses are present, they are always in that section of cord 3 cm from the placenta (*Altshuler* et al., 1975). Careful dissection of the umbilical cord at each end should be supplemented by histologic examination, and this has been done in most series reported.

VIII. Relationship to Acardiac Twin

Bryan and *Kohler* (1974) found the incidence of SUA in twins to be no greater and even marginally less than that of singletons, but SUA is common in the twin affected by acardia (*Benirschke* and *Driscoll,* 1967): It could be held that in acardiac monsters it is the vitelline vessels which persist, as is the case in sympodia. In most reported acardiacs, unfortunately, the major vessels cannot be studied in detail because of the marked degree of fetal malformations (Fig. 3).

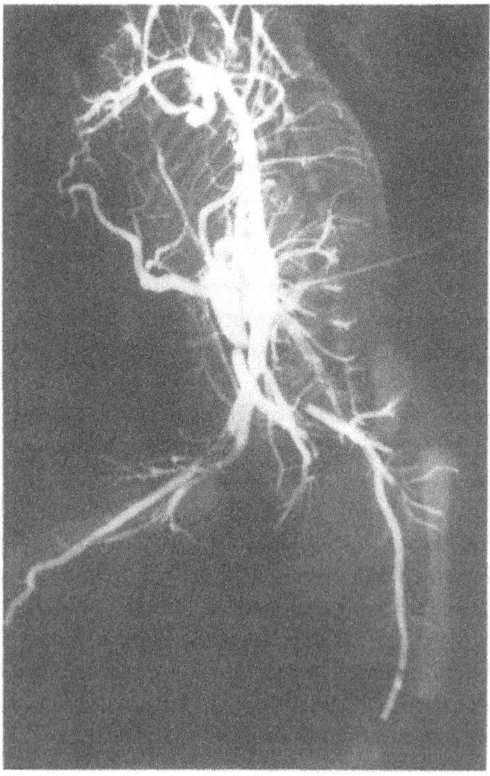

Fig. 3. Angiography of an acardiac monster. Note lack of common and internal iliac artery on the left side where umbilical artery is absent

Severn and *Holyoke* (1973) have studied in some detail the abnormal vasculature of an acardiac fetus with SUA. On the arterial side the SUA joined the left iliac artery and the bilateral iliac arteries were derived from a single dorsal aorta which also gave off branches to both upper extremities. *Benirschke* and *Harper* (1977) have recently reported that the umbilical cord of an acardiac twin possessed one artery near the fetus and an atrophic secondary artery near the placenta, a vein with a small mural thrombus, and remnants of allantoic and omphalomesenteric ducts. Thus, little support exists for preservation of omphalomesenteric vessels in these anomalous twins.

Wharton et al. (1968) described aplasia of the umbilical artery in one monoamniotic twin and found the anomaly in 2 cases of a total of 18 monoamniotic pregnancies. In one case it was an acardiac monster, where SUA is common. *Moestrup* (1970) reported that the second case with SUA, one of a pair of monoamniotic twins, survived without demonstrable malformations. We have already described a fetus papyraceous found with a diamniotic, monochorionic twin placenta who had coexistence of a SUA and amnion nodosum (*Soma* et al., 1963) (Fig. 4).

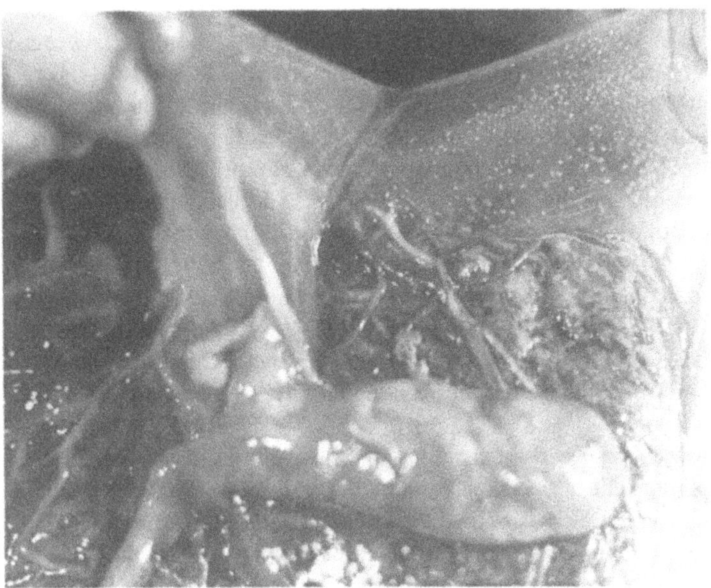

Fig. 4. A fetus papyraceus who had one umbilical artery is encircled by amnion nodosum of the membrane

Very little information is recorded about the cords of higher multiple births and in only a few cases of triplets, quintuplets and septuplets has SUA been detected (*Neubecker* et al., 1962; *Turksoy* et al., 1967; *Benirschke* and *Driscoll,* 1967; *Soma* and *Yoshida,* 1976); more attention should be paid to this area. Absence of one umbilical artery in multiple pregnancies can be regarded as a response to increased functional demands and perhaps to an abnormally large area of implantation. Its presence with apparently normal fetuses may be considered as a potentially abnormal condition (*Bhargava* et al., 1971).

IX. Follow-up Studies

It has been suggested that SUA in infants leads to hypoxia which, in turn, causes an embryonic abnormality. However, there remain a considerable number of infants in whom SUA is the only detectable anomaly. There has been some question whether SUA infants can survive the perinatal period, and particularly, whether they would develop normally.

A follow-up study of infants up to 4 years of age was undertaken which compared 266 SUA survivors with 798 matched controls (*Froehlich* and *Fujikura*, 1973). Among malformations found in the survivors, only inguinal hernia was significantly higher in SUA children. The incidence of other specific abnormal conditions was not significantly different in the two groups. The mean values of body weight, body length, and head circumference at 4 months, 1 year, and 4 years of age were almost equal in the two groups, as were the mental and motor scores at 8 months and the I.Q. at 4 years of age. *Bryan* and *Kohler* (1975) reported the follow-up of 112 SUA survivors in an attempt to ascertain whether their development was in any way abnormal over a 7-year period and whether any unsuspected congenital abnormality had appeared. Of the 112 infants with SUA and without major abnormalities in the neonatal period, 14 could not be located, 2 had died, 78 were normal and 18 had abnormalities. Most of the abnormalities now detected were less severe and conspicuous than those of the other group whose anomalies were found at birth Therefore, these abnormalities might have been diagnosed in only a few cases by a much more thorough examination in the perinatal period. Recently, *Nishimura* and *Iwatsubo* (1977) reported on a follow-up study of SUA survivors with the longest interval above 13 years; of malformations, only inguinal or umbilical hernia were found, and no retardation of their development was noted.

From these follow-up studies, it is concluded that the majority of SUA infants with severe malformations die in the neonatal period. Those with SUA surviving the perinatal period appear to develop as normally as children without malformations. As *Benirschke* (1973) has expressed, these various studies appear to reaffirm the notion that SUA is probably part of a complex of malformations rather than their cause.

Acknowledgements: The author wishes to thank Dr. Kurt Benirschke, University of California, San Diego, Department of Pathology for correcting the manuscript. This present paper was supported by the grant from Ministry of Health and Welfare of Japan for research on handicapped children.

References

Altshuler, G., Tsang, R.C., Ermocilla, R.: Single umbilical artery: Correlation of clinical status and umbilical cord histology. Am. J. Dis. Child. *129*, 697 (1975)

Benirschke, K.: Major pathologic features of the placenta, cord and membranes. Birth Defects *1*, 52 (1965)

Benirschke, K.: The final answers to single umbilical artery? Pediatrics *52*, 116 (1973)

Benirschke, K., Bourne, G.L.: The incidence and prognostic implication of congenital absence of one umbilical artery. Am. J. Obstet. Gynecol. *79*, 251 (1960)

Benirschke, K., Brown, W.H.: A vascular anomaly of the umbilical cord. The absence of one umbilical artery in the umbilical cords of normal and abnormal fetuses. Obstet. Gynecol. *6*, 300 (1955)

Benirschke, K., Driscoll, S.G.: The pathology of the human placenta, pp. 169. New York, Heidelberg, Berlin: Springer 1967

Benirschke, K., Harper, V. de R.: The acardiac anomaly. Teratology *15*, 311 (1977)

Benirschke, K., Sullivan, M.M., Marin-Padilla, M.: Size and number of umbilical vessels. A study of multiple pregnancy in man and the armadillo. Obstet. Gynecol. *24*, 819 (1964)

Berry, C.L., Gosling, R.G., Laogun, A.A., Bryan, E.: Anomalous iliac compliance in children with a single umbilical artery. Br. Heart J. *38*, 510 (1976)

Bhargava, I., Chakravaty, A., Raja, P.T.K.: Anatomy of foetal blood vessels on the chorial surface of the human placenta. IV. With absence of one umbilical artery. Acta Anat. (Basel) *30*, 620 (1971)

Bourne, G.L., Benirschke, K.: Absent umbilical artery. A review of 113 cases. Arch. Dis. Child. *35*, 534 (1960)

Bryan, E.M., Kohler, H.G.: The missing umbilical artery. I. Prospective study based on a maternity unit. Arch. Dis. Child. *49*, 844 (1974)

Bryan, E.M., Kohler, H.G.: The missing umbilical artery. II. Paediatric follow-up. Arch. Dis. Child. *50*, 714 (1975)

Cederqvist, L.: Die Bedeutung des Fehlens einer Arterie in der Nabelschnur. Acta Obstet. Gynecol. Scand. *49*, 113 (1970)

Chaurasia, B.D.: Single umbilical artery with caudal defects in human fetuses. Teratology *9*, 287 (1974)

Cipparone, J.R.: Absence of one umbilical artery. Analysis of 20 cases in a 5-year study. Am. J. Clin. Pathol. *45*, 247 (1966)

Emmanouilides, G.C., Townsend, D.E., Bauer, R.A.: Effects of single umbilical artery ligation in the lamb fetuses. Pediatrics *42*, 919 (1968)

Feingold, M., Fine, R.N., Ingall, D.: Intravenous pyelography in infants with single umbilical artery. A preliminary report. N. Engl. J. Med. *270*, 1178 (1964)

Finley, W.H., Finley, S.C., Carte, E.: 17–18 trisomy snydrome. Am. J. Dis. Child. *106*, 591 (1963)

Froehlich, L.A., Fujikura, T.: Significance of a single umbilical artery. Report from the collaborative study of cerebral palsy. Am. J. Obstet. Gynecol. *94*, 274 (1966)

Froehlich, L.A., Fujikura, T.: Follow-up of infants with single umbilical artery. Pediatrics *53*, 6 (1973)

Fujikura, T.: Single umbilical artery and congenital malformations. Am. J. Obstet. Gynecol. *88*, 829 (1964)

German, J., Rankin, J., Harrison, P.A.: Autosomal trisomay of a group 16–18 chromosome. J. Pediatr. *60*, 503 (1962)

Gömöri, Z., Koller, Th.: Über das Fehlen einer Arterie in der Nabelschnur. Gynaecologia *157*, 177 (1964)

Hack, M., Brish, M., Sen, D.M., Insler, V., Luenfeld, B.: Outcome of pregnancy after induced ovulation. JAMA *211*, 791 (1970)

Harris, R.J., Van Leeuwen, G.: Single umbilical artery. J. Pediatr. *72*, 98 (1968)

Hendrickx, A.G., Katzberg, A.A.: A single umbilical artery in the baboon. Folia Primatol. (Basel) *5*, 295 (1967)

Itoh, H., Nishimura, K., Iwatsubo, T.: Single umbilical artery: A review of 37 cases. Acta Obstet. Gynaecol. Jap. *23*, 96 (1976)

Johnsonbaugh, R.E.: Unilateral short lower extremity and single umbilical artery. Absence of a relationship. Am. J. Dis. Child. *126*, 186 (1973)

Kajii, T., Shinohara, M., Kikuchi, K., Dohmen, S., Akichika, M.: Thalidomide and the umbilical artery. Lancet *1963 II*, 889

Kelber, R.: Gespaltene „solitäre" Nabelschnurarterie. Arch. Gynäk. *220*, 319 (1976)

Khudr, G., Benirschke, K.: Pure gonadal dysgenesis associated with a single umbilical artery. A case report. Obstet. Gynecol. *38*, 697 (1971)

Kristoffersen, K.: The significance of absence of one umbilical artery. Acta Obstet. Gynecol. Scand. *48*, 195 (1969)

Krone, H.A.: Pathologische Fruchtentwicklung bei Placentaanomalien. Arch. Gynäk. *198*, 224 (1963)

Lenoski, E., Medory, H.: Single umbilical artery: Incidence, clinical significance and relation to autosomal trisomy. Can. Med. Assoc. J. *87*, 1229 (1962)

Lewis, A.J.: Autosomal trisomy. Lancet *1962 I*, 866

Little, W.A.: Umbilical artery aplasia. Obstet. Gynecol. *17*, 695 (1961)

Marin-Padilla, M., Hoefnagel, D., Benirschke, K.: Anatomic and histopathologic study of 2 cases of D trisomy. Cytogenetics *3*, 758 (1964)

Matayoshi, K.: Pathologic features of the human placenta associated with fetal congenital malformations. J. Tokyo Med. Coll. *35*, 325 (Japanese) (1977)

Matayoshi, K., Yoshida, K., Soma, H., Miyabara, S., Okamoto, N.: Placental pathology associated with chromosomal anomalies of the human neonate. A survey of seven cases. Congenital Anomalies *17*, 507 (1977)

Meyer, W.W., Lind, J.: Iliac arteries in children with a single umbilical artery. Structure, calcification, and early atherosclerotic lesions. Arch. Dis. Child. *49*, 671 (1974)

Miller, J.Q., Picard, F., Alkan, M.: A specific congenital brain defect (arhinencephaly) in 13–15 trisomy. N. Engl. J. Med. *268*, 120 (1963)

Moestrup, J.K.: Monoamniotic twins. A case with vessel anomaly in one twin's umbilical cord. Acta Obstet. Gynecol. Scand. *49*, 85 (1970)

Molz, G.: Fehlbildungen bei reduzierter und bei vollständiger Zahl der Nabelarterien. Obduktionsbefunde bei 955 Reif-, Früh- oder Mangelgeborenen. Schweiz. Med. Wochenschr. *101*, 824 (1971)

Monie, I.W.: Genesis of single umbilical artery. Am. J. Obstet. Gynecol. *108*, 400 (1970)

Monie, I.W., Khemmani, M.: Absent and abnormal umbilical arteries. Teratology 7, 135 (1973)

Neubecker, R.D., Blumberg, J.M., Townsend, F.M.: A human monozygotic quintuplet placenta. Report of a specimen. J. Obstet. Gynaecol. Br. Commonw. *69*, 137 (1962)

Nishimura, K., Iwatsubo, T.: Clinical observation on children with single umbilical artery. Symposium on correlation between fetal congenital malformations and placenta, 17th Annual Meeting, Japanese Congenital Anomalies Research Association, July 1977. Teratology *16*, 86 (Abstract) (1977)

Papadatos, C., Paschos, A.: Single umbilical artery and congenital malformations. Obstet. Gynecol. *26*, 367 (1965)

Peckham, G.H., Yerushalmy, J.: Aplasia of one umbilical artery: Incidence by race and certain obstetric factors. Obstet. Gynecol. *26*, 359 (1965)

Phillipe, E.: Histopathologic Placentaire, pp. 90. Pairs: Masson 1974

Pinto, W., Jr., Gardner, L.I., Rosenbaum, P.: Abnormal genitalia as a presenting sign in two male infants with hydantoin embryopathy syndrome. Am. J. Dis. Child. *131*, 452 (1977)

Richart, R., Benirschke, K.: Gonadal dysgenesis in a newborn infant. N. Engl. J. Med. *258*, 974 (1958)

Satoh, Y.: The relation between single umbilical artery and associated anomalies. Symposium on correlation between fetal congenital malformations and placenta, 17th Annual Meeting, Japanese Congenital Anomalies Research Association, July 1977. Teratology *16*, 86 (Abstract) (1977)

Seki, M., Strauss, L.: Absence of one umbilical artery. Analysis of 60 cases with emphasis on associated development aberrations. Arch. Pathol. *78*, 446 (1964)

Severn, C.B., Holyoke, E.A.: Human acardiac anomalies. Am. J. Obstet. Gynecol. *116*, 358 (1973)

Solnitzky, O.: Absence of one umbilical artery: An important clue to hidden congenital malformations. Georgetwon Univ. Med. Bull. *20*, 142 (1967)

Soma, H., Yoshia, K.: Absence of one umbilical artery. Jap. J. Pediat. Surg. Med. *2*, 1065 (Japanese) (1970)

Soma, H., Yoshida, K.: Observations on placentas of higher multiple births. Obstet. Gynecol. Jap. *43*, 935 (Japanese) (1976)

Soma, H., Yoshida, K.: Fetal congenital malformations and placental structural abnormalities. Symposium on correlation between fetal congenital malformations and placenta, 17th Annual Meeting, Japanese Congenital Anomalies Research Association, July 1977. Teratology *16*, 85 (Abstract) (1977)

Soma, H., Yoshida, K., Sashida, T., Nakai, S.: Fetus papyraceus in the light of placenta. Clin. Gynecol. Obstet. Jap. *17*, 709 (Japanese) (1963)

Soma, H., Yoshida, K., Tateoka, S., Nakai, S., Okamoto, R.: Correlation between umbilical vascular anomaly and fetal abnormalities. Acta Obstet. Gynaecol. Jap. *15*, 1050 (Japanese) (1963)

Tanimura, T.: Abnormalities of embryos and their membranes. Symposium on correlation between fetal congenital malformations and placenta, 17th Annual Meeting, Japanese Congenital Anomalies Research Association, July 1977. Teratology *16*, 86 (Abstract) (1977)

Thomas, J.: Die gestörte Vaskularisation der menschlichen Placenta und ihre Auswirkungen auf die Frucht. Geburtshilfe Frauenheilkd. *19*, 801 (1959)

Thomas, J.: Die Entwicklung von Fetus und Placenta bei Nabelgefäßanomalien. Arch. Gynäk. *198*, 216 (1963)

Turksoy, R.N., Toy, B.L., Rogers, J., Papageorge, W.: Birth of septuplets following human gonadotropin administration in Chiari-Frommel syndrome. Obstet. Gynecol. *30*, 692 (1967)

Uchida, I., Bowman, J.M., Wang, H.C.: The 18-trisomy snydrome. N. Engl. J. Med. *266*, 1198 (1962)

Van Leeuwen, G., Glenn, L.: Single umbilical artery. J. Pediatr. *71*, 103 (1967)

Vlietinck, R.F., Thiery, M., Orye, E., DeClercq, A., Van Vaerenbergh, P.: Significance of the single umbilical artery. A clinical, radiological, chromosomal and dermatoglyphic study. Arch. Dis. Child. *47*, 639 (1972)

Wharton, B., Edwards, J.H., Cameron, A.H.: Monamniotic twins. J. Obstet. Gynaecol. Br. Commonw. *75*, 158 (1968)

C-Type Virus Expression in the Placenta

SANDRA PANEM

I. Introduction 175
II. Ultrastructural Detection of C-Type Virus in Placentas 176
III. Biochemical Detection of C-Type Viruses 181
IV. Isolation of C-Type Virus from Placentas 183
V. Possible Function of C-Type Virus in Placentas 183
VI. Transplacental Infection 185
VII. Conclusions 185

References 187

I. Introduction

During the last decade, interest in C-type RNA viruses has expanded with observations
that virus may participate in normal host functions (i.e., embryogenesis, development,
speciation) in addition to their role in the pathogenesis of some malignant and immune
complex diseases. By the late 1960s, the correlation of C-type virus with leukemias and
sarcomas in diverse animal species was well documented. Genetic breeding experiments
provided evidence that, in some species (e.g., murine, avian), viral associated disease was
apparently transmitted vertically whereas the epidemiology of leukemia in other species
(e.g., feline, bovine) suggested horizontal spread (*Tooze*, 1973). The discovery in 1970
that all C-type viruses contain an RNA-directed DNA polymerase (i.e., reverse transcriptase) provided a molecular mechanism to explain the different patterns of C-type virus
associated disease (*Mitzutani* and *Temin*, 1970; *Baltimore*, 1970).

It is now generally accepted that C-type viruses replicate by synthesizing a DNA
copy of their RNA genome using the virion reverse transcriptase. This DNA "provirus"
is then integrated into the host chromosomal DNA. Progeny virus production occurs
via transcription of proviral DNA into virion RNA. Following integration, viral information can be transmitted as a host gene. Two modes of virus transmission are therefore
possible: first, horizontal transmission requires infection of the host by exogenous
virus; second, viral information already present in the host can be vertically transmitted
in chromosomal DNA. Operationally, an endogenous virus of a species is defined as one
whose provirus is present in at least one copy per haploid genome in all members of
the species. If a virus is transmitted horizontally as an exogenous virus of the species,
an infected individual will have some cells harboring proviral DNA and others which
do not. If horizontal infection of germ cells occurs, the host's progeny will inherit
viral genes vertically. If this event occurs frequently, an exogenous virus of the species
may become endogenous.

A number of species have been shown to harbor both endogenous and exogenous viruses. In some well studied examples, as many as 11 distinct proviruses may exist in the same cell. It has been suggested that perhaps 0.4% of the mouse genome is represented by C-type proviral DNA (*Callaghan* and *Todaro*, 1978).

Cells may harbor proviral DNA in the absence of viral gene transcription and translation (i.e., latent infection). Endogenous virus gene expression may be transient and correlate with normal processes. Expression of some endogenous virus genes may occur in the absence of virus progeny production (i.e., nonproductive infection). The frequency of proviral genes in mammalian cells is far greater than the disease with which C-type viruses are associated. Therefore, virus mediated diseases are probably the tip of an iceberg and the currently unexplored regions may provide answers to questions concerning what, if any, functions these viruses play in normal processes and by which mechanisms normal functions are perverted to result in disease.

Particular interest in C-type virus expression in placentas develops from two observations: First, C-type viruses become increasingly difficult to demonstrate and isolate as one climbs the phylogenetic tree. Secondly, replication of several C-type viruses has been found to be augmented by steroid hormones. In primates, it is now thought that the most common virus-cell interaction is nonproductive. However, it appears that the tissue in which a complete virus can be most frequently demonstrated is the placenta.

Several reviews have been concerned with the basic virology and replication of C-type viruses and should be consulted (*Tooze*, 1973; *Weinberg*, 1977; *Verma*, 1977; *Eisenman* and *Vogt*, 1977; *Aaronson* and *Stephenson*, 1976). In this paper I have attempted to review what is currently known concerning C-type virus expression in placentas of humans and other animal species. The literature concerning expression of non-C-type retroviruses in placentas has not been included. This review is written from the perspective that the placenta provides a model system to isolate human C-type viruses, understand their regulation, and generate information on the mode of virus transmission and function in normal individuals.

II. Ultrastructural Detection of C-Type Virus in Placentas

C-type virus has been detected in placentas of eight species of primates, including man (Tables 1, 2). In addition, particles have been found in placentas of mice, guinea pigs, and rabbits (*Kalter* et al., 1975; *Hsuing* et al., 1974; *Bedigian* et al., 1976). Electron microscopy is the technique which has most frequently demonstrated virus.

C-type viruses have a distinctive ultrastructural appearance (*De Harven*, 1974). On cross section, a complete spherical particle (1000–1200 A) has an icosahedral nucleoid surrounded by a double membrane envelope with projecting surface spikes. The viral envelope is derived from the host plasma membrane during maturation. Extracellular particles have either electron lucent (i.e., immature particles) or electron opaque (i.e., mature particles) cores. The opacity of the core reflects the configuration of the virion RNA within the nucleoid (*Yoshinaka* and *Luftig*, 1977). The concentric location of the nucleoid within the particles, the clarity of surface spikes, and the location of membranes where the virus matures allow C-type viruses to be morphologically distinguished from other retroviruses.

Table 1. Detection of C-type virus in subhuman primate placenta

Primate species	Technique	Reference
Old World primates		
Rhesus (M. mulatta)	Electron microscopy	*Schidlovsky* and *Ahmed*, 1973; *Kalter* et al., 1973a; *Feldman*, 1975
	Reverse transcriptase assay	*Mayer* et al., 1974
Baboon (P. cynocephalus)	Electron microscopy	*Kalter* et al., 1973b
	Hybridization following virus isolation by cocultivation	*Benveniste* et al., 1974
	Isolation by cocultivation	*Kalter* and *Heberling*, 1974; *Benveniste* et al., 1974; *Heberling* et al., 1976
	CF detection of interspecies-antigen and reverse transcriptase assay	*Strickland* et al., 1973
Patas (E. patas)	Electron microscopy	*Kalter* et al., 1975
Cynomologus (M. fascicularis)	Electron microscopy	*Kalter* et al., 1975
Chimpanzee (Pan sp.)	Electron microscopy	*Kalter* et al., 1975
New World primates		
Marmoset (S. fuscicollis)	Electron microscopy	*Kalter* et al., 1975
(S. oedipus)	Electron microscopy	*Kalter* et al., 1975; *Seman* et al., 1975

When particles observed in primate placenta are compared with those propagated in tissue culture, several differences are apparent (*Dalton* et al., 1974). Tissue culture grown virus displays an electron lucent area between the nucleoid and envelope. C-type viruses observed in placentas have envelopes which appear to be applied directly to the nucleoid without an intervening electron lucent space. When the M7 virus, isolated from a baboon placenta (*Benveniste* et al., 1974) is grown in culture, all particles exhibit an electron lucent space (*Dalton* et al., 1974). In contrast, predominant particle morphology observed in the placenta is that of the closely applied envelope (*Kalter* et al., 1973b; *Dalton* et al., 1974). This suggested that either the morphological differences resulted from differential fixation of virions in vitro and in vivo or that there were at least two morphologically distinct particles in vivo (*Dalton* et al., 1974). There is no precedence for differential fixation in view of the experience with avian and murine C-type viruses. Furthermore, both viral forms could be demonstrated in vivo. In addition, a C-type virus recently isolated from a human testicular tumor metastasis and grown in vitro appears to have a closely applied envelope (*Bronson* et al., 1978). Considering the multiplicity of C-type viruses which can be present in an individual, it is probable that only viruses with electron lucent areas between core and envelope have, to date, been isolated in vitro from baboons. Without the use of molecular probes specific for each morphologic form, the

178

question remains unresolved whether the two particles are different forms of the same virus or biologically distinct. Recognizing this question, we have used the term "C-type virus" rather than "C-type virus-like" throughout this manuscript for simplicity.

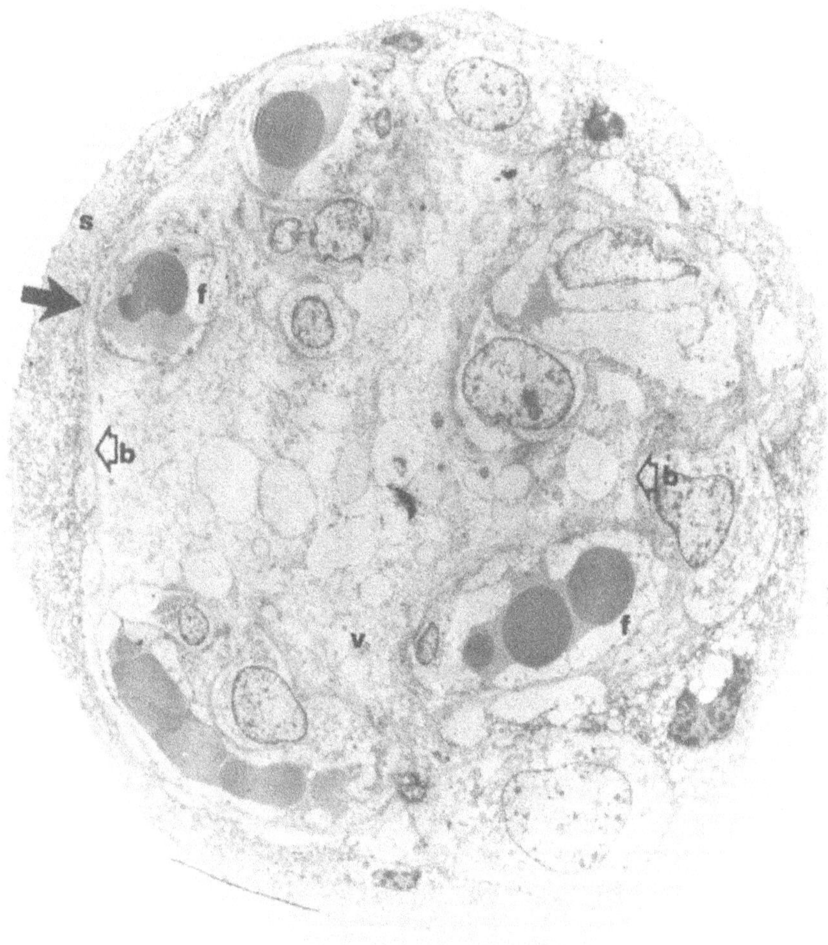

Fig. 1. A chorionic villous in cross section of a normal human term placenta. The syncytial trophoblast *(s)*, basal lamina *(b)*, villous stroma *(v)*, and fetal capillaries are marked. An arrow indicates the position of a maturing virion. (x 3,500)

The predominant morphology of C-type virions in human placentas are of particles with closely applied envelopes. However, particles with the appearance of tissue culture grown virus can also be found and both virus forms can be observed within the same placenta. Figures 1–4 demonstrate the morphologic forms found in a normal human term placenta compared with virus propagated in human cells in vitro.

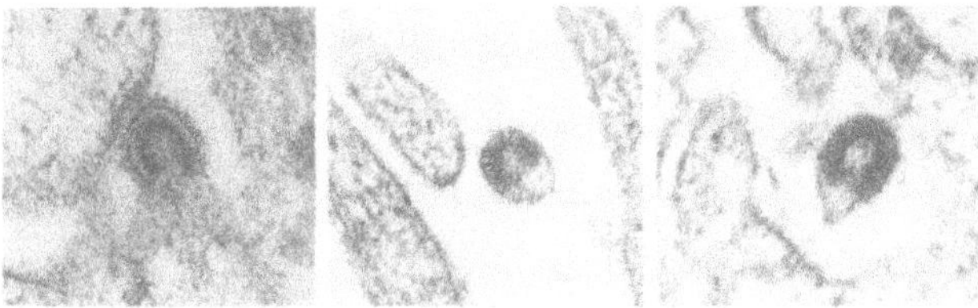

Fig. 2. Comparative morphology of virions in vitro and in vivo. *Left*, HEL-12 virus is maturing at the plasma membrane of cells propagated in vitro (x 90,000). An electron lucent space between core and envelope, condensed nucleoid, and surface spikes are evident. *Center*, a particle maturing in a human term placenta (x 90,000). The condensed core and spikes are apparent and the lucent area between core and envelope can be discerned. *Right*, a particle maturing in a human term placenta (x 97,500). The layers surrounding the core are tightly applied. Three distinct layers can be discerned.

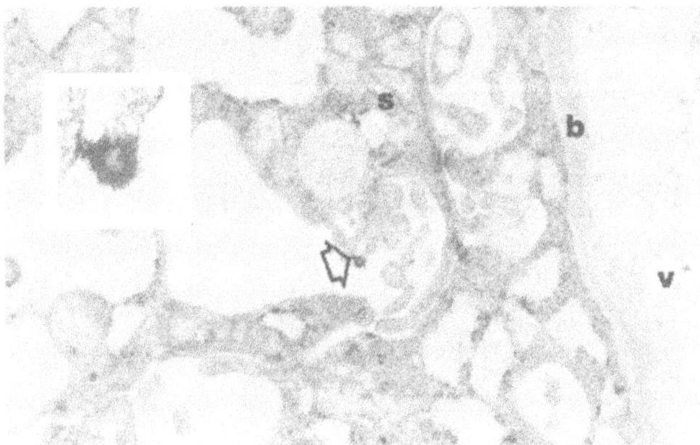

Fig. 3. C-type virion budding from a syncytiotrophoblast. The position of the virion budding from a syncytiotrophoblast *(s)* near the basal lamina *(b)* is evident (x 30,000). The insert shows an enlargement of the virion (x 100,000)

The C-type virions detected in placentas of all species studied to date have been found at the same location. Usually, budding virions are located at the convoluted plasma membrane of the basal or inner border of the syncytiotrophoblast. Occasionally, C-type particles have been observed budding from the cytotrophoblast. Particles have not been observed at the brush border or outer surface of the chorionic *villi*. *Kalter* et al. reported that in an early gestation baboon placenta, virions could be found maturing from mesenchymatous embryonic cells (*Kalter* et al., 1975). It is of interest to note that in placentas of subhuman primates, the frequency of detecting C-type virus is often greater at early stages of gestation than at term. In man, more term placentas have been examined than those of the 1st or 2nd trimesters. However, in those studies where placentas of varying gestational age were included, virus was not detected with greater frequency in early gestation samples than those compared with term specimens (*Imamura* et al., 1976; *Dirksen* and *Levy*, 1977). Figures 1, 2, and 4 demonstrate the position of C-type virus in normal human term placenta.

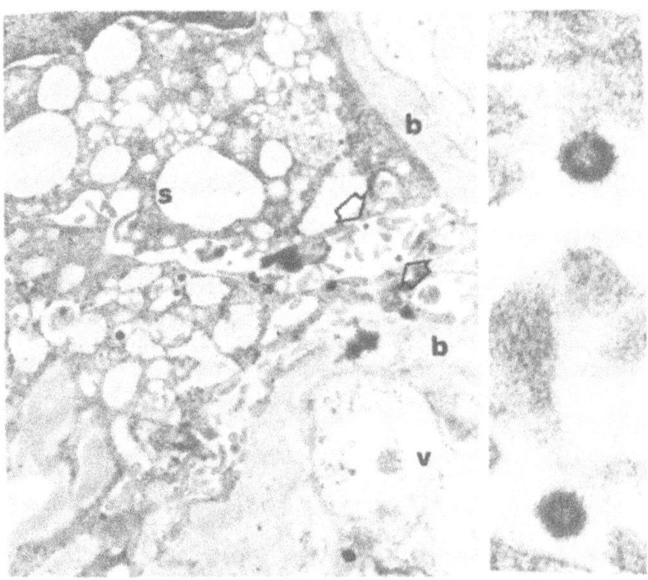

Fig. 4. Extracellular virions. A complete and a budding virion located near the basal lamina *(b)* (x 9,000). The two virions are seen enlarged at the *right* (x 90,000)

Table 2. Detection of C-type virus in human placenta by electron microscopy

No. placentas positive / No. placentas examined (%)	Reference
7/11 (62.8%)	*Kalter* et al., 1973a
15/32 (46.9%)	*Kalter* et al., 1975
12/15 (80%)	*Vernon* et al., 1974
6/12 (50%)	*Imamura* et al., 1976
7/19 (36.7%)	*Dirksen* and *Levy*, 1977
15/31 (48.5%)	*Raineri* and *Panem*, this paper

Table 2 lists the electron microscopic surveys performed with human placentas. Particles were detected in 36.7–80% of the specimens. In two studies, placentas of normal women were compared with placentas of women with systemic lupus erythematosus (SLE). Although SLE patients express readily detectable C-type viral antigen (*Mellors* and *Mellors,* 1976; *Panem* et al., 1976), there was no difference in the proportion of SLE and normal placentas with regard to the expression of morphologic C-type virus (*Imamura* et al., 1976; *Dirksen* and *Levy,* 1977). In view of the biochemical evidence described below, our opinion is that all the electron microscopic surveys are underestimates of the proportion of human placentas which contain C-type viral information. However, the time required to demonstrate particles by electron microscopy (10–20 h of continuous scanning per placenta) indicates that progeny virus production is limited. The time and luck factors involved in ultrastructural surveys probably explain differences in frequency of virion detection seen in Table 2. Nevertheless, ultrastructural surveys of placentas have been more successful in demonstrating viruses than surveys of other human tissues. Although these studies are limited by the size of each specimen examined, it is not surprising that the most consistent and compelling evidence for the presence of C-type virus in man is ultrastructural. It is the only technique that does not depend on prior knowledge of unique antigenic or nucleic acid configurations for positive virus identification.

III. Biochemical Detection of C-Type Viruses

Several biochemical techniques have been employed to detect C-type virus in placentas (Table 1, 3). Four techniques directed toward the identification of viral proteins have been successfully employed. Virion reverse transcriptase can be distinguished from cellular enzymes on the basis of template preference, divalent cation preference, and antigenic specificity. *Strickland* et al. (1973) detected reverse transcriptase in extracts of a baboon placenta. Similarly, *Mayer* et al. (1974) confirmed electron microscopic observations of C-type virus in rhesus monkey placentas by demonstrating enzyme in microsomal pellets of two early gestation placentas. The reverse transcriptase of rhesus placentas had the template and cation characteristics of the primate C-type virus enzyme and was inhibited by antisera raised to M7 baboon endogenous virus reverse transcriptase, but not by control sera or sera raised to enzymes of Mason-Pfizer monkey virus (MPMV) or simian sarcoma virus (SiSV). These data indicate that rhesus

Table 3. Biochemical detection of C-type virus expression in human placenta

Technique	No. positve placentas / No. placentas examined (%)	Reference
Viral proteins		
Competition radioimmuno-assay for mammalian interspecies antigen	3/3 (100)	*Strand* and *August,* 1974
Reverse transcriptase assay	65/72 (90.5)	*Leong* et al., 1978
Immunofluorescence with antisera to HEL-12 virus and SiSV	24/24 (100)	*Sawyer* et al., 1978
Proviral sequences		
Hybridization of placenta DNA and SiSV RNA	7/7 (100)	*Prochownik* et al., unpublished observations
	1/3 (33.3)	*Wong-Staal* et al., 1978

monkey placentas contain antigen which is cross-reactive with the gene product of an endogenous virus of old world primates. Reverse transcriptase has also been found in human placenta (*Leong* et al., 1978). Homogenates of human placenta contain particles which band in sucrose at the bouyant density characteristic of C-type viruses (1.15–1.17 g/cm) and generate particles of nucleoid density (1.22–1.25 g/cm) when treated with detergent. Detergent treated particles contain Mn^{++} dependent enzyme which prefers poly rC.oligo dG and can be distinguished from terminal transferase and human cellular DNA polymerases. Of interest was the finding that placentas from multiparous woman had the highest levels of reverse transcriptase (*Leong* et al., 1978).

Mammalian C-type viruses have antigenic determinants (i.e., interspecies antigens) which have been conserved during evolution. These determinants can be detected by complement fixation (CF) and competition radioimmunoassay (RIA). *Strickland* et al. (1973) detected interspecies antigen in baboon placenta by CF. *Strand* and *August* (1974) detected antigen in three human placentas in RIA between labeled Rauscher murine leukemia virus p30 antigen and an antiserum raised to RD114 virus, an endogenous virus of cats.

Immunofluorescence has also been used to detect C-type virus antigen in human placenta (*Sawyer* et al., 1978). Using antisera raised to HEL-12 virus, antigen was detected in 24 of 24 human term placentas. The antibody reaction could be specifically blocked by purified virus but not by fetal calf serum, human immunoglobulin, or serum albumin. An extract of placentas which was enriched in 70,000 mol. wt. glycoprotein was found to block the reaction. An antiserum made from the placenta extract reacted with HEL-12 virus infected cells of several species.

Studies using reverse transcriptase assays, CF, RIA, and indirect immunofluorescence (Table 1) indicate that antigens related to known C-type viruses are present in the majority, if not all, human placentas. The experiments do not yet distinguish whether an endogenous human virus is responsible for the reactivity and/or if the placentas are a target organ for frequent horizontal infection by exogenous C-type viruses.

Molecular hybridization technics have also been used to detect C-type virus in placentas. The M7 baboon virus was isolated following cocultivation of a baboon placenta with human and canine cells (*Benveniste* et al., 1974). A DNA transcript of M7 virus RNA was prepared with reverse transcriptase. This cDNA hybridized with cellular DNA from a normal baboon placenta and other tissues indicating that M7 was an endogenous baboon virus. To date, an endogenous human C-type virus has not been isolated. However, several primate C-type viruses including SiSV are thought to exogenously infect man (*Prochownik* and *Kirsten*, 1977; *Kurth* et al., 1977; *Snyder* et al., 1977). Hybridization experiments between normal human placenta DNA and labeled SiSV-RNA (*Prochownik* et al., unpublished observations; *Wong-Staal* et al., 1978) suggest human placentas contain proviral sequences which are very closely related to SiSV. However, these experiments do not distinguish between the presence of complete SiSV-like virus in a small number of cells and an endogenous human virus which is only partially homologus with SiSV.

IV. Isolation of C-Type Virus from Placentas

A C-type virus was first isolated from a baboon placenta (*Kalter* and *Heberling*, 1974; *Benveniste* et al., 1974). This so-called baboon virus was recovered after 36–90 days of cocultivation of primary placenta cells with human rhabdomyosarcoma, fetal canine thymus, and bat lung cells. M7 was shown to be derived from baboon cells by hybridization of M7 cDNA with DNA extracted from normal baboon tissues. In similar experiments with other baboon placentas, virus isolation was independent of treatment with halogenated pyrimidines, agents known to enhance the isolation of C-type virus in several species (*Aaronson* and *Stephenson*, 1976). The available data indicate that M7 is an endogenous virus of baboons. When hybridization studies were performed between M7 viral RNA and RNA extracted from normal baboon tissues, the placenta was found to transcribe M7 nucleotide sequences, whereas the liver did not (*Benveniste* et al., 1974). These experimentes confirmed the implication of ultrastructural studies that subhuman primates preferentially express C-type virus information in placentas.

Attempts to isolate virus from human placentas have, to date, been unsuccessful. In view of the previously summarized data on virus expression in human placentas, these failures most probably reflect inappropriate culture conditions for virus isolation. Some C-type viruses show augmented expression following treatment with steroid hormones in vitro (*Schaller* et al., 1976; *Wu* et al., 1977) as well as in vivo (*Fowler* et al., 1972). It is therefore probable that successful virus isolation from human placentas requires the addition of appropriate hormones to the culture milieu. The isolation of a C-type virus from a human testicular tumor metastasis was accomplished following treatment of cells with both halogenated pyrimidines and dexamethasone (*Bronson* et al., 1978).

An additional consideration concerns the cell type in placentas which appears to be productively infected with C-type virus. The syncytiotrophoblasts most frequently appear to contain maturing C-type virus. These cells can be isolated and maintained for short periods in vitro, but cannot be propagated (*Kaspi* and *Nebel,* 1974). Although immunofluorescence studies demonstrated that cells of the villous stroma can express C-type viral antigen (*Sawyer* et al., 1978), it is unclear whether or not these cells can support the production of progeny virus. Cocultivation experiments with susceptible host cells are therefore logical. As the host range characteristics of placental C-type virus (e.g., xenotropic, amphotropic, ecotropic) are unknown, use of a wide range of cells is warranted. Based on host range studies with subhuman primate C-type viruses, the most likely cell candidates are fetal, canine, human, and human tumor cell lines.

V. Possible Function of C-Type Virus in Placentas

Two possibilites present themselves to explain the observations reviewed so far. In general, C-type virus expression appears to be augmented in placentas as compared with normal adult tissues. First, the expression in placentas may reflect the participation of C-type viruses in embryologic development; second, the hormonal milieu and immunologic status may allow placentas to be highly susceptible to C-type virus infection and/ or derepression of proviral information. These two possibilities are not mutually exclusive.

The protovirus hypothesis suggests that C-type virus may act as a mechanism for intercellular information transfer (*Temin*, 1971). The necessity for information exchange between cells during development has been documented (*Slavkin* and *Bringas*, 1976; 1976; *Slavkin*, 1972). Experimental evidence for virus activation during cell-cell contact derives from experimental graft versus host disease of mice (*Hirsch* et al., 1972).

A model for virus mediated information transfer can easily be envisioned. Virions could encapsidate host RNA for transfer to other cells. On infection, the host RNA might be transcribed into DNA and integrated into chromosomal DNA or translated into protein. It has been known for a long time that C-type viruses incorporate host transfer RNA into virions (*Erikson* and *Erikson*, 1969) and can also form pseudo-virions with nonretroviruses (*Huang* et al., 1973). These findings suggest C-type viruses can act as stable vehicles for transfer of nonvirion nucleic acids between cells.

In support of the hypothesis that C-type viruses participate in development are experiments which suggest that viral gene products can act as tissue specific antigens. This work derives from correlating the appearance of the GIX cell surface antigen of mice with lymphoid cell differentiation and from the isolation of viral glycoproteins with idiotypic differences from several tissues within strains of inbred mice (*Tung* et al., 1975; *Elder* et al., 1977). Cell surface marker antigens have been detected for differentiating lymphocytes. One marker, the GIX antigen, appears on AKR mouse thymocytes. GIX is antigenically identical to the 70,000 molecular weight glycoprotein of an endogenous AKR virus. 70,000 molecular weight glycoproteins were isolated from several tissues of inbred mice and compared by tryptic fingerprint technique with envelope proteins of viruses present in the same mice. The tissue antigens and viral proteins were remarkably similar and the data were interpreted as evidence for viral related antigens acting as tissue specific markers. Additional evidence for this hypothesis stems from studies on the effects of virus expression during differentiation of murine and human myeloid cells in vitro (*Friend* et al., 1971; *Ruscetti* et al., 1978).

The possibility that virus expression is augmented in placentas due to hormonal factors is based on observations that cells producing C-type virus may produce more virus following hormonal treatment (*Schaller* et al., 1976; *Wu* et al., 1977). Augmentation of virion production is transient and dependent on the continuing presence of hormones. Experiments on the mechanism of dexamethasone induced enhancement of virus expression suggests that, in at least one virus-cell system, dexamethasone acts following transcription (*Wu* et al., 1977).

Since autologous antibody production to C-type viruses is widespread (*Tooze*, 1973), it has been suggested that the circulating antibody may play a role in regulating C-type virus expression. One can therefore postulate that C-type virus expression in placentas is a reflection of a lack of an antiviral immunity in placentas. For example, the antiviral antibody may not cross the placenta. However, the complete abrogation of the antiviral antibody during pregnancy cannot explain elevated virus gene expression in man. In fact, it has recently been found that both cell mediated and humoral immunity to SiSV and BaEV-like viruses is elevated during pregnancy (*Hirsch* et al., 1978; *Thiry* et al., 1978).

VI. Transplacental Infection

The expression of C-type virus in placentas may reflect activation of endogenous viruses and/or de novo infection. The reasons why placentas might be a tissue in which virus is activated are discussed in the preceding section. The arguments explaining why placentas may be a privileged site for endogenous C-type virus expression are equally valid for explaining placentas as a site for exogenous infection (i.e., hormonal milieu, immune status, maternal/paternal interactions). Several sources of infection with C-type virus are: (1) activation of endogenous virus in maternal cells, (2) expression of exogenous virus in maternal cells, (3) activation of endogenous virus of maternal or paternal virus following fertilization, (4) expression of exogenously infecting virus in egg or sperm, and (5) de novo exogenous virus infection.

These possibilities indicate that either parent may provide a source of C-type virus for infection. However, it is equally plausible that virus activated in the placenta of paternal origin or de novo infection of the placenta may result in infection of the mother.

Table 4 lists observations of C-type virus in germinal tissue. These data provide evidence that both exogenous infection and activation of endogenous virus can occur in germ cells.

It remains unclear whether exogenous virus infection has positive, negative, or neutral consequences for the host. However, the feasibility of in utero infection suggests that infection with a potentially pathogenic virus may occur under conditions where the host may become immunologically tolerant of the virus. This possibility may have implications for understanding diseases in which C-type viruses are thought to participate.

VII. Conclusions

Morphologic and biochemical data indicate that expression of C-type virus in placentas is widespread. Hormonal and immunologic factors may explain why C-type virus is readily detected in the placenta. Most probably, several distinct species of virus are expressed. The activation of endogenous virus may reflect the participation of this virus in normal developmental processes. In utero infection by exogenous virus may allow a latent virus-cell interaction to be established whereby a potentially pathogenic virus enters the host and the host becomes immunolgically tolerant of the virus. Finally, the placenta may be the tissue from which human C-type viruses can best be isolated.

Acknowledgements: This work was supported by grants from the Elsa U. Pardee Foundation, the National Foundation — March of Dimes, and the National Cancer Institute (CA 19264). Electronmicroscopy of human placenta done in our laboratory was expertly performed by C. Raineri. I thank W.H. Kirsten and R. Black for a critical reading of the manuscript.

Table 4. Germinal tissue in which C-Type viruses have been detected

Species	Tissue	Technique	Reference
Rabbit	Blastocyts and uterine lining cells	Electron microscopy	*Daniels*, 1976
	Uterine fluid	Reverse transcriptase assay	*Bedigian* et al., 1976
Guinea pig	Oogonia and oocytes; developing testis; whole embryo	Electron microscopy	*Andersen* and *Jeppesen*, 1972; *Black*, 1974; *Hsuing* et al., 1974
Mouse	One-cell embryo to blastocyst; embryos at all stages; embryos at all stages	Electron microscopy Complement fixation Hybridization	*Chase* and *Piko*, 1973; *Huebner* et al., 1970; *Jaenisch*, 1976
	Uterus	Radioimmunoassay, reverse transcriptase assay	*Strickland* et al., 1974
	Yolk sac	Electron microscopy	*Feldman* et al., 1976
Baboon	Preimplantation embryos	Electron microscopy	*Kalter* et al., 1974b
	follicular oocytes and tubal ova	Electron microscopy	*Kalter* et al., 1974a
Man	Sperm	Electron microscopy, reverse transcription assay	*Witkin* et al., 1978
		Electron microscopy	*Bronson* et al., 1978

References

Aaronson, S.A., Stephenson, J.: Endogenous C-type viruses of mammalian cells.
Biochem. Biophys. Acta *458*, 323–354 (1976)

Anderson, H.K., Jeppesen, T.: Virus like particles guinea pig oogonia and oocytes.
J. Natl. Cancer Inst. *49*, 1403–1410 (1972)

Baltimore, D.: Viral RNA-dependent DNA polymerase. Nature *226*, 209–211 (1970)

Bedigian, H.G., Fox, R.R., Meier, H.: Evidence for a particle-associated RNA-directed
DNA polymerase in rabbit placental and uterine tissues. Cancer Res. *36*, 4687–
4692 (1976)

Benveniste, R.E., Lieber, M.M., Livingston, D.M., Sherr, C.J., Todaro, G.J., Kalter, S.S.:
Infectious C-type virus isolated from a baboon placenta. Nature *248*, 17–20
(1974)

Black, V.H.: Gonocytes in fetal guinea pig testes. Am. J. Anat. *131*, 415–426 (1971)

Bronson, D.L., Ritzi, D.M., Fraley, E.E., Dalton, A.J.: Morphologic evidence for retrovirus production by epithelial cells derived from a human testicular tumor metastasis.
(In press) (1978)

Callaghan, R., Todaro, G.: Four major endogenous retrovirus classes of the genus mus.
RNA Tumor Virus Workshop 1978, Cold Spring Harbour Laboratory, N.Y.

Chase, D.G., Piko, L.: Expression of A- and C-type particles in early mouse embryos.
Natl. Cancer Inst. *51*, 1971–1975 (1973)

Dalton, A.J., Hellman, A., Kalter, S.S., Helmke, R.J.: Ultrastructural comparison of
placental virus with several type-C oncogenic viruses. J. Natl. Cancer Inst. *52*,
1379–1381 (1974)

Daniels, J.C.: The uterus as an agent for informational exchange between mother and
early embryo. Annual Meeting Amer. Soc. Zool. (1973)

De Harven, E.: Remarks on the ultrasturcture of type A, B, and C virus particles.
Adv. Virus Res. *19*, 221–264 (1974)

Dirksen, E.R., Levy, J.A.: Virus like particles in placentas from normal individuals and
·patients with systemic lupus erythematosus. J. Natl. Cancer Inst. *59*, 1187–1192
(1977)

Eisenman, R., Vogt, V.M.: The biosynthesis of oncovirus proteins. Biochem. Biophys.
Acta *473*, 187–239 (1977)

Elder, J.H., Jensen, F.C., Bryant, M.L., Lerner, R.A.: Polymorphism of the major
envelope glycoprotein (gp70) of murine C-type viruses: virion associated and differentiation antigens encoded by a multi-gene family. Nature *267*, 23–28 (1977)

Erikson, E., Erikson, R.I.: Association of 4S rubonucleic acid with oncornavirus
ribonucleic acids. J. Virol. *8*, 24–30 (1971)

Feldman, D.: An electron microscopic study of virus particles in rhesus monkey
placenta. Proc. Natl. Acad. Sci. USA *72*, 118–121 (1975)

Feldman, D., Gross, L., Swarm, R.L.: Electron microscopic study of virus particles in
yolk sac and placenta and in hematopoietic organs of newborn C3HF mice. Cancer
Res. *36*, 1814–1820 (1976)

Fowler, A.K., Reed, C.D., Todaro, G.J., Hellman, A.: Activation of C-type RNA virus
markers in mouse uterine tissue. Proc. Natl. Acad. Sci. USA *69*, 2254–2257 (1972)

Friend, C., Scher, W., Holland, J.G., Soto, T.: Hemoglobin synthesis in murine virus-
induced leukemic cells in vitro: stimulation of erythroid differentiation by dimethyl-
sulfoxode. Proc. Natl. Acad. Sci. USA *68*, 378–381 (1971)

Heberling, R.L., Kalter, S.S., Barker, S.T., Weislow, O.S.: Isolation and biological
properties of endogenous baboon (Papio Cynocephalus) type C viruses. Bibl.
Haematol. *43*, 158–160 (1976)

Hirsch, M.S., Kelly, A.P., Chapin, D.S., Kurth, R.: Immunity to antigens associated
with primate C-type oncoviruses in pregnant women. Science *199*, 1337–1340
(1978)

Hirsch, M.S., Phillips, S.M., Solnik, C., Black, P.H., Schwartz, R.S., Carpenter, C.B.: Activation of leukemia viruses by graft-versus-host and mixed lymphocyte reactions in vitro. Proc. Natl. Acad. Sci. USA *69*, 1069–1072 (1972)

Hsiung, G.D., Fong, C.K., Evans, C.H.: Prevalence of endogenous oncornavirus in guinea pigs. Intervirology *3*, 319–331 (1974)

Huang, A.S., Besmer, P., Chu, L., Baltimore, D.: Growth of pseudo-types of vesicular stomatitis virus with N-tropic murine leukemia virus coats in cells resistant to N-tropic viruses. J. Virol. *12*, 659–662 (1973)

Huebner, R.J., Kelloff, G.J., Sarma, P.S., Lane, W.T., Turner, H.C., Gilden, R.V., Oroszian, S., Meier, H., Myers, D.D., Peters, R.L.: Group-specific antigen expression during embryogenesis of the genome of the C-type RNA tumor virus: implications for ontogenesis and oncogenesis. Proc. Natl. Acad. Sci. USA *67*, 366–376 (1970)

Imamura, M., Phillips, P.E., Mellors, R.C.: The occurrence and frequency of type C virus-like particles in placentas from patients with systemic lupus erythematosus and from normal subjects. Am. J. Pathol. *83*, 383–394 (1976)

Jaenisch, R.: Germ line integration and Mendelian transmission of the exogenous moloney leukemia virus. Proc. Natl. Acad. Sci. USA *73*, 1260–1264 (1976)

Kalter, S.S., Heberling, R.L.: Isolation of C-type viruses from baboon (papio cynocephalus) placental tissue. Abstracts of the Annual Meeting, American Society for Microbiology, 233 (1974)

Kalter, S.S., Helmke, R.J., Heberling, R.L., Panigel, M., Fowler, A.K., Strickland, J.E., Hellman, A.: C-type particles in normal human placentas. J. Natl. Cancer Inst. *50*, 1081–1084 (1973a)

Kalter, S.S., Helmke, R.J., Panigel, M., Felsburg, P.J., Axelrod, L.R.: Observations of apparent C-type particles in baboon (papio cynocephalus) placentas. Science *179*, 1332–1333 (1973b)

Kalter, S.S., Heberling, R.L., Smith, G.C., Panigel, M., Kraemer, D.C., Helmke, R.J., Hellman, A.: Vertical transmission of C-type viruses: their presence in baboon follicular oocytes and tubal ova. J. Natl. Cancer Inst. *54*, 1173–1176 (1974a)

Kalter, S.S., Panigel, M., Kraemer, D.C., Heberling, R.L., Helmke, R.J., Smith, G.C., Hellman, A.: C-type particles in baboon (papio cynocephalus) pre-implantation embryos. J. Natl. Cancer Inst. *52*, 1927–1928 (1974b)

Kalter, S.S., Heberling, R.L., Helmke, R.J., Panigel, M., Smith, G.C., Kraemer, D.C., Hellman, A., Fowler, A.K., Strickland, J.E.: A comparative study on the presence of C-type viral particles in placentas from primates and other animals. Bibl. Haematol. *40*, 391–401 (1975)

Kaspi, T.K., Nebel, L.: Isolation of syncytiotrophoblast from human term placenta. Obstet. Gynecol. *43*, 549–557 (1974)

Kurth, R., Teich, N., Weiss, R., Oliver, R.T.D.: Natural human antibodies reactive with primate type-C viral antigens. Proc. Natl. Acad. Sci. USA *74*, 1237–1240 (1977)

Leong, J., Nelson, J., Levy, J.A.: Reverse transcriptase like activity in extracts of human placenta. Annual Meeting of The American Society for Microbiology, 223 (1978)

Mayer, R.J., Smith, R.G., Gallo, R.C.: Reverse transcriptase in normal rhesus monkey placenta. Science *185*, 864–867 (1974)

Mellors, R.C., Mellors, J.W.: Antigen related to mammalian type-C RNA viral p30 proteins is located in renal glomeruli in human systemic lupus erythematosus. Proc. Natl. Acad. Sci. USA *73*, 233–237 (1976)

Mitzutani, S., Temin, H.: RNA-dependent DNA polymerase in virions of Rous sarcoma virus. Nature *226*, 1211–1213 (1970)

Panem, S., Ordonez, N.G., Kirsten, W.H., Katz, A.I., Spargo, B.H.: C-type virus expression in systemic lupus erythematosus. N. Engl. J. Med. *295*, 470–475 (1976)

Prochownik, E.V., Kirsten, W.H.: Nucleic acid sequences of primate type C viruses in normal and neoplastic human tissues. Nature *267*, 175–176 (1977)

Ruscetti, F., Collins, S., Gallagher, R., Gallo, R.: Inhibition of human myeloid differentiation in vitro by primate type-C retroviruses. To be published

Sawyer, M.H., Nachlas, N.E., Jr., Panem, S.: C-type virus antigen expression in normal human placenta. Nature *275*, 62–64 (1978)

Schaller, J.P., Milo, G.E., Blakeslee, J.R., Jr., Olsen, R.C., Yohn, D.S.: Influence of glucocorticoid, estrogen, and androgen hormones on transformation by feline sarcoma virus. Cancer Res. *36*, 1980–1987 (1976)

Schidlovsky, G., Ahmed, M.: C-type virus particles in placentas and fetal tissues of rhesus monkeys. J. Natl. Cancer Inst. *51*, 225–233 (1973)

Seman, G., Levy, B.M., Panigel, M., Dmochowski, L.: Type-C virus particles in placenta of the cottontop marmoset (saguinus oedipus). J. Natl. Cancer Inst. *54*, 251–252 (1975)

Slavkin, H.C.: Intercellular communication during epidermal organ formation. In: Epidermal wound healing. Maibach, H., Rovee, D.T. (eds.). Chicago: Yearbook Medical Publishers 1972

Slavkin, H.C., Bringas, P.: Epithelial-mesenchyme interactions during odontogenesis IV. morphological evidence for direct cell cell contacts. Dev. Biol. *50*, 428–442 (1976)

Snyder, W.H., Jr., Pincus, T., Fleissner, E.: Specificities of human immunoglobulins reactive with antigens in preparations of several mammalian type C viruses. Virology *75*, 60–73 (1977)

Strand, M., August, J.T.: Type-C RNA virus gene expression in human tissue. J. Virol. *14*, 1584–1596 (1974)

Strickland, J.E., Fowler, A.K., Kind, P.P., Hellman, A., Kalter, S.S., Heberling, R.L., Helmke, R.J.: Group specific antigen and RNA-directed DNA polymerase activity in normal baboon placenta. Proc. Soc. Exp. Biol. Med. *144*, 256–258 (1973)

Strickland, J.E., Kind, P.D., Fowler, A.K., Hellman, A.: Comparison of viral marker proteins in murine leukemia virus and mouse uterus. Natl. Cancer Inst. *52*, 1161–1165 (1974)

Temin, H.: The protovirus hypothesis: speculations on the significance of RNA-directed-DNA synthesis for normal development and for carcinogenesis. J. Natl. Cancer Inst. *46*, 3–4 (1971)

Thiry, L., Sprecher-Goldberger, S., Bossens, M., Neuray, F.: Cell mediated immune response to simian oncoviruses in pregnant women. J. Natl. Cancer Inst. *60*, 527–532 (1978)

Tooze, J.: The molecular biology of tumor viruses. Cold Spring Harbor Laboratory, N.Y. (1973)

Tung, J.S., Vitetta, E.S., Fleissner, E., Boyse, E.A.: Biochemical evidence linking the G-IX thymocyte surface antigen to the gp69/71 envelope glycoprotein of murine leukemia virus. J. Exp. Med. *141*, 198–205 (1975)

Verma, I.M.: The reverse transcriptase. Biochem. Biophys. Acta *473*, 1–38 (1977)

Vernon, M.L., McMahon, J.M., Hackett, J.J.: Additional evidence of type-C particles in human placentas. J. Natl. Cancer Inst. *52*, 987–989 (1974)

Weinberg, R.A.: Structure of the intermediates leading to the integrated provirus. Biochem. Biophys. Acta *473*, 39–56 (1977)

Witkin, S.S., Higgins, P.J., Bendich, A.: Antibodies to baboon retrovirus reverse transcriptase in sera from infertile humans. J. Supramol. Struc. Suppl. *2*, 255 (1978)

Wong-Staal, F., Josephs, S., Gallo, R.C.: Hybridization of simian sarcoma virus RNA to endonuclease restricted human DNA: selection of endogenous and acquired viral related fragments. RNA Tumor Virus Workshop, Cold Spring Harbor Laboratory, p. 71 (1978)

Wu, A.M., Reitz, M.S., Paran, M., Gallo, R.C.: Mechanism of stimulation of murine type C RNA tumor virus production by glucocorticoids post-transcriptional effects. J. Virol. *14*, 808–812 (1977)

Yoshinaka, Y., Luftig, R.B.: Murine leukemia virus morphogenesis: clevage of P70 can be accompanied by a morphological conversion from an immature to a mature form of the core. Proc. Natl. Acad. Sci. USA *74*, 3446–3450 (1977)

Transplacental Effects of Diethylstilbestrol

M. BIBBO

I. Introduction 191
II. Neonatal Data 192
III. Female Offspring 193

    1. Anatomical Abnormalities 193

        a) Vaginal Adenosis 193

            α) Pathology 193
            β) Colposcopy 195
            γ) Cytology 196

        b) Cervicovaginal Ridges 199
        c) Clear Cell Adenocarcinoma 201

            α) Pathology 201
            β) Cytology 202

        d) Pathogenesis of Vaginal Adenosis, Cervicovaginal Ridges, and Clear
           Cell Adenocarcinoma 202

    2. Functional Abnormalities 204

IV. Male Offspring 204

    1. Anatomical Abnormalities 204
    2. Functional Abnormalities 206
    3. Psychological Effects 208

V. Conclusions 209

References 209

I. Introduction

Diethylstilbestrol (DES) was the most widely administered estrogen for maintenance of pregnancy, in part because of its inexpensiveness, its activity when given in oral form, and its potency. The action and effects of DES were comparable to those of the natural estrogens (*Noller* and *Fish,* 1974).

In 1946, *Smith* et al. recommended that DES be given for some of the complications of pregnancy, beginning with 5 mg/day as early in gestation as possible, increasing the dose by 5 mg/day every second week up to a maximum daily dose of 150 mg by the 34th week, and discontinuing the drug at the 35th week.

In the decade 1945–1955, it has been estimated that 500,000–3,000,000 women received DES (*Noller* and *Fish,* 1974) and *Heinonen* (1973) calculated that during the period 1960–1970, 33,000–100,000 children were exposed to DES each year.

Interestingly enough, in 1953, *Dieckmann* et al. reported the results of a double blind placebo controlled investigation directed at determining the value of DES in pregnancy. It was concluded that DES did not reduce the incidence of abortion, prematurity, postmaturity, prenatal mortality, and toxemia of pregnancy. Nevertheless, DES continued to be used for pregnancy maintenance until *Herbst* et al. reported, in 1971, a possible relationship between prenatal exposure to DES and clear cell adenocarcinoma of the vagina in the adolescent woman.

In 1972, *Noller* et al. and *Herbst* et al. showed that clear cell adenocarcinoma of the cervix was also related to prenatal exposure to DES. A registry of Research on Hormonal Transplacental Carcinogenesis has been created, and to date more than 300 cases of clear cell adenocarcinoma have been entered.

Since the original studies by *Herbst* et al., many other studies have been published on transplacental effects of DES in the female showing that numerous benign abnormalities of the vagina and cervix (e.g., adenosis, cervicovaginal ridges) are more common than the development of adenocarcinoma of the vagina and cervix (*Antonioli* and *Burke*, 1975; *Bibbo* et al., 1977; *Herbst* et al., 1975; *Ng* et al., 1977; *Sandberg*, 1976). In 1974, *Stafl* and *Mattingly* reported an increase in squamous neoplasia in DES-exposed female offspring. In 1977, *Kaufman* et al. discovered a number of anomalies involving the corpus and tube by performing hysterosalpingograms on DES-exposed women. These anomalies included T-shaped uterus, constricting bands in the uterine cavity, hypoplasia, polypoid defects, and synechiae.

In 1975(a), *Bibbo* et al. reported benign anatomical abnormalities (e.g., epididymal cysts, undescended testis, hypoplastic testis) in males exposed to DES in utero. In 1976, *Gill* et al. reported severely pathologic changes in semen analyses of DES-exposed male offspring.

Research continues in this area, but to date many questions still remain unanswered (e.g., the risk for clear cell adenocarcinoma and squamous neoplasia in the female offspring with the advance of age, fertility impairment in female and male offspring, risk for testicular carcinoma in the male offspring, effects on human development due to the interaction of postnatal environmental variables with prenatal hormone influence). A slight but statistically not significant increase in the breast cancer rate in mothers exposed to DES has brought some concern and has caused the extension of the DES research to the mothers themselves (*Bibbo* et al., 1978a).

II. Neonatal Data

Scarce data are available on the neonatal period of DES-exposed offspring. The assessment of neonatal medical records of DES-exposed subjects born at the University of Chicago shows that the babies' conditions at birth, as well as postnatally, were normal for most male and female subjects; a few cases of congenital malformations were reported in the charts at birth. The rate of premature babies was slightly higher in the male DES-exposed group, and the average weight in the female DES-exposed group was smaller when compared to unexposed subjects. There were no differences in the childhood medical histories of the DES-exposed and unexposed groups, none of whom had malignancy or endocrine disease. The deaths of the deceased offspring had no relationship to genital cancer or endocrine disease (*Bibbo* et al., 1977).

III. Female Offspring

Most data pertaining to physical examination of DES-exposed females were obtained in subjects after adolescence (*Bibbo* et al., 1977; *Herbst* et al., 1975; *Stafl* et al., 1974; *Townsend,* 1978). It is generally agreed that the gynecologic examination of the female offspring should include inspection of the vulva, vagina, and uterine cervix; vaginal and cervical cytology; colposcopy (optional); iodine stain; biopsy, when indicated; vaginal palpation; and bimanual examination.

1. Anatomical Abnormalities

Numerous benign abnormalities (e.g., vaginal adenosis; gross structural abnormalities of the cervix and vagina consisting of transverse ridges, collars, protuberances or cock's combs, sulci, pseudopolyps of the cervix, and hypoplasia of the cervix) are more prevalent than clear cell adenocarcinoma of the vagina in the female DES-exposed offspring (*Bibbo* et al., 1977; *Herbst* et al., 1975; *Ng* et al., 1975; *Sandberg,* 1976).

a) Vaginal Adenosis

α) Pathology

Vaginal adenosis is the presence of columnar epithelium lining the surface of the vagina or glands in the lamina propria. Often these glands are lined with metaplastic epithelium (Fig. 1). The frequency of this finding in the DES-exposed population is 35%–90% (*Antonioli* and *Burke,* 1975; *Bibbo* et al., 1977; *Herbst* et al., 1975). It is most commonly seen on the anterior wall of the upper portion of the vagina. According to *Bibbo* et al. (1977), vaginal adenosis was found in 66.8% of a DES-exposed female group and in 3.7% of a control group not exposed to DES. The epithelial changes reflecting the presence of adenosis were localized in the anterior wall of the vagina in 17.6% of the patients; in the anterior and posterior walls in 42.5%; in the anterior, posterior, and one of the lateral walls in 15%; and in all four quadrants in 25%. In the subjects with adenosis, 92.8% had lesions in the upper third of the vagina, 5.8% in the middle third, and 1.3% in the lower third.

The columnar epithelium of vaginal adenosis may be composed of mucin rich cells, resembling those of the endocervix, or of mucin free cells with dense cytoplasm, resembling those of the endometrium and fallopian tube. Histologic studies of specimens of adenosis have shown that mucinous epithelium is found alone in 85% of the specimens, endometrial tubal-type alone in 4%–6%, and mixtures of the two epithelial cell

194

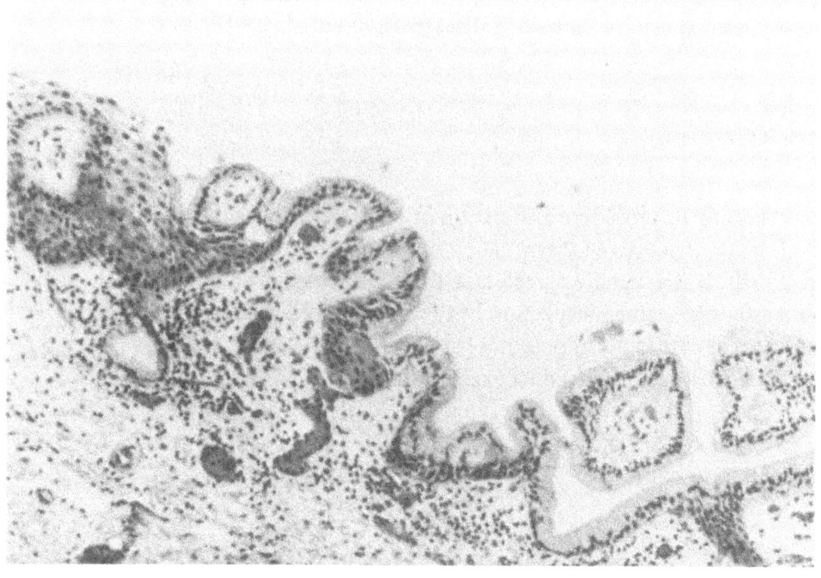

Fig. 1. Vaginal adenosis. Columnar and immature metaplastic epithelium line surface of vagina and glands (H & E x 100)

types in the remainder (*Antonioli* and *Burke*, 1975; *Ng* et al., 1977). In most cases of vaginal adenosis, a chronic inflammatory infiltrate is present, usually in mild to moderate degree, and may be associated with an increased vascularity of the lamina propria.

It seems that most of the lesions classified as adenosis undergo involution as time elapses and, as a result, the columnar epithelium is replaced by squamous metaplasia. Not a single case of vaginal adenosis progressing to clear cell carcinoma has been observed. The involution starts as reserve cell proliferation and may go through the stages of immature squamous metaplasia, mature metaplasia, and fully glycogenated squamous epithelium that is indistinguishable from the normal native squamous epithelium (*Ng* et al., 1977).

Dysplastic changes and carcinoma in situ have been reported in a small number of DES-exposed women (*Bibbo* et al., 1977; *Hart* et al., 1976; *Mattingly* and *Stafl*, 1976; *Robboy* et al., 1976, 1978). These findings have led some investigators to speculate that the incidence of carcinoma in situ and invasive squamous cell carcinoma of the lower genital tract will rise greatly as the exposed population reaches the peak age when these lesions are encountered in the cervix of the unexposed woman (*Mattingly* and *Stafl*, 1976; *Stafl* and *Mattingly*, 1974). The validity of this prediction, however, has been challenged. Several investigators have pointed out the relatively common misinterpretation of mature and immature metaplastic epithelium for dysplastic or neoplastic squamous epithelium (*Richart* et al., 1978). It seems that only a long term follow up of the DES-exposed female could elucidate the true incidence of dysplasia, carcinoma in situ, and invasive squamous cell carcinoma in this population.

Histologically, the grades of dysplasia and carcinoma in situ reflect both the qualitative and quantitative degrees to which each of the following abnormalities is found:
1) a deficiency of cellular maturation from the basement membrane toward the surface;
2) crowding of the nuclei; 3) variation in nuclear size and shape, nuclear hyperchromatism, mitoses, particularly abnormal forms, disturbances of nuclear polarity; 4) and a decrease of cytoplasm toward the surface. In mild dysplasia the cellular atypicality involves a small focus of basally located cells whereas in carcinoma in situ it involves cells from all layers of the epithelium (*Robboy* et al., 1978).

β) Colposcopy

Colposcopically, true adenosis is characterized by the presence of columnar epithelium (Fig. 2) and transformed adenosis by white epithelium and fine mosaic (Fig. 3). Punctation and coarse mosaic are associated with dysplastic epithelium.

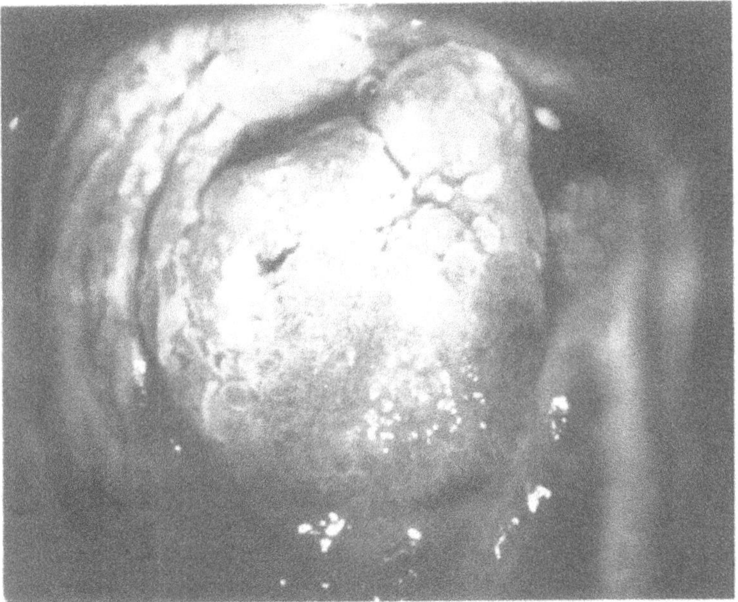

Fig. 2. Colposcopical picture of vaginal adenosis. Columnar epithelium is present on the surface of vagina and uterine cervix. The grape-like structures become visible after application of acetic acid

The shades of whiteness of white epithelium vary due to several factors and the histologic findings in the white epithelium also differ greatly. In our study, we used the term "white epithelium" for all epithelial changes in the vagina which became distinct after application of acetic acid and had more or less definite borders. The Schiller

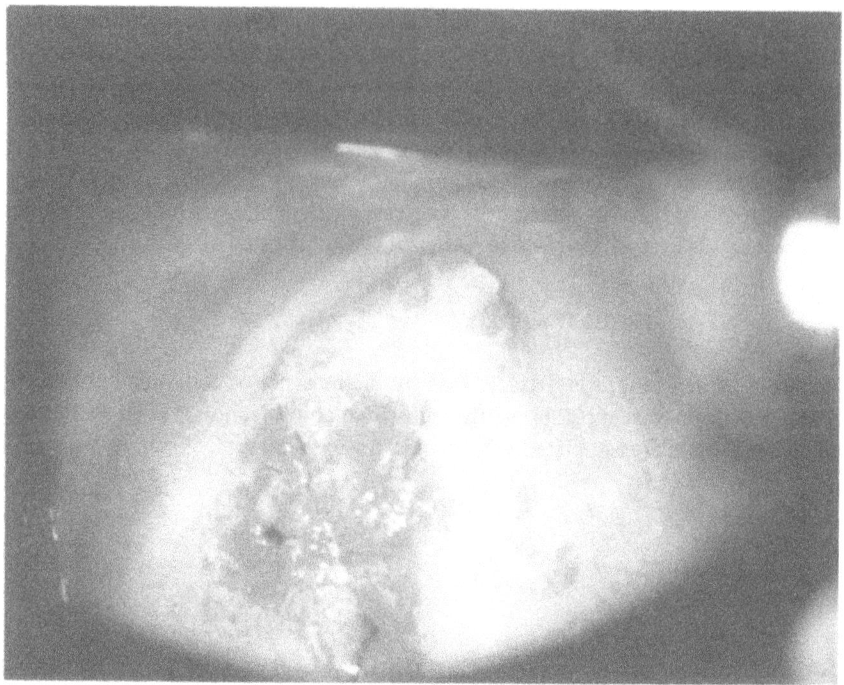

Fig. 3. Colposcopical picture of transformed vaginal adenosis. White epithelium is present on the surface of the vagina and on the deformity of the cervix which has been referred to as "cock's comb"

test was performed only for confirmation of these findings. The terms "punctation" and "mosaic" in the vagina were used in the same sense as used in routine colposcopy of the cervix. It should be mentioned that both of these focal changes were fine and smooth with relatively small intercapillary distances in all our cases. Of interest in our study was the lack of a statistically significant difference in the occurrence of columnar epithelium in the cervix between the control group and the DES-exposed group, in contrast to other reports in the literature (*Sonek* et al., 1976).

Analysis of the correlation between the commencement of DES treatment and the incidence of vaginal adenosis showed that the earlier the DES treatment is initiated during pregnancy, the higher is the incidence of vaginal adenosis (P < 0.001) (Fig. 4) (*Bibbo*, 1978b). This may explain the variations in the reports of vaginal adenosis by different authors (*Antonioli* and *Burke,* 1975; *Bibbo* et al., 1977; *Herbst* et al., 1975).

γ) Cytology

Several cellular sampling techniques have been used in females exposed in utero to DES in order to provide information about the vaginal epithelium. A comparison of the diagnostic accuracy of several types of vaginal samples showed negative cellular findings of 9% when the lesions of the vagina were directly scraped, 12% in the four quadrant

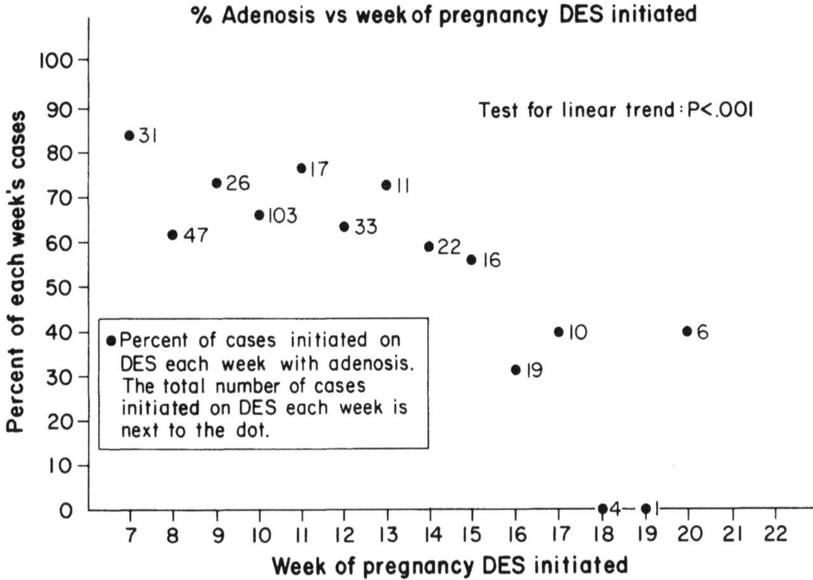

Fig. 4. Plot of the data shows a relatively constant proportion of adenosis cases over starting times prior to the 16th week of pregnancy followed by a sharp drop in subsequent weeks

sample, and 82% in a single vaginal sample (*Ng* et al., 1975). Using circumvaginal scraping, adenosis was detected in 45% of DES-exposed patients and 88% of patients with confirmed adenosis (*Hart* et al., 1976). By means of four-smear vaginal samples, *Bibbo* et al. (1975b) detected vaginal adenosis in 90% of DES-exposed patients with colposcopic evidence of adenosis. The method of collection of vaginal smears in DES-exposed females has, as an important step, the removal of the excess mucus or secretions from the uterine cervix and vagina before the smears are taken. In order to prepare the four-smear vaginal sample, the scrapings are taken from the upper to the lower third of the vagina, using four wooden tongue blades, and each sample is spread onto a glass slide labeled anterior, posterior, right lateral, and left lateral. In addition to the vaginal smears, routine ecto- and endocervical smears are taken with Ayre spatulas. The specimens are immediately fixed in 95% ethyl alcohol and stained according to the Papanicolaou method (*Bibbo* et al., 1975b).

True adenosis in the vagina is associated with columnar cells in the cellular sample. Most columnar cells resemble the tall endocervical cells which one frequently observes in samples taken from the uterine cervix (Fig. 5). Fewer columnar cells are of the small columnar type and resemble endometrial cells. Both cell types exhibit granular or vacuolated cytoplasm and a round or oval nucleus in the base of the cell. Honeycomb arrangements are frequently observed.

Transformed adenosis is associated with metaplastic cells. The metaplastic cells are similar to those observed in samples from the uterine cervix and are seen in sheets or singly. Vacuolization of the cytoplasm is a common feature. Transitional forms between columnar and metaplastic cells may be present. Anucleated squames reflecting

198

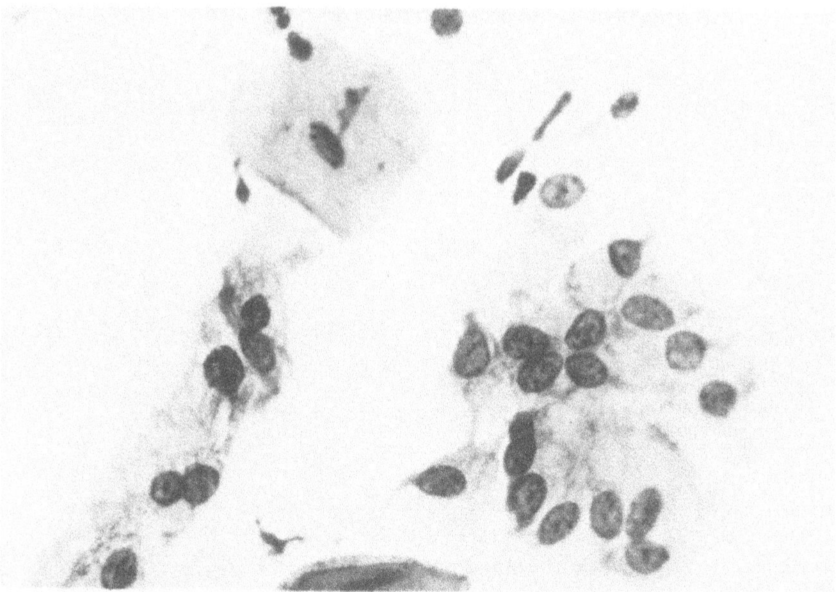

Fig. 5. Vaginal smear of patient with adenosis exhibiting columnar cells (Papanicolaou x 400)

the presence of hyperkeratosis in the epithelium and parakeratotic cells, which may reflect the presence of parakeratosis in the epithelium, may also be observed.

Squamous dysplastic cells and carcinoma in situ can be observed in the vaginal samples from DES-exposed patients. Dysplastic cells are characterized by an increased nucleo/cytoplasmic ratio, nuclear hyperchromasia, and irregular nuclear borders. In the mild dysplasias, the abnormal cells are of the superficial or intermediate type, whereas in moderate and severe dysplasias, they are usually of the intermediate and parabasal types. Dysplastic cells of all grades are observed more frequently in clusters than as isolated cells (*Robboy* et al., 1978). Carcinoma in situ is characterized by round or oval cells with a markedly increased nucleo/cytoplasmic ratio, coarsely granular chromatin, and hyperchromasia.

Table 1 shows the breakdown of cellular findings in DES-exposed patients with confirmed adenosis. These results were obtained by our group in a follow-up study of offspring of mothers who were part of a double-blind placebo investigation (*Bibbo* et al., 1977). The average age of the patients was 24 years. Metaplastic cells were the most common cytologic finding, suggesting that in this age group the columnar epithelium is replaced by metaplastic epithelium in approximately 75% of the patients. In a study by *Ng* et al. (1975), the cellular findings in the offspring of women exposed in utero varied in relation to age — metaplastic cells increased in frequency in vaginal scrapings from women with adenosis over age 15. In our study, mild dysplasias were observed in the vaginal scrapings in eight cases, confirmed by histology in five cases and all three cases of moderately dysplastic lesions were evident in the biopsy specimen. In other studies the prevalence of dysplastic changes has also been low (*Hart* et al., 1976; *Robboy* et al., 1976, 1978).

Table 1. DES-exposed females with adenosis-four-smear vaginal sample

Cellular findings	Number	Percent
Negative	17	7.4
Columnar cells	17	7.4
Metaplastic cells	140	61.1
Anucleated squames, metaplastic and parakeratotic cells	44	19.2
Mild dysplastic cells	8	3.5
Moderately dysplastic cells	3	1.3
Total	229	100.0

b) Cervicovaginal Ridges

Reports on the incidence of gross structural abnormalities of the cervix and vagina were 22%–58% of cases of DES exposure (*Bibbo* et al., 1977; *Herbst* et al., 1975; *Sandberg*, 1976). These abnormalities consist of transverse ridges; collars; deformities of the cervix, which vary from a very small protuberance on the anterior lip to a typical cock's comb formation or complete cervical deformity; and hypoplastic cervix (Figs. 6 and 7).

Investigation into the relationship between the time of commencement of the DES treatment (i.e., week of pregnancy) and the incidence of ridging also showed evidence

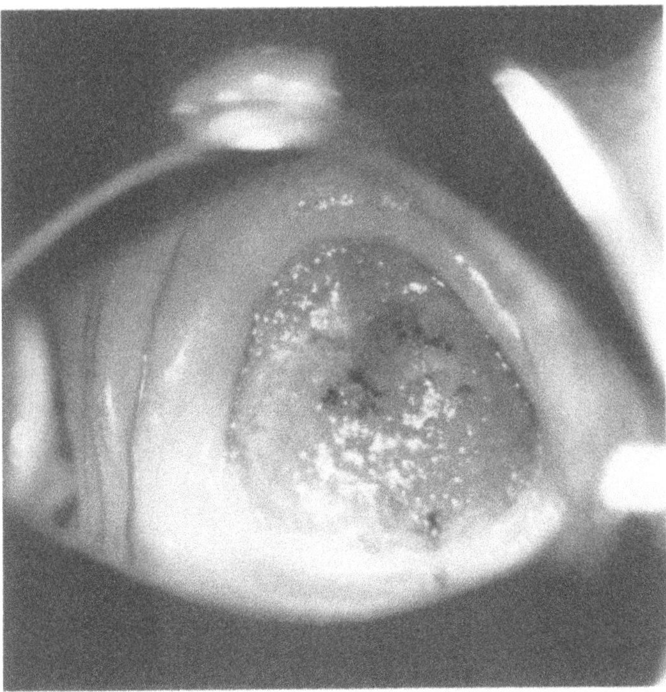

Fig. 6. Colpophotograph of cervix of a DES-exposed offspring demonstrating a complete cervical collar

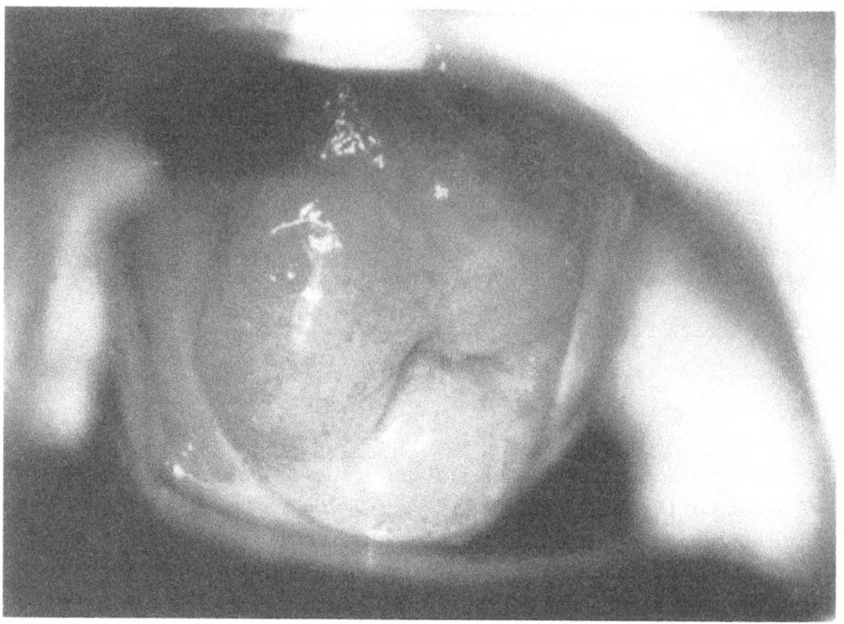

Fig. 7. Colpophotograph of a lobulated cervix of a DES-exposed female covered by columnar epithelium

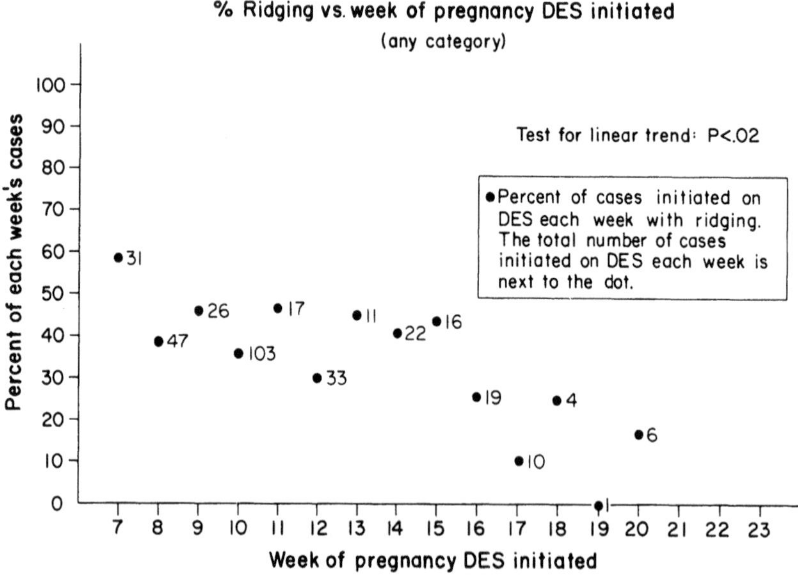

Fig. 8. Plot of data shows that the earlier the DES treatment is initiated during pregnancy, the higher is the incidence of ridging

that the higher incidences were associated with initiation in the earlier weeks, except that the nominal significance was not as great as for the incidence of vaginal adenosis (P < 0.02) (Fig. 8) (*Bibbo*,1978b).

There appears to be a definite correlation between adenosis and ridging or cervical deformity. In one study of 218 patients with adenosis, 109 (50%) also had ridging or cervical deformity while only 22 (17%) of the 128 patients without adenosis had ridging or cervical deformity (*Bibbo*, 1978b).

c) Clear Cell Adenocarcinoma

It has been shown that the risk of clear cell adenocarcinoma is small in the population exposed to DES (*Herbst* et al., 1977; *Lanier* et al., 1973). The adenocarcinoma of the vagina or cervix appears 7–27 years after intrauterine exposure to DES or chemically related nonsteroidal estrogens (*Herbst* and *Cole*, 1978).

α) Pathology

In the Registry for Research on Hormonal Transplacental Carcinogenesis, about 60% of the clear cell adenocarcinomas have been designated as vaginal and 40% as cervical. The cervical carcinomas are situated predominantly on the exocervix and the vaginal tumors are most often located on the anterior wall, usually in the upper third of the vagina. The smallest carcinoma in the Registry measured 0.3 cm in diameter and the largest over 10 cm. The tumors were described as polypoid or nodular predominantly, but some were flat or ulcerated with an indurated or granular surface. One carcinoma was confined to the lamina propria and was covered by the squamous epithelium of the vagina or cervix (*Scully* et al., 1978).

Microscopically, three predominant patterns and three predominant cell types have been described. The most common pattern has tubule and cyst formation (Fig. 9); the second most common pattern is characterized by solid nests or masses of cells; and the least common pattern has numerous papillae within the tubules and cysts. Often the three patterns are combined in a single lesion. The predominant cell type is the clear cell, the second most common is the hobnail, and the third is the flat. The clear cell type is characterized by large polyhedral cells with clear cytoplasm, the hobnail has a bulbous nucleus protruding into the lumen beyond the cytoplasmic limits of the cell, and the flat is characterized by neoplastic cells which are flat and line cysts. The lumens of the tubules and cysts often contain mucus, but the cytoplasm is almost always mucin free (*Scully* et al., 1978).

In addition to local spread, clear cell adenocarcinomas metastasize via lymphatics and blood vessels.

The size and depth of invasion of the primary tumor are significant in relation to prognosis. The tubulocystic pattern is the most favorable in contrast to the papillary pattern which is associated with the worst prognosis (*Scully* et al., 1978).

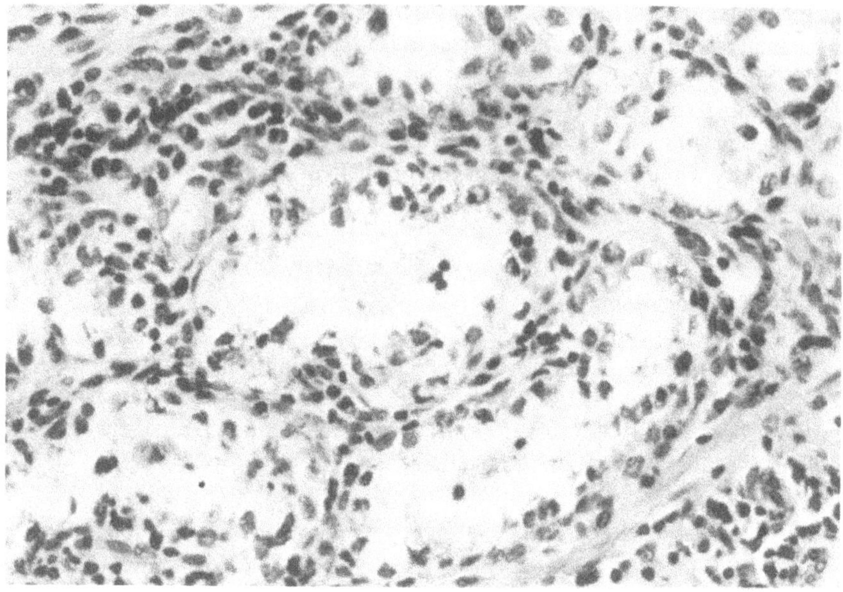

Fig. 9. Clear cell adenocarcinoma of vagina (H & E x 250)

β) Cytology

The cellular abnormalities observed in the presence of clear cell adenocarcinoma are different from those associated with adenosis. The cells resemble those of cervical adenocarcinoma since they are larger than the cells of most endometrial adenocarcinomas. The tumor cells occur singly and in clumps and have delicate cytoplasm, large nuclei, and a prominent nucleolus (Fig. 10). Bare nuclei are frequently observed. In the well differentiated tumors, the degree of atypia is less pronounced, which makes the recognition of the tumor cells more difficult (*Taft* et al., 1974). Cytology plays an important role in the detection of both the primary and recurrent tumors, provided that adequate cell samples are obtained.

d) Pathogenesis of Vaginal Adenosis, Cervicovaginal Ridges, and Clear Cell Adenocarcinoma

Most investigators believe that embryologically the vagina has a double origin from the fused lower ends of the Müllerian ducts and the urogenital sinus (*Bulmer*, 1957; *Forsberg*, 1973; *Ulfelder*, 1976). The primitive vagina is first lined by Müllerian columnar epithelium, which is transformed into stratified squamous epithelium before a second type of squamous epithelium grows upward from the urogenital sinus to replace it (*Forsberg*, 1973). It is believed that DES interferes in some manner with the replacement of the Müllerian columnar epithelium by squamous epithelium. The administration of estrogens to the neonatal mouse inhibits mitotic activity in the columnar epithelium and,

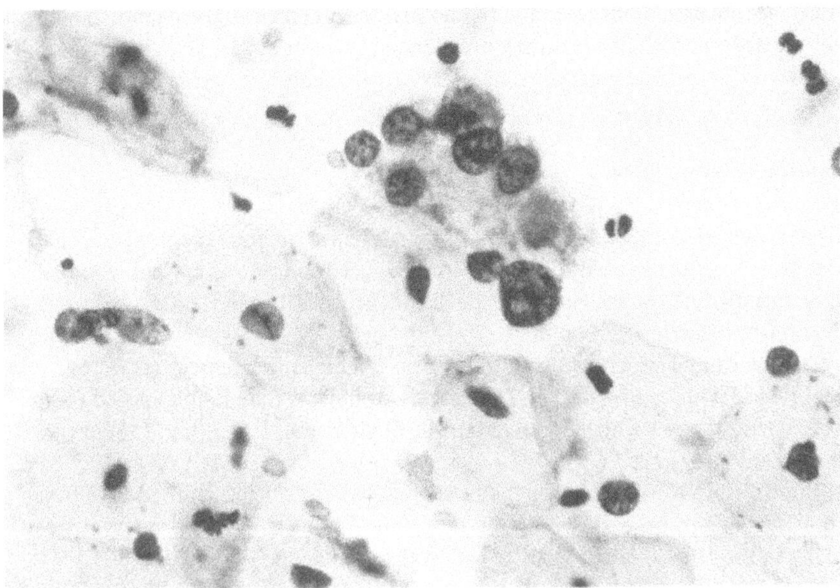

Fig. 10. Vaginal smear in a case of vaginal clear cell adenocarcinoma. Tumor cells exhibit clear cytoplasm, enlarged nuclei, chromatin clumping and macronucleoli (Papanicolaou x 400)

according to *Forsberg* (1973), this phenomenon is essential for the transformation of columnar epithelium into squamous epithelium. *Forsberg* (1975, 1976) has produced in this animal model a glandular lesion similar to human adenosis. There is a possibility that the estrogens may act primarily on the stroma with secondary abnormal induction of epithelial changes. A direct action on the stroma might also explain the various gross structural abnormalities of the cervix and vagina which are largely due to deficiencies or overgrowths of connective tissue (*Scully* et al., 1978).

The histogenesis of the clear cell adenocarcinoma of the female genital tract was originally linked to the mesonephros and its derivatives (*Schiller*, 1939; *Teilum*, 1954). The reasons for postulating the mesonephric origin have been refuted and in recent years the Müllerian nature of the tumor has gained more support. This interpretation was first introduced in 1967 by *Scully* and *Barlow* and this theory was subsequently confirmed with additional evidence by others (*Aure* et al., 1971; *Kurman* and *Scully*, 1976). The study of small clear cell adenocarcinomas of the cervix and vagina in the Registry on Hormonal Transplacental Carcinogenesis has revealed their origin in the superficial layers of these organs where epithelium of the Müllerian-type is found in over 90% of the cases in the form of cervical ectropion and vaginal adenosis. Meso-nephric remnants lie deeply situated in the wall of the cervix and vagina, except for the openings of their ducts. In addition, most clear cell adenocarcinomas of the vagina in-volve primarily the anterior wall where adenosis is predominantly situated, whereas mesonephric remnants are in an anterolateral or lateral location (*Herbst* et al., 1974).

Existing evidence links the clear cell adenocarcinoma to the endometrial or endo-metrioid type of cell. Light and electron microscopic studies have shown that the cells of clear cell adenocarcinomas resemble the hobnail cells and clear glycogen rich cells found in the endometrial glands during pregnancy (*Lewis* et al., 1973; *Scully* et al., 1978). However, more investigation is necessary to elucidate the nature of this tumor.

2. Functional Abnormalities

It has been shown that 18% of DES-exposed females have irregular menstrual cycle compared to 10% of unexposed females. With the exception of one patient who had secondary amenorrhea, all patients with menstrual irregularities in the DES-exposed group had oligomenorrhea (*Bibbo* et al., 1977).

In reference to menstrual flow duration, there is a higher percentage (60%) of menstrual flows lasting 1 to 4 days in DES-exposed subjects than in unexposed females (43%) who present a higher percentage of flows lasting 5 to 7 days (55% vs 26%) (*Bibbo* et al., 1977).

How these different patterns of menstrual cycles will affect the reproductive function is not clear at this time. However, an important finding is the lower percentage of pregnancies in the DES-exposed females (18%) than in unexposed females (33%) (*Bibbo* et al., 1977).

In 40 women exposed to DES, *Kaufman* et al. (1977) reported changes in the uterus, detected by means of hysterosalpingograms, which differed significantly from those seen in the past in unexposed individuals. These changes consisted of a T-shaped appearance of the uterus; constricting bands in the uterine cavity; hypoplastic uterus; and less frequently intrauterine polypoid defects, synechiae, and unicornuate uterus. In 36 of the 40 women, gross defects were also noted in the cervix.

Most investigators agree that it is too early to evaluate the clinical significance of the cervical and uterine abnormalities because, to date, few of the DES-exposed women have been pregnant. It will be very interesting to observe in the coming years the pregnancy outcome of DES-exposed females, especially the ones with uterine abnormalities.

IV. Male Offspring

The transplacental effects of DES on the human male fetus were originally reported by our group (*Bibbo* et al., 1975a; *Gill* et al., 1976). Both anatomical abnormalities (e.g., epididymal cysts, undescended testes, hypoplastic testes) and functional abnormalities (e.g., abnormal semen) of the genital tract were significantly greater in the DES-exposed males compared to unexposed control males whose mothers were all participants in a prospective, randomized, and double blind study of the effects of DES on pregnancy at the Chicago Lying-in Hospital during the early 1950s (*Dieckmann* et al., 1953).

1. Anatomical Abnormalities

DES-exposed offspring have a significantly increased incidence of epididymal cysts (Fig. 11) (20.8%) and testicular hypoplasia (testis < 3.6 cm) (8.4%) compared to unex-

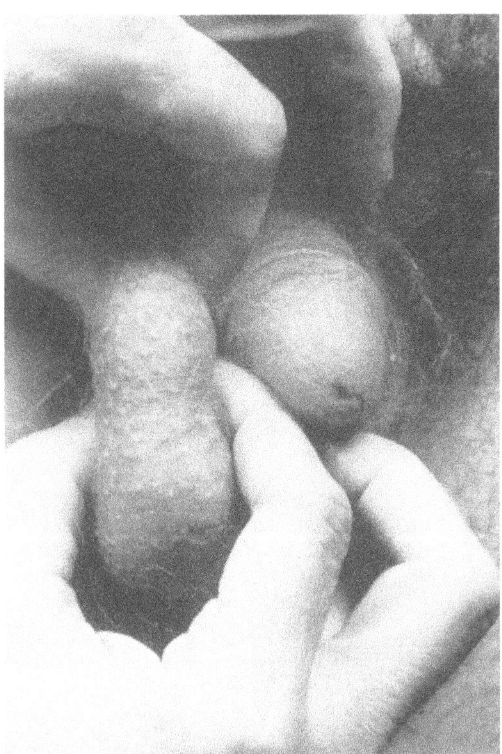

Fig. 11. External genitalia of a DES-exposed male with a right epididymal cyst superior to testis

posed males. The exact nature of abnormal physical findings in the testis and epididymal areas is difficult to ascertain since biopsies have not been performed in the affected organs. One could speculate that the cysts in the area of the efferent ductules and superior epididymis may be abnormally DES-stimulated Müllerian duct remnants. Aspirates of the epididymal masses in nine DES-exposed patients revealed a straw-colored fluid that did not contain spermatozoa in six cases and a slightly milky fluid that did contain sperm in three cases. Cytologic examination revealed only epithelial cells and amorphous precipitates without any material suggestive of malignancy (*Gill* et al., 1977).

Table 2 summarizes the abnormal physical findings in our study where the males were examined 2 1/2 decades after in utero exposure to placebo or DES (*Bibbo*, 1978b). A history of cryptorchidism is evident in 65% of the patients with hypoplastic testes in the DES-exposed group, which raises the risk of testicular carcinoma.

These findings in human beings are quantitatively in agreement with old and new studies in animals. In 1940, *Greene* et al. reported that the effects on rats of in utero exposure to estradiol or diethylstilbestrol were cryptorchidism, hypoplastic testes, and underdeveloped epididymis. *Dunn* and *Green* (1963) reported the occurrence of cysts of the epididymis in male mice and cancer of the cervix in female mice after subcutaneous DES injections to these mice at birth. *McLachlan*'s group (1975) has published data on the reproductive tract lesions in male mice exposed prenatally to DES.

Table 2. Genital tract abnormalities in the adult males 25 years after in utero exposure to DES

	Control	DES-exposed	P values
Total number of men	307	308	
Epididymal cysts	15 (4.9%)	64 (20.8%)	<0.0005
Unilateral			
Left	9	29	
Right	3	20	
Bilateral	3	15	
Testicular abnormalities	9 (2.9%)	35 (11.4%)	<0.0005
Hypoplastic testis	6 (1.9%)	26 (8.4%)	<0.0005
Unilateral			
Left	3	14	
Right	1	7	
Bilateral	2	5	
Cryptorchidism[a]	1	17	<0.0005
Capsular induration	3	9	<0.100
Microphallus	0	4	<0.050
Total number of patients with one or more of above abnormalities	24 (7.8%)	97 (31.5%)	<0.0005

[a] Cryptorchidism history in patients with hypoplastic testes.

These workers found in the male mice studied that 60% were sterile, 33% had epididymal cysts, 25% had undescended testes, and 25% had nodular enlargement of the seminal vesicles and/or coagulating glands which were associated with squamous metaplasia. *Nomura* and *Kanzaki* (1977) have shown that DES given to mice only later in pregnancy produced undescended testes and testicular hypogenesis in addition to lung tumors.

Although carcinogenesis has not been demonstrated in human males, it has been demonstrated that prenatal exposure to DES produces detectable anatomical changes in the male reproductive tract. The following factors raise the question of potential malignancy in the adult male exposed to DES in utero: 1) the increased incidence of cryptorchidism and hypoplastic testes increases the risk of testes carcinoma (*Mostofi*, 1973); 2) the prostatic utricle, which is the Müllerian duct remnant homologous to the female vagina, has been found to be the site of endometrial carcinoma in older human males (*Melicow* and *Pachter*, 1967); and 3) the natural history of prostatic carcinoma, which occurs largely in the 7th and 8th decades of life, may be related to changes in the steroid environment.

2. Functional Abnormalities

DES-exposed males show a decreased average sperm density when compared to unexposed males (*Bibbo* et al., 1977). Table 3 shows the up-to-date results of sperm counts of DES-exposed male offspring obtained by our group. The subsets of hypoplastic

Table 3. Sperm counts

	Control	DES-exposed
Average sperm density x 10^6/ml		
Hypoplastic testes (n)	47 (4)	42 (21) p<0.001
Total group (n)	115 (87) (p<0.05)	91 (134)
Azoospermia		
Hypoplastic testes	0	2
Total group	0	3
$\leq$ 10 million sperm/ml		
Hypoplastic testes	1	5
Total group	4	9
< 20 million sperm/ml		
Hypoplastic testes	2	7
Total group	8	20

testes in both groups showed considerable depression of the average sperm concentration as compared to the total groups. The azoospermics and oligospermics also showed a positive correlation with testicular hypoplasia (*Bibbo*, 1978b).

The distribution of spermatozoa analyses is given in Table 4 by *Eliasson*'s method (1975), which combines the sperm count, the sperm motility, the motility grade, and the sperm morphology into one quantitative number. Note that the average Eliasson Score is significantly higher in the DES-exposed group (4.9) compared to the unexposed group (2.5). Further, the hypoplastic testes subset of the DES-exposed group has a considerable further increase in the average Eliasson Score to 10.3. Table 4 also shows a further clustering of patients with abnormal semen (Eliasson Scores $\geq$ 5,

Table 4. Eliasson scores of semen analyses

	Control	DES-exposed
Average Eliasson score		
Hypoplastic testes (n)	6.2 (4)	10.3 (21) p<0.001
Total group (n)	2.5 (87) p<0.01	4.9 (134)
Eliasson score $\geq$ 5 "pathological semen"		
Hypoplastic testes	2 (50%)	14 (67%)
Total group	14 (16%) p<0.025	43 (32%)
Eliasson score > 10 "severely pathological semen"		
Hypoplastic testes	2 (50%)	7 (33%)
Total group	7 (8%) p< 0.050	24 (18%)

208

"pathological semen"; and > 10, "severely pathological semen") in the DES-exposed
males. Also, the hypoplastic testis subgroups have an increased incidence in the pathological semens.

Administration of DES during pregnancy appears to be followed by effects on the
fetal male genital tract that have shown up in the form of structural and functional
changes that may well impair fertility in a certain number of patients. With the delays
in family planning prevalent today, it will probably be another decade before the
actual infertility rate is known. However, since semen analyses give insight into the
probability of male infertility (*Amelar,* 1966), one needs to follow these and expanded
numbers of patients carefully with regard to the association of DES-exposure and subnormal fertility.

3. Psychological Effects

Data related to the hypothesis that steroid hormones affect neural (CNS) tissue during
development and thereby influence intelligence and personality come primarily from
experimental animal research and human clinical studies. It has been demonstrated that
during critical periods in development the presence of exogenously introduced or endo-
genously produced steroids affects both reproduction linked (i.e., mating) behavior and
dimorphically expressed nonmating behavior (e.g., aggression, play, wheel running,
open-field activity). This has been shown in rats, guinea pigs, mice, hamsters, and rhesus
monkeys. Furthermore, studies spanning the last 35 years have demonstrated that CNS
tissue is modified functionally, anatomically, histologically, and in metabolic activity
by the presence or absence of androgen during critical periods of early development.
Many of these effects, which occur normally under the influence of androgen, can be
mimicked by administration of estrogen (*Reinisch,* 1974, 1976, 1977).

Given the large number of individuals exposed to DES in utero, it is interesting to
note that only a few studies of the possible psychological effects of prenatal DES have
been carried out. *Yalom* et al. (1973) evaluated nondiabetic male offspring of diabetic
mothers who received DES during pregnancy. The results revealed that 16-year-old sons
of hormone treated diabetic mothers were less aggressive, less assertive, had less athletic
skill and grace, and performed less well on the embedded figure task than the control
group. The authors suggested, albeit tentatively, that "it is not the diabetes but the hormone administration which influenced the psychosocial development to move in the
direction we have described." Analysis of the data on the DES-exposed older subjects
showed a trend toward "low dose, late initiation of hormone to be related to feminine
behavior." This finding of a relationship between "feminized" behavior and prenatal
treatment with estrogen in human males parallels the results of animal studies. *Reinisch*
and *Karow,* in 1977, found differences in personality between hormone exposed subjects and their unexposed siblings and felt that the finding strongly suggests a relationship between prenatal treatment with hormones and personality.

V. Conclusions

In conclusion, in the short period of 8 years, much has been learned on transplacental effects of diethylstilbestrol. Many questions still remain unanswered, but continuing investigation will hopefully increase our knowledge in this area.

References

Amelar, R.D.: Infertility in men: diagnosis and treatment. Philadelphia: Davis 1966

Antonioli, D., Burke, L.: Vaginal adenosis. Analysis of 325 biopsy specimens from 100 patients. Am. J. Clin. Pathol. *64*, 625–638 (1975)

Aure, J.C., Høeg, K., Kolstad, P.: Carcinoma of the ovary and endometriosis. Acta Obstet. Gynecol. Scand. *50*, 63–67 (1971)

Bibbo, M., Al-Naqeeb, M., Baccarini, I., Gill, W., Newton, M., Sleeper, K.M., Sonek, M., Wied, G.L.: Follow-up study of male and female offspring of DES-treated mothers. A preliminary report. J. Reprod. Med. *15*, 29–32 (1975a)

Bibbo, M., Ali, I., Al-Naqeeb, M., Baccarini, I., Climaco, L.A., Gill, W., Sonek, M., Wied, G.L.: Cytologic findings in female and male offspring of DES treated mothers. Acta Cytol. *19*, 568–572 (1975b)

Bibbo, M., Gill, W.B., Azizi, F., Blough, R., Fang, V.S., Rosenfield, R.L., Schumacher, G.F.B., Sleeper, K., Sonek, M.G., Wied, G.L.: Follow-up study of male and female offspring of DES-exposed mothers. Obstet. Gynecol. *49*, 1–8 (1977)

Bibbo, M., Haenszel, W.M., Wied, G.L., Hubby, M., Herbst, A.L.: A twenty-five-year follow-up study of women exposed to diethylstilbestrol during pregnancy. N. Engl. J. Med. *298*, 763–767 (1978a)

Bibbo, M.: Unpublished data (1978b)

Bulmer, D.: The development of the human vagina. J. Anat. *91*, 490–509 (1957)

Dieckmann, W.J., Davis, M.E., Rynkiewicz, L.M., Pottinger, R.E.: Does the administration of diethylstilbestrol during pregnancy have therapeutic value? Am. J. Obstet. Gynecol. *66*, 1062–1081 (1953)

Dunn, T.B., Green, A.W.: Cysts of the epididymis, cancer of the cervix, granular cell myoblastoma, and other lesions after estrogen injection in newborn mice. J. Natl. Cancer Inst. *31*, 425–438 (1963)

Eliasson, R.: Analysis of semen. In: Progress in infertility. Behrman, S.J., Kistner, R.W. (eds.), 2nd ed., p. 691. Boston: Little, Brown and Co. 1975

Forsberg, J.-G.: Cervicovaginal epithelium: Its origin and development. Am. J. Obstet. Gynecol. *115*, 1025–1043 (1973)

Forsberg, J.-G.: Late effects in the vaginal and cervical epithelia after injections of diethylstilbestrol into neonatal mice. Am. J. Obstet. Gynecol. *121*, 101–103 (1975)

Forsberg, J.-G.: Animal model of human disease. Adenosis and clear cell carcinomas of vagina and cervix. Animal model: Estrogen-induced adenosis of vagina and cervix in mice. Am. J. Pathol. *84*, 669–672 (1976)

Gill, W.B., Schumacher, G.F.B., Bibbo, M.: Structural and functional abnormalities in the sex organs of male offspring treated with diethylstilbestrol (DES). J. Reprod. Med. *16*, 147–153 (1976)

Gill, W.B., Schumacher, G.F.B., Bibbo, M.: Pathological semen and anatomical abnormalities of the genital tract in human male subjects exposed to diethylstilbestrol in utero. J. Urol. *117*, 477–480 (1977)

Greene, R.R., Burril, M.W., Ivy, A.C.: Experimental intersexuality: the effects of estrogens on the antenatal sexual development of the rat. Am. J. Anat. *67*, 305–345 (1940)

Hart, W.R., Zaharov, I., Kaplan, B.J., Townsend, D.E., Aldrich, J.O., Henderson, B.E., Roy, M., Benton, B.: Cytologic findings in stilbestrol exposed females with emphasis on detection of vaginal adenosis. Acta Cytol. *20*, 7–14 (1976)

Heinonen, O.P.: Diethylstilbestrol in pregnancy: Frequency of exposure and usage patterns. Cancer *31*, 573–577 (1973)

Herbst, A.L., Ulfelder, H., Poskanzer, D.C.: Adenocarcinoma of the vagina: association of maternal stilbestrol therapy with tumor appearance in young women. N. Engl. J. Med. *284*, 878–881 (1971)

Herbst, A.L., Kurman, R.J., Scully, R.E., Poskanzer, D.C.: Clear-cell adenocarcinoma of the genital tract in young females: Registry report. N. Engl. J. Med. *287*, 1259–1264 (1972)

Herbst, A.L., Robboy, S.J., Scully, R.E., Poskanzer, D.C.: Clear-cell adenocarcinoma of the vagina and cervix in girls: Analysis of 170 Registry cases. Am. J. Obstet. Gynecol. *119*, 713–724 (1974)

Herbst, A.L., Poskanzer, D.C., Robboy, S.J., Friedlander, L., Scully, R.E.: Prenatal exposure to stilbestrol: a prospective comparison of exposed female offspring with unexposed controls. N. Engl. J. Med. *292*, 334–339 (1975)

Herbst, A.L., Cole, P., Colton, T., Robboy, S.J., Scully, R.E.: Age-incidence and risk of diethylstilbestrol-related clear cell adenocarcinoma of the vagina and cervix. Am. J. Obstet. Gynecol. *128*, 43–50 (1977)

Herbst, A.L., Cole, P.: Epidemiologic and clinical aspects of clear cell adenocarcinoma in young women. In: Intrauterine exposure to diethylstilbestrol in the human. Proceedings of "Symposium on DES," 1977. Herbst, A.L. (ed.), pp. 2–7. Chicago: The American College of Obstetricians and Gynecologists 1978

Kaufman, R.H., Binder, G.L., Gray, P.M., Jr., Adam, E.: Upper genital tract changes associated with exposure in utero to diethylstilbestrol. Am. J. Obstet. Gynecol. *128*, 51–56 (1977)

Kurman, R.J., Scully, R.E.: Clear cell carcinoma of the endometrium. Cancer *37*, 872–882 (1976)

Lanier, A.P., Noller, K.L., Decker, D.G., Elveback, L.R., Kurland, L.T.: Cancer and stilbestrol: A follow-up of 1,719 persons exposed to estrogens *in utero* and born 1943–1959. Mayo Clin. Proc. *48*, 793–799 (1973)

Lewis, J.L., Jr., Nordquist, S.R.B., Richart, R.M.: Studies of nuclear DNA in vaginal adenosis and clear cell adenocarcinoma. Am. J. Obstet. Gynecol. *115*, 737–746 (1973)

Mattingly, R.F., Stafl, A.: Cancer risk in diethylstilbestrol-exposed offspring. Am. J. Obstet. Gynecol. *126*, 543–548 (1976)

McLachlan, J.A., Newbold, R.R.: Reproductive tract lesions in male mice exposed prenatally to diethylstilbestrol. Science *190*, 991–992 (1975)

Melicow, M.M., Pachter, M.R.: Endometrial carcinoma of the prostatic utricle (Uterus Masculinus). Cancer *20*, 1715–1722 (1967)

Mostofi, F.K.: Testicular tumors: epidemiologic, etiologic, and pathologic features. Cancer *32*, 1186–1201 (1973)

Ng, A.B.P., Reagan, J.W., Hawliczek, S., Wentz, W.B.: Cellular detection of vaginal adenosis. Obstet. Gynecol. *46*, 323–328 (1975)

Ng, A.B.P., Reagan, J.W., Nadji, M., Greening, S.: Natural history of vaginal adenosis in women exposed to diethylstilbestrol in utero. J. Reprod. Med. *18*, 1–13 (1977)

Noller, K.L., Decker, D.C., Lanier, A.P., Kurland, L.T.: Clear-cell adenocarcinoma of the cervix after maternal treatment with synthetic estrogens. Mayo Clin. Proc. *47*, 629–630 (1972)

Noller, K.L., Fish, C.R.: Diethylstilbestrol usage: Its interesting past, important present, and questionable future. Med. Clin. North Am. *58*, 793–810 (1974)

Nomura, T., Kanzaki, T.: Induction of urogenital anomalies and some tumors in the progeny of mice receiving diethylstilbestrol during pregnancy. Cancer Res. *37*, 1099–1104 (1977)

Reinisch, J.M.: Fetal hormones, the brain, and human sex differences: a heuristic integrative review of the literature. Arch. Sex. Behav. *3*, 51–90 (1974)

Reinisch, J.M.: Effects of prenatal hormone exposure on physical and psychological development in humans and animals. With a note on the state of the field, pp. 69–93. In: Hormones, behavior and psychopathology. Sachar, E.J. (ed.). New York: Raven Press 1976

Reinisch, J.M.: Prenatal exposure of human foetuses to synthetic progestin and estrogen affects personality. Nature *266*, 561–562 (1977)

Reinisch, J.M., Karow, W.G.: Prenatal exposure to synthetic progestins and estrogens: effects on human development. Arch. Sex. Behav. *6*, 257–288 (1977)

Richart, R.M., Fu, Y.S., Reagan, J.W., Barron, B.A.: The problem of squamous neoplasia in female DES progeny. In: Intrauterine exposure to diethylstilbestrol in the human. Proceedings of "Symposium on DES," 1977. Herbst, A.L. (ed.), pp. 45–52. Chicago: The American College of Obstetricians and Gynecologists 1978

Robboy, S.J., Friedlander, L.M., Welch, W.R., Keh, P.C., Taft, P.D., Barnes, A.B., Scully, R.E., Herbst, A.L.: Cytology of 575 young women with prenatal exposure to diethylstilbestrol. Obstet. Gynecol. *48*, 511–515 (1976)

Robboy, S.J., Keh, P.C., Nickerson, R.J., Helmanis, E.K., Prat, J., Szyfelbein, W.M., Taft, P.D., Barnes, A.B., Scully, R.E., Welch, W.R.: Squamous cell dysplasia and carcinoma in situ of the cervix and vagina after prenatal exposure to diethylstilbestrol. Obstet. Gynecol. *51*, 528–535 (1978)

Sandberg, E.C.: Benign cervical and vaginal changes associated with exposure to stilbestrol in utero. Am. J. Obstet. Gynecol. *125*, 777–788 (1976)

Schiller, W.: Mesonephroma ovarii. Am. J. Cancer *35*, 1–21 (1939)

Scully, R.E., Barlow, J.F.: "Mesonephroma" of ovary. Tumor of mullerian nature related to the endometrioid carcinoma. Cancer *20*, 1405–1417 (1967)

Scully, R.E., Robboy, S.J., Welch, W.R.: Pathology and pathogenesis of diethylstilbestrol-related disorders of the female genital tract. In: Intrauterine exposure to diethylstilbestrol in the human. Proceedings of "Symposium on DES," 1977. Herbst, A.L. (ed.), pp. 8–22. Chicago: The American College of Obstetricians and Gynecologists 1978

Smith, O.W., Smith, G. van S., Hurwitz, D.: Increased excretion of pregnanediol in pregnancy from diethylstilbestrol with special reference to the prevention of late pregnancy accidents. Am. J. Obstet. Gynecol. *51*, 411–415 (1946)

Sonek, M., Bibbo, M., Wied, G.L.: Colposcopic findings in offspring of DES-treated mothers as related to onset of therapy. J. Reprod. Med. *16*, 65–71 (1976)

Stafl, A., Mattingly, R.F.: Vaginal adenosis: a precancerous lesion? Am. J. Obstet. Gynecol. *120*, 666–673 (1974)

Taft, P.D., Robboy, S.J., Herbst, A.L., Scully, R.E.: Cytology of clear-cell adenocarcinoma of genital tract in young females: review of 95 cases from the Registry. Acta Cytol. *18*, 279–290 (1974)

Teilum, G.: Histogenesis and classification of mesonephric tumors of the female and male genital system and relationship to benign so-called adenomatoid tumors (mesotheliomas). A comparative histological study. Acta Pathol.Microbiol. Scand. *34*, 431–481 (1954)

Townsend, D.E.: Techniques of examination and screening of the DES-exposed female. In: Intrauterine exposure to diethylstilbestrol in the human. Proceedings of "Symposium on DES," 1977. Herbst, A.L. (ed.), pp. 23–28. Chicago: The American College of Obstetricians and Gynecologists 1978

Ulfelder, H.: Robboy, S.J.: The embryologic development of the human vagina. Am. J. Obstet. Gynecol. *126*, 767–773 (1976)

Yalom, I.D., Green, R., Risk, N.: Prenatal exposure to female hormones: Effect on psychosexual development in boys. Arch. Gen. Psychiatry *28*, 554–561 (1973)

Subject Index

The numbers set in *italics* refer to those pages on which the respective catch-word is discussed in detail.

abnormal chord insertion 27, 48, 165
– length of cord 165
– placental configurations 6, *8*, 48
abruptio placentae 10, 73
acardiac twin *168*
–twins and single umbilical artery *168*
accessory lobes 8, 21, 24
adenosis, vaginal 192, *193*, 201
allantoic duct remnants 169
allantochorial vessels *14*
allantochorionic arteries 13, *14*, 18
alloantibodies 85
alloantigens 87, 91, 92
amnion nodosum 169
aneurysm, intervillous 67, 68, 71
angiogram, dispersed type 14
angiography of placenta 5, *13*
–, transumbilical 166, 167, 168, 169
angiomatosis 65, 66
angiomatous hyperplasia 66
angiopathy, obliterating 60, 66, 72
anomalies, congenital 168, 170
–, multiple 161, 166
antibody-independent lympholysis 86
antigenic determinants 182
– specifity 181
antigens, bacterial 87
–, T-cell independent 87
antiviral immunity, lack of 184
aplasia of umbilical artery 160, 166
appropriate for gestion age (AGA) 3, 10, 11, 19, 23, 26, 40, 44, 48
arrested ramification 59, 60, 61
arterial compliance 167
asynchronous maturation 3
atherosclerosis of iliac artery 167
atrophy of umbilical artery 160, 166
atypical trisomy 164
autosomal chromosomal aberration 163
azoospermia 207

B lymphocytes (B cells) 87, 94, 95, 97, 132, *145*, 148
bacterial antigens 87
basal attachment area 58
basement membrane, thick 3
battledore placenta 9, 26
bilobate placenta 20, 22, 26
bilobation 8
biochemical detection of C-type viruses *181*
birth, premature 74, 75
–, retarded 75
birthweight, low (LBW) *1*, 160, 163
– and single umbilical artery *160*, 163
blastocyst 86
blood group antigens 87
brain damage 2
breast cancer 192
"buds" 30

C-type proviral DNA 176
– virus, biochemical detection *181*
– –, isolation from placentas *183*
– –, possible function in placenta *183*
– –, ultrastructural detection *176*
– – and diseases 176
– – and leukemia 175
– – and sarcoma 175
– viruses in germinal tissue 185, *186*
calcification 12, 67, 75, 165
– of iliac arteries 167
carcinoma in situ 194, 195, 198
Cathepsin 125
cell-mediated lympholysis 86
central cord insertion 14
cervicovaginal ridges 192, *199*
chorangioma 4, 5, 8, 12, 27, 33
chorangiomatosis 60, 63, 64
chord insertion, abnormal 27, 48
chorioamnion 109
chorionic artery 17
– cyst 167

chorionic plate 58
– villus, ultrastructure *28*
chromosomal anomalies and single
    umbilical artery 161, *163*
chromosome anomaly 161, *163*
– errors and single umbilical artery
    160
chronic fetal distress 2, 12, 166
circulation disorders *66*
circummargination 165
circumvallation 165
clear cell adenocarcinoma *201*
– – – of the cervix 192, *201*
– – – of the vagina 192, *201*
coated-vesicle mediated transport *127*
collapse of villi, focal 67, 68, 70, 73
complement fixation 182
compliance, arterial 167
concanavalin A 146
concordant retardation 60, 62, 63
congenital anomalies 168, 170
– malformations *162*, 192
cord abnormalities 5
–, abnormal insertion 165
–, – length 165
– insertion *9*
– –, central 14
– –, marginal 9, 20, 22, 23, 26, 27, 48
– –, velamentous 4, 9, 12, 21, 27, 48
corticosteroids 139
cotyledons 13, 14, 15, 16, 17, 18, 19,
    20, 21, 22, 23, 24, 25, 26, 27, 28,
    29, 40, 41, 42, 43, 45, 46, 48
–, types 15, 16, 18, 19, 23
criterial of placental maturation *58*
cryptorchidism 192, 204, 205, 206
cyclophosphamide 88, 139
cytotoxicity 86, 87, 89, 91, 97, 98
– assays 91, 93
cytotoxic antibodies 139
cytotrophoblast 38, 116, 179

decidua necrosis 165
delivery, premature 2
dermatoglyphics 163
dexamethasone 183, 184
diabetes mellitus 68, 73, 76, 77, 79,
    165
diamniotic monochorionic twin
    placenta 169
diffuse fibrinosis 10
DNA "provirus" 175
discontinued centroperipheral vascular-
    ity 63
discordant retardation 59, 61, 79

disorders of gestation period *74*
dispersed pattern 13, 14, 26
divalent cation preference 181
Doppler technique 167
"dormant" viruses 99
Down-syndrome 163
dysgenesis, gonadal 163, 164
dysmaturity 2, 3, 10, 43, 45
dysplasia 194, 195, 198
dysplastic epithelium 194, 195, 198, 199
dystrophy, fetal 74, 75

E-trisomy syndrome 163, 164
effector cells 86, 91
Eliasson Score 207
embryonic villi, persisting 59, 78
endocytosis 108, 109, 111, 112, 115,
    117, 122, *125*, 134, 135
endogenous viruses 175, 176, 185
endometrial carcinoma in males 206
– cells 203
endometrioid type of cell 203
endothelium, fetal *38*
EPH gestosis 67, 68, 73, 76, 77, 79
epididymal cysts 192, 204, 205, 206
"error in outline" 8
erythroblasts in fetal blood 77
erythroblastosis 136, 139
excentric insertion 165
exocytosis 112, 125, 127
exogenous viruses 175, 176, 185
extrachorial implantation 27
– placenta 5, 6, 8, 20, 23, 24, 25, 27,
    48, 165

Fc receptors 108, 111, 113, 117, *123*,
    126, 128, 13o, 148
fetal death in utero 73
– distress, chronic 2, 12
– –, subacute 2
– dystrophy 74, 75
– hypotrophy 74, 75
– hypoxia 162, 165, 170
– underweight *74*
fetal-placental weight ratio 7, 58, 74, 77
α-fetoprotein 84, 98
fetus papyraceus 169
fibrin deposition, intervillous (IVFD)
    5, 77
– precipitation, intervillous 5, 77
fibrin, subchorial 5
fibrinoid changes 3
fingerprints 163
focal collapse of villi 67, 68, 70, 73

gene expression 176
- transcription 176, 184
- translation 176
gestation period, disorders *74*
"ghost villi" 70
glycocalyx *46*, 87
gonadal dysgenesis 163, 164
gonadotropin 36
graft-versus-host reactions (GVH)
   88, 89, 97, 139
gridlike infarktion 67, 68, 69, 75
"growing ends" 30
growth retardation, intrauterine
   47, 48, 163

Hauptbezirke 17
HEL-12 virus 179, 182
hematoma, retroplacental 73
hemolytic disease of newborn 76, 77, 78
hemorrhage, intervillous 67, 71
-, marginal 165
hemorrhagic infarction 67, 68
hernia, inguinal 170
-, umbilical 170
herpes virus 99
HL-A antigen 86, 87
Hofbauer cells 38, 45, 59, 61
horizontal transmission 175
human chorionic gonadotropin (HCG)
   85, 137
- placental lactogen (HPL) 85
hyaluronic acid 47
hydantoin embryopathy 163
hydramnion 73, 165
hyperkeratosis 198
hypertension, maternal 10
hypogammaglobulinemia 97
hypotrophy, fetal 74, 75
hypoxia, fetal 12, 45, 162, 165, 170

"immature" villi 48
Immune complexes 85, 98
- complex diseases 175
immunocompetence of the fetus *86*
- of the pregnant individual *84*
immunodeficiency 97
immunglobulin G, structure *123*
IgA 116, 117, 124, 129, 130, 131, 132,
   134, 135, 145
IgD 87
IgE 87
IgG 85, 98, 108, 109, 111, 112, 113, 114,
   115, 116, 117, 118, 119, 122, 123, 124,
   125, 126, 127, 128, 131, 134, 138, 139,
   148

IgM 87, 116, 117, 124, 128, 130
immunofluorescence 182
infarction *9*, 48
infarkt, acute (fresh) 5, 6, 7, 10, 11, 48
-, - brown 10
-, anemic 66, 67
-, mixed 10, 11
-, old 5, 7, 10, 11
-, red 67
-, subacute 5, 6, 7, 10, 11
-, white 66, 67
infarktion, gridlike 67, 68, 69, 75
infection, transplacental *185*
inguinal hernia 170
injection-corrosion technique 165
insertion, abnormal, of cord 165
-, excentric 165
-, velamentous 164, 165
insufficiency, placental *57*, 166
"insufficient vascular pattern" 24
intercalary defective ramification 60,
   63, 64, 78
intercotyledonary zone 18
intervillous aneurysma 67, 68, 71
- fibrin depositon (IVFD) 5, 77
- hemorrhage 67, 71
- thrombosis 5, 12, 67, 68, 79, 165
intracotyledonary arteries *17*, 19, 23
- -, types 19
intrauterine growth retardation 163
- malnutrition 2, 9, 48

K cells 86
killer cells 86, 91

labor, prolonged 45
α lactalbumin 115
lactoferrin 115
Langhans' cells 45
"last field" 68
latent infection 176
- viruses 99
leukemia and C-type virus 175
ligation of umbilical artery 166
lobes, accessory 8
low birth weight (LBW) *1*, 160, 163
low density lipoprotein (LDL) receptor
   system 128
lupus erythematosus 180
lymphocyte reactions, mixed 85, 86, 87,
   89, 91, 92
lympholysis, antibody-independent 86
-, cell-mediated 86
lysosomes 113, 114, 115, 122, *125*, 145

M 7 baboon virus 177, 181, 182, 183
macrophages 87, 88, 140, 142, 146, 147
magistral pattern 13, 14, 15, 23, 26
malformations 11, 12, 192
– and single umbilical artery *162*
malignant melanoma 138
malnutriton, intrauterine 2, 9, 48
marginal cord insertion 9, 20, 22, 23, 26 26, 27, 48
– hemorrhage 165
Mason-Pfitzer monkey virus 181
maturation, asynchronous 3
maturitas praecox 74, 75
– retardata 74, 75, 77
melanoma, malignant 138
membranous placentation 8
mesonephric remnants 203
mesonephros 203
microfibrin deposits 67, 68
β_2 microglobulin 86
microphallus 206
microvilli 110, 125, 126
mitogens 85, 87, 88, 89, 92, 94, 96, 98
mixed lymphocyte reactions (MLR) 85, 86, 87, 89, 92
– – – –, one-way 85, 91
– – – –, two-way 89, 91
molecular hybridization technic 182*
monoamniotic twin 169
monocytes 94, 95
monocytic cells in milk 145
morphallaxis 73
mortality, perinatal 161, *162*, 168
–, –, and single umbilical artery *162*
mucoproteins 87
Müllerian ducts 202, 203
– duct remnants 205, 206
multiple anomalies 161, 166
– pregnancy 2, 4, 73, 165, 169

Na-clearance studies 43
nanism, placental 74, 75
necrosis of villi 5, 10, 67, 70, 73
neuraminidase 87
nonproductive infection 176

obliterating angiopathy 60, 66, 72
occlusive changes in uteroplacental vessels 10
oligomenorrhea 204
oligospermia 207
omphalomesenteric duct remnants 169

one-way MLR 85, 91
oxygen tension 42

parakeratotic cells 198, 999
pattern, dispersed 13, 14, 26
–, magistral 13, 14, 15, 23, 26
perfusion, placental 57
perinatal death 2, 11
– mortality 161, *162*, 168
– – and single umbilical artery *162*
permeability of the placental barrier *88*
persisting embryonic villi 59, 78
pervillous fibrin deposition 10
phagocytosis 129, 134, 145
phagolysosome-mediated transport *125*
phagolysosomes *125*
phagosomes 125, 126, 127
phenytoin 163
phytohemagglutinin (PHA) 85, 86, 87, 89, 91, 92, 93, 98, 145, 146
pinocytosis 111, 148
placenta, bilobata 20, 22, 26
– circummarginata 8, 9
– circumvallata 8, 9, 11, 12, 20, 21, 48
– duplex 164
– extrachorialis 5, 6, *8*, 20, 23, 24, 25, 27, 48
– praevia 7
placental anomalies *164*
– arterial vasculature *13*
– configurations, abnormal 6, *8*, 48
– infarction 67, 68, 70, 165
– infarcts 3, 5, 44, 164, 165
– insufficiency 2, 7, 9, 10, *57*, 166
– –, acute 73, 74
– –, chronic 73, 74, 75
– –, subacute 74, 75
– lobes 13
"– membrane" 3
– nanism 74, 75
– perfusion 57
placentation disorders 59, 77
– –, primary 60
– –, secondary 60
–, membranous 8
placentofetal ratio 7, 58, 74, 77
placentomaternal unit ("placenton") 58, 66, 68
"placenton" (= placentomaternal unit) 58, 66, 68
plasma cells, IgA secreting *131*
pokeweed mitogen (PWM) 145, 146
postnatal runt disease 88, 89
pre-eclampsia 3, 45, 79

"pregnancy-zone protein" 84, 98
premature birth 74, 75
– delivery 2
– labor 8, 9, 10
– separation 73
prematurity 11, 74, 75
primary cotyledonary artery 13, 15
– trunc 13
primordial embryonic connective
   tissue 59
prolonged labor 45
prostatic carcinoma 206
– utricle 206
protovirus hypothesis 184
proviral DNA 176
– genes 176
"provirus" 175, 176
pseudoinfarction, subchorionic
   67, 68, 69
pseudoprematurity 2
pyelography, intravenous 167
pyrimidine, halogenated 183

radioimmunoassay 182
ramification, arrested 59, 60, 61
–, intercalary defective 60, 63, 64, 78
recanalized thrombus 72
reserve cell proliferation 194
respiratory insufficiency 73, 74, 77
retardation, concordant 60, 62, 63
–, discordant 59, 61, 79
retarded birth 75
– maturation 74, 75, 77
retinoic acid 166
retroplacental hematoma 5, 6, *11*, 73
reverse transcriptase 175, 181, 182
– – assay 186
Rh-erythroblastosis 76, 77, 78
Rh incompatibility 136, 139
rhabdomyosarcoma 183
ridges, cervico-vaginal *199*
RNA-directed DNA polymerase 175
runting disease 138, 139, 140, *147*

sarcoma and C-type virus 175
Schiller test 195, 196
"seaweed" cotyledons *27*, 48
secondary cotyledonary artery 15
secretory immune system *129*
– immunoglobulins *130*
– IgA antibody 130
semen, abnormal 192, 204
seminal vesicles, nodular enlargement
   206
Shigella paradysenteriae 97

simian sarcoma virus 181
single umbilical artery (SUA) 4, 5, 9, *12*,
   22, 23, 27, 48, *159*
– – –, chromosomal anomalies 161,
   163
– – –, requency *160*
– – –, pathogenesis *166*
– – –, placental features *164*
– – – and acardiac twins *168*
– – – and birthweight, *160*, 163
– – – and malformations *162*
– – – and perinatal mortality *162*
– – – and twins 160, 161
sinusoidal differentiation 59, 61
small for date baby (SFD) 2, 3, 75
– – gestation age (SGA) 5, 9, 10, 11, 19,
   25, 26, 27, 40, 41, 42, 43, 44, 46, 47,
   48
spiral arteries 26, 27, 42, 43, 48, 58, 68,
   73, 76
squamous cell carcinoma invasive 194
– metaplasia 165, 194, 197, 198, 199
steroid hormones 176, 183
subacute fetal distress 2
subchorial fibrin 5
– thrombosis 48
subchorionic artery 13, 17
– pseudoinfarction 67, 68, 69
– thrombus *11*
subcotyledonary vessels 17
subcotyledons 13, 15, *17*, 18, 20, 21, 22,
   23, 27, 41, 42, 46
succenturiate lobe 165
suppressor T lymphocytes *94*, 97, 98
sympodia 168
syncytial adhesions 29, 30, 32, 33, 41
– crests 32, 35, 39
– knots 3
– microvilli *33*, 38, 39, *43*, 45, 46
– ridges 33
– sprout 41
– trophoblast 28, 45
syncytiocapillary membranes 3
syncytiotrophoblast 28, *31*, 45, 110, 111,
   124, 126, 137, 179, 183

T lymphocytes (T cells) 84, 85, 88, 94,
   95, 97, 98, 99, 132, 139, *145*, 148
T-cell independent antigens 87
target cells 87, 91, 93
– –, labeled 86
– –, xenogeneic 87
template preference 181
terminal transferase 182

tertiary cotyledonary artery 15
testicular carcinoma 205, 206
testis, hypoplastic 192, 204, 205, 206, 207, 108
–, undescended 192, 204, 205, 206
thalidomide embryopathy 163
thrombosis, intervillous 12, 67, 68, 79, 165
–, subchorial 48
thrombus, recanalized 72
–, subchorionic *11*
toxemia 5, 10, 45, 48
transcriptase assay 186
transfer of humoral immunity *106*
transmission, horizontal 175
–, vertical 175
transplacental infection *185*
transplantation antigens 86, 87, 136
transumbilical angiography 166, 167, 168, 169
Trisomy D 164
– D-1 164
– E 163, 164
– 13-15 164
– 16-18 164
– 17-18 164
– 18 164
–, atypical 164
– syndrome 163
trophectoderm 86
trophoblast 59, 84, 86, 87, 99, 109, 136
trophoblastic basement membrane 85
– layer *31*, 35, *43*
trophotropism 9, 166
truncus chorii 13
tuberculin 85
twins 4, 5, 6, 9, 12, 21, 22, 76, 168
–, monoamniotic 169
– and single umbilical artery 160, 161
two-way MLR 89, 91

ultrasonic Doppler technique 167
umbilical arteries 14
– artery, aplasia 160, 166
– –, atrophy 160, 166

– –, single (SUA) 4, 5, 9, *12*, 22, 23, 27, 48, *159*
– –, –, frequency *160*
– –, –, pathogenesis *166*
– –, –, and acardiac twins *168*
– –, –, and birth weight *160*, 163
– –, –, and chromosomal anomalies 161, *163*
– –, –, and malformations *162*
– –, –, and perinatal mortality *162*
– –, –, and placental features *164*
– –, –, and twins 160, 161
– cord arterial anastomoses 168
– hernia 170
underweight, fetal *74*
urinary abnormalities 162, 167
urogenital sinus 202
utero-placental unit 4

vaginal adenosis 192, *193*, 201
vascularity, discontinued centroperipheral 63
velamentous cord insertion 4, 9, 12, 21, 27, 48, 164, 165
vertical transmission 175
villitis *4*, 48
villous core *38*
– inflammation 5
virion detection, frequency 181
– reverse transcriptase 175, 181, 182
virus activation 99
– transmission 175
viruses, "dormant" 99
–, endogenous 175, 176, 185
–, exogenous 175, 176, 185
–, latent 99
vitelline vessels 168
vitello-umbilical anastomoses 166

"watershed infarkt" 68

xenogeneic target cells 87

yolk sac 106, 107, 109, 111, 112, 123, 124, 125, 126, 128, 148
"young villi" 30
"youthful" chorionic villi 42

Index to Volumes 59–65 Current Topics in Pathology

Volume 59

J. Torhorst, Studies on the Pathogenesis and Morphogenesis of Glomerulonephrosis 1
L. Damjanov, D. Solter, Experimental Teratoma 69
W. Meier-Ruge, Hirschsprung's Disease: Its Aetiology, Pathogenesis and Differential Diagnosis 131
U.N. Riede, Experimental Aspects of Growth Plate Disorders 181

Volume 60

F. Huth, M. Kojimahara, T. Franken, P. Rhedin, K.A. Rosenbauer, Aortic Alterations in Rabbits Following Sheathing with Silastic and Polyethylene Tubes 1
K. Bürki, J.C. Schaer, P. Grétillat, R. Schindler, Radioactively Labelled Iododeoxyuridine in the Study of Experimental Liver Regeneration 33
G. Altshuler, P. Russel, The Human Placental Villitides. A Review of Chronic Intrauterine Infection 63
H. Mitschke, W. Saeger, Ultrastructural Pathology of the Adrenal Glands in Cushing's Syndrome 113
N. Böhm, W. Sandritter, DNA in Human Tumors: A Cytophotometric Study 151

Volume 61

A. Okabayashi, Y. Kondo, H. Shigematsu, Cellular and Histopathologic Consequences of Immunologically Induced Experimental Glomerulonephritis 1
Ch. Witting, The Terminology of Glomerulonephritis – A Review 45
G.H. Toenes, The Immunohistology of Glomerulonephritis – Distinctive Marks and Variability 61
J. Churg, E. Grishman, Electron Microscopy of Glomerulonephritis 107
H. Fischbach, The Morphologic Course of Different Glomerulonephritides (Examination of Repeat Biopsies in 264 Patients) 155
U. Helmchen, U. Kneissler, Role of the Renin-Angiotensin System in Renal Hypertension. An Experimental Approach 203
H. Loew, A. Samizadeh, E. Heilmann, New Clinical Syndromes under Regular Intermittent Hemodialysis 239

Volume 62

C.R. Austin, Developmental Anomalies Arising from Errors of Fertilization and Cleavage 3
D. Szöllösi, Oocyte Maturation and Paternal Contribution to the Embryo in Mammals 9
W. Engel, W. Franke, Maternal Storage in the Mammalian Oocyte 29
Ch. Epstein, The Genetic Activity of the Early Mammalian Embryo 53
H.W. Denker, Formation of the Blastocyst: Determination of Trophoblast and Embryonic Knot 59
C. Lutwak-Mann, The Response of the Preimplantation Embryo to Exogenous Factors 83

H. Spielmann, Embryo Transfer Technique and Action of Drugs on the Preimplantation Embryo 87
H.M. Beier, Uterine Secretion Protein Patterns Under Hormonal Influences . 105
L. Saxén, M. Karkinen-Jääskeläinen, I. Saxén, Organ Culture in Teratology . 123
V.H. Ferm, Teratogenic Effects and Placental Permeability of Heavy Metals . 145
O. Bomsel-Helmreich, Experimental Heteroploidy in Mammals 155
A. Gropp, B. Putz, U. Zimmermann, Autosomal Monosomy and Trisomy
  Causing Developmental Failure 177
J.G. Boué, A. Boué, Chromosomal Anomalies in Early Spontaneous Abortion 193

Volume 63

Aa. Johansen, Early Gastric Cancer 1
H. Thompson, Pathology of Coeliac Disease 49
K. Elster, Histologic Classification of Gastric Polyps 77
*H.T. Enterline,*Polyps and Cancer of the Large Bowel 95
M.I. Filipe, A.C. Branfoot, Mucin Histochemistry of the Colon 143
R.H. Riddell, The Precarcinomatous Phase of Ulcerative Colitis 179
Dawson, I.M.P., The Endocrine Cells of the Gastro-Intestinal Tract and the
  Neoplasms which Arise from Them 221
J.M. Skinner, R. Whitehead, Immunological Aspects of Gastro-Intestinal
  Pathology 259
D.M. Goldenberg, Oncofetal and Other Tumor-Associated Antigens of the
  Human Digestive System 289

Volume 64

S. Widgren, Pulmonary Hypertension Related to Aminorex Intake (Histologic,
  Ultrastructural, and Morphometric Studies of 37 Cases in Switzerland) . . . 1
J.L. van Lancker, DNA Injuries, Their Repair, and Carcinogenesis 65
C. Thomas, H.J. Steinhardt, K. Küchemann, D. Maas, U.N. Riede, Soft Tissue
  Tumors in the Rat (Pathogenesis and Histopathology) 129
K. Salfelder, K. Ueda, E.L. Quiroga, J. Schwarz, Visceral Candidosis (Anatomic
  Study of 34 Cases) 177

Volume 65

*H.-V. Gärtner, T. Watanabe, V. Ott, A. Adam, A. Bohle, H.H. Edel, R. Kluthe,
  E. Renner, F. Scheler, R.M. Schmülling, H.G. Sieberth*, Correlations Between
  Morphologic and Clinical Features in Idiopathic Perimembranous
  Glomerulonephritis 1
J. Thiele, Human Parathyroid Gland: A Freeze Fracture and Thin Section
  Study 31
*A. Bohle, U. Helmchen, K.E. Grund, H.-V. Gärtner, D. Meyer, K.D. Bock,
  M. Bulla, P. Bünger, L. Diekmann, U. Frotscher. K. Hayduk, W. Köster,
  M. Strauch, F. Scheler, H. Christ*, Malignant Nephrosclerosis in Patients
  with Hemolytic Uremic Syndrome 81
A.M. Novi, Liver Carcinogenesis in Rats After Aflatoxin B_1 Administration . . 115
J. Schwarz, K. Salfelder, Blastomycosis 165

GPSR Compliance
The European Union's (EU) General Product Safety Regulation (GPSR) is a set
of rules that requires consumer products to be safe and our obligations to
ensure this.

If you have any concerns about our products, you can contact us on

ProductSafety@springernature.com

In case Publisher is established outside the EU, the EU authorized
representative is:

Springer Nature Customer Service Center GmbH
Europaplatz 3
69115 Heidelberg, Germany